meds Publishing

NCLEX-PN EXAM ESSENTIALS REVIEW

Complete Source of Vital NCLEX Exam Information

SIXTH EDITION

PATRICIA A. HOEFLER, M.S.N., R.N.

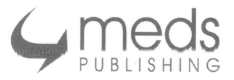

PUBLISHING

4000 BLACKBURN LANE, SUITE 260
BURTONSVILLE, MARYLAND 20866
WWW.MEDSPUB.COM

SIXTH EDITION

Editor: Mark Williams-Abrams

Copies of this book may be obtained from:
MEDS PUBLISHING
4000 Blackburn Lane
Suite 260
Burtonsville, MD 20866
www.medspub.com

ISBN 1-56533-049-8
Printed in the United States of America

CONTRIBUTING AUTHORS

Jennifer Burks, M.S.N., R.N.
Consultant

Janet Gysi, M.S.N., R.N.
Associate Professor

Carol Jernigan, M.S.N., R.N.
Clinical Nurse Specialist

Elizabeth Kassel, M.S.N., R.N.
Associate Professor

Marian Kovatchitch, M.S.N., R.N.
Associate Professor

Laura McQueen, M.S.N., R.N., C.S.
Ph.D. Candidate
Clinical Specialist

Michele Michael, Ph.D., R.N.
Professor of Nursing

Cherralene Peer, M.S.N., R.N.
Associate Professor

May Phillips, Ph.D., R.N.
Professor

Karyn Plante, M.S.N., R.N.
Associate Professor

Sandra Schuler, M.S.N., R.N.
Professor

Donna Snelson, M.S.N., R.N.
Associate Professor

Eleanor Walker, Ph.D., R.N.
Professor

Lois Walker, Ph.D., R.N.
Psychotherapist

TABLE OF CONTENTS

AN INTRODUCTION TO THE SIXTH EDITION V

INTRODUCTION
   REVIEW OF TEST-TAKING STRATEGIES FOR THE NCLEX-PN EXAM I
      SECTION I   PREPARING FOR THE EXAM 3
      SECTION II   ANSWERING QUESTIONS 5
      SECTION III   PREPARING FOR EXAM TIME 7

UNIT ONE
   MEDICAL-SURGICAL NURSING 9
      SECTION I   REVIEW OF FLUIDS AND ELECTROLYTES, ACID-BASE BALANCE II
      SECTION II   REVIEW OF RESPIRATORY SYSTEM DISORDERS I5
      SECTION III   REVIEW OF GENERAL PREOPERATIVE AND POSTOPERATIVE CARE 23
      SECTION IV   REVIEW OF GASTROINTESTINAL, HEPATIC, AND PANCREATIC DISORDERS 24
      SECTION V   REVIEW OF MUSCULOSKELETAL DISORDERS 34
      SECTION VI   REVIEW OF ENDOCRINE SYSTEM FUNCTIONS AND DISORDERS 38
      SECTION VII   REVIEW OF BLOOD DISORDERS 46
      SECTION VIII REVIEW OF CARDIOVASCULAR SYSTEM DISORDERS 48
      SECTION IX   REVIEW OF GENITOURINARY SYSTEM DISORDERS 56
      SECTION X   REVIEW OF NEUROLOGICAL SYSTEM DISORDERS 63
      SECTION XI   REVIEW OF ONCOLOGY NURSING 70
      SECTION XII   REVIEW OF IMMUNOLOGIC DISORDERS 72
      SECTION XIII REVIEW OF BURNS 73

UNIT TWO
   PSYCHIATRIC NURSING 77
      SECTION I   OVERVIEW 79
      SECTION II   ANXIETY 85
      SECTION III   SCHIZOPHRENIA 89
      SECTION IV   MOOD DISORDERS AND ASSOCIATED BEHAVIORS 91
      SECTION V   PERSONALITY DISORDERS 95
      SECTION VI   CHEMICAL DEPENDENCE/ABUSE 100
      SECTION VII   ORGANIC MENTAL DISORDERS 103
      SECTION VIII EATING DISORDERS 105
      SECTION IX   DEVELOPMENTAL DISABILITIES 105
      SECTION X   FAMILY VIOLENCE 107
      SECTION XI   RAPE 108
      SECTION XII   LEGAL ASPECTS OF PSYCHIATRIC NURSING 109

UNIT THREE
   WOMEN'S HEALTH NURSING III
      SECTION I   REVIEW OF FEMALE REPRODUCTIVE NURSING II3
      SECTION II   REVIEW OF LABOR AND DELIVERY II8
      SECTION III   REVIEW OF POSTPARTAL ADAPTATIONS AND NURSING ASSESSMENT 124
      SECTION IV   REVIEW OF REPRODUCTIVE RISKS AND COMPLICATIONS 125
      SECTION V   NURSING CARE OF THE NEONATE 128
      SECTION VI   REVIEW OF HIGH-RISK NEWBORN 130
      SECTION VII   NURSING CARE OF THE GYNECOLOGIC CLIENT 131

TABLE OF CONTENTS

UNIT FOUR

PEDIATRIC NURSING 135

    SECTION I   GROWTH AND DEVELOPMENT 137

    SECTION II   THE HOSPITALIZED CHILD 145

    SECTION III   NURSING CARE OF THE CHILD WITH CONGENITAL ANOMALIES 147

    SECTION IV   NURSING CARE OF THE CHILD WITH AN ACUTE ILLNESS 154

    SECTION V   NURSING CARE OF THE SURGICAL CHILD 159

    SECTION VI   NURSING CARE FOR PEDIATRIC ACCIDENTS 160

    SECTION VII   NURSING CARE OF THE CHILD WITH CHRONIC OR LONG-TERM PROBLEMS ... 162

    SECTION VIII   NURSING CARE OF THE CHILD WITH AN ONCOLOGY DISORDER 166

    SECTION IX   NURSING CARE OF THE CHILD WITH AN INFECTIOUS DISEASE 170

UNIT FIVE

COORDINATED CARE 175

    SECTION I   MANAGEMENT 177

    SECTION II   DELEGATION 179

    SECTION III   ETHICAL ISSUES 179

    SECTION IV   LEGAL ISSUES 180

UNIT SIX

ALTERNATE TEST ITEM FORMATS 183

    SECTION I   OVERVIEW 185

    SECTION II   FILL-IN-THE-BLANK 185

    SECTION III   MULTIPLE RESPONSE 186

    SECTION IV   HOT SPOT 186

    SECTION V   CHARTS, TABLES, GRAPHIC IMAGES 187

APPENDICES 189

    APPENDIX A   REVIEW OF CALCULATIONS AND CONVERSIONS 191

    APPENDIX B   NUTRITION 193

    APPENDIX C   POSITIONING CLIENTS 195

    APPENDIX D   PSYCHIATRIC TERMS 196

    APPENDIX E   PHARMACOLOGY 198

INDEX 213

LIST OF TABLES & GRAPHICS

TABLE I-1	MAJOR ELECTROLYTES: IMBALANCE/INTERVENTIONS	13
TABLE I-2	ACIDOSIS/ALKALOSIS	14
TABLE I-3	INHALER THERAPY	22
TABLE I-4	COMMON POSTOPERATIVE COMPLICATIONS	25
TABLE I-5	COMPARISON OF CHRONIC DUODENAL AND CHRONIC GASTRIC ULCERS	28
TABLE I-6	COMPARISON OF CROHN'S DISEASE AND ULCERATIVE COLITIS	29
TABLE I-7	COMPARISON OF COLOSTOMY AND ILEOSTOMY	30
TABLE I-8	TYPES OF INTESTINAL OSTOMIES	32
TABLE I-9	COMPARISON OF HEPATITIS A; HEPATITIS B; HEPATITIS NON-A, NON-B; HEPATITIS C	32
TABLE I-10	COMPARISON OF RHEUMATOID ARTHRITIS AND OSTEOARTHRITIS	36
TABLE I-11	PITUITARY GLAND: HORMONES PRODUCED AND FUNCTIONS	39
TABLE I-12	ADRENAL GLAND: HORMONES PRODUCED AND FUNCTIONS	40
TABLE I-13	THYROID GLAND: HORMONES PRODUCED AND FUNCTIONS	42
TABLE I-14	PARATHYROID GLAND: HORMONES PRODUCED AND FUNCTIONS	43
TABLE I-15	PANCREAS: HORMONES PRODUCED AND FUNCTIONS	44
TABLE I-16	INSULIN	45
TABLE I-17	BLOOD VALUES	46
TABLE I-18	SURGICAL APPROACHES FOR PROSTATECTOMY	62
TABLE I-19	NURSING INTERVENTIONS FOR CLIENT ON CHEMOTHERAPY	72
TABLE II-1	ERIKSON'S STAGES OF DEVELOPMENT	80
TABLE II-2	ERIKSON'S STAGES DEFINED	80
TABLE II-3	MASLOW'S PYRAMID	81
TABLE II-4	MENTAL HEALTH/ILLNESS CONTINUUM	83
TABLE II-5	LEVELS OF ANXIETY	86
TABLE II-6	ANTIANXIETY AGENTS AND ADVERSE REACTIONS	88
TABLE II-7	ANTIPSYCHOTIC AGENTS AND ADVERSE REACTIONS	92
TABLE II-8	CONTINUUM OF EMOTIONAL RESPONSES	94
TABLE II-9	ANTIDEPRESSANT AGENTS	96
TABLE II-10	ANTIDEPRESSANT AGENTS: MAOI'S	97
TABLE II-11	ANTIMANIA AGENTS AND MOOD STABILIZERS	99
TABLE II-12	SUBSTANCE ABUSE	101
TABLE II-13	ANOREXIA/BULIMIA CONTRASTED	106
TABLE II-14	SIGNS OF ABUSE IN CHILDREN	108
TABLE III-1	ADAPTATIONS TO PREGNANCY	115
TABLE III-2	STAGES OF LABOR	120
TABLE III-3	MEDICATIONS USED IN LABOR AND DELIVERY	121
TABLE III-4	ANALGESIA/ANESTHESIA FOR LABOR AND DELIVERY	122
TABLE IV-1	SCHEDULE OF PRIMARY TOOTH ERUPTION	137
TABLE IV-2	SCHEDULE OF PERMANENT TOOTH ERUPTION	143
TABLE IV-3	REVIEW OF ACYANOTIC CONGENITAL HEART ANOMALIES	148
TABLE IV-4	REVIEW OF CYANOTIC CONGENITAL HEART ANOMALIES	149
TABLE IV-5	OVERVIEW OF COMMON ACCIDENTAL INGESTION	161
TABLE IV-6	COMPARISON OF INSULIN SHOCK AND DIABETIC COMA GUIDE	165
TABLE IV-7	RENAL DISORDERS	167

LIST OF TABLES & GRAPHICS

TABLE IV-8   COMPARISON OF CYSTIC FIBROSIS AND CELIAC DISEASE 168
TABLE IV-9   NURSING CARE OF THE CHILD WITH CANCER 169
TABLE IV-10   RECOMMENDED IMMUNIZATION SCHEDULE 170
TABLE IV-11   COMMUNICABLE DISEASES GUIDE 171

GRAPHIC VI-1   FILL-IN-THE-BLANK CALCULATION ITEM 185
GRAPHIC VI-2   FILL-IN-THE-BLANK ORDERED RESPONSE ITEM 186
GRAPHIC VI-3   MULTIPLE RESPONSE ITEM 186
GRAPHIC VI-4   HOT SPOT ITEM 186
GRAPHIC VI-5   CHARTS, TABLES, & GRAPHIC IMAGES ITEM 187

TABLE APP-1   POSITIONING CLIENTS 195
TABLE APP-2   PSYCHIATRIC TERMS 196

NCLEX-PN EXAM ESSENTIALS REVIEW

Complete Source of Vital NCLEX Exam Information

Sixth Edition

Welcome to MEDS *NCLEX-PN EXAM ESSENTIALS REVIEW!* MEDS Publishing is a professional organization directed by nurse educators and dedicated to excellence in nursing education. MEDS Publishing was the first to offer review courses for the NCLEX-PN Exam and to introduce unique test-taking strategies and original methods for reviewing nursing information.

If you are now beginning a MEDS Publishing comprehensive review - in live or video format - you are in good company! Students reviewing with MEDS Publishing have experienced a 99.5% NCLEX Exam pass rate. MEDS Publishing is the leader in NCLEX-PN Exam reviews.

This MEDS Publishing Review outline, previously available only to students enrolled in the 3-Day Review Course, is now being offered independently "by popular demand."

This sixth edition features:

✓ A unit on the new NCLEX Exam Alternate Test Item Formats
✓ Critical information on the new NCLEX Exam computerized format
✓ Expanded and updated outlines for each of the five clinical areas
✓ An outline of MEDS Publishing's unique test-taking strategies
✓ Easy-to-understand charts and graphs
✓ Expanded appendices covering the areas of calculations and conversions, nutrition, and pharmacology
✓ An easy-to-use pharmacology guide

We hope this outline will facilitate your review of nursing information for the NCLEX exam. You have our best wishes for success on the exam and for success and fulfillment in your career as a professional nurse.

For more information about MEDS software, books, video tapes, audio tapes, and eLearning Center products, contact MEDS Publishing at (800) 200-9191 or visit our website at www.medspub.com. We always are pleased to assist you.

INTRODUCTION

REVIEW OF TEST-TAKING STRATEGIES FOR THE NCLEX-PN EXAM

UNIT CONTENT

SECTION I.   Preparing for the Exam 3
SECTION II.   Answering Questions 5
SECTION III. Preparing for Exam Time 7

SYMBOLS

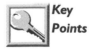 **Key Points**

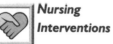 **Nursing Interventions**

! **Points to Remember**

SECTION I

PREPARING FOR THE EXAM

A. What You Should Know About the NCLEX-PN Exam

1. General information
   a. The first integrated exam was given in July 1982
   b. The purpose of the exam is to determine that a candidate is prepared to practice entry-level nursing safely
   c. The exam is designed to test essential knowledge of nursing and a candidate's ability to apply that knowledge to clinical situations
   d. The purpose of the new test plan is to bring the exam in line with current nursing behaviors (the nursing process and decision making)
   e. Exam is "pass/fail," and no other score is given

2. Computerized Adaptive Testing
   a. Computer program continuously scores answers and selects questions suitable for each candidate's competency level for a more precise measurement of competency
   b. A higher weight is assigned to difficult questions so a passing score can be obtained by answering a lot of easier questions-or a smaller number of more difficult questions
   c. Special screen design is used (see SCREEN DESIGN below)
   d. Use the mouse to move the cursor on the screen to the desired location.

   Single-click your mouse to select an option as your answer.
   e. A drop-down calculator also is featured. Double-click your mouse on the calculator icon, and the drop-down calculator will appear.
   f. After you have confirmed your selection, click on "next" to input your answer and proceed to the next screen
   g. After you proceed to the next screen, you CANNOT go back to a previous question to change your answer.

3. Exam schedule
   a. Given year-round
   b. Retake policy: The exam can only be repeated every 45 days

4. Number of questions and time allowed
   a. No minimum amount of time; however, a candidate must answer a minimum of 85 test questions
   b. Maximum time is five hours, with a maximum of 205 test questions
   c. About one out of three candidates completes the exam in less than two hours; one in three will use the complete five hours
   d. The computer will automatically stop as soon as one of the following occurs:
      1) Candidate's measure of competency is determined to be above or below the passing standard
      2) Candidate has answered all 205 test questions
      3) Maximum amount of time (five hours) has expired

5. A candidate will pass by either:

Case Scenario and Stem

SCREEN DESIGN

On the psychiatric unit, a nurse observes a client standing near a window and touching the glass. The client also mutters from time to time. Which comment by the nurse indicates the best understanding of the client's behavior?

1. "Why are you standing by the window and touching the glass?"

2. "There you are. I came to see if you wanted to see the video we are showing on the unit?"

3. What are you looking at through the window?"

4. "Are you hearing voices or seeing things?"

Choices 1, 2, 3, and 4

    a. Answering 85 to 205 questions above the passing standard (the required weighted score) for all questions answered, within the time allowed; or

    b. Answering at least 85 questions within the time allowed and achieving the passing standard for the last 60 questions answered

6. Types of questions
    a. The majority of the questions are standard multiple choice
      1) Each question has four options
      2) The best option is the only correct answer
    b. Exam includes 25 unmarked experimental or "try-out" questions
    c. A small percentage of the questions are alternative format questions including:
      1) Fill-in-the-blank items
      2) Calculation items
      3) Ordered response (sequencing) items
      4) Hot Spot (point and click) items
      5) Multiple Response items
      6) Items with graphs, tables, or charts

7. Exam procedure:
    a. Look for the BEST answer to each question
    b. It is not possible to skip questions or return to previous questions
    c. Mandatory 10-minute break after first two hours and after another one-and-one-half hours
    d. Scratch paper provided for calculations must be returned at end of exam

8. Structure of the test plan *
    a. Safe, Effective Care Environment
      1) Coordinated Care   6 - 12%
      2) Safety and Infection Control   7 - 13%
    b. Health Promotion and Maintenance
      1) Growth & Development Through the Life Span   4 - 10%
      2) Prevention & Early Detection of Disease   4 - 10%
    c. Psychosocial Integrity
      1) Coping & Adaptation   6 - 12%
      2) Psychosocial Adaptation   4 - 10%
    d. Physiological Integrity
      1) Basic Care and Comfort   10 - 16%
      2) Pharmacological Therapies   5 - 11%
      3) Reduction of Risk Potential   11 - 17%
      4) Physiological Adaptation   13 - 19%
    Information courtesy of the National Council of State Boards of Nursing, Inc., Test Plan April 2002.

B. Schedule Your Study Time

1. The minimum time for preparation is two hours a day for six to eight weeks
    a. Spend 1/3 of your time reviewing content
    b. Spend 2/3 of your time answering test questions
2. For content review, use an NCLEX-PN exam review book such as this one, which outlines content
3. Begin with areas that are most difficult for you, or the areas that are least familiar
4. For more detailed information on your difficult or less familiar areas, use a good nursing reference manual
5. Review medical-surgical, pediatric, women's health, and psychiatric nursing, as well as nursing management and alternate test item formats
6. Use a body systems approach for medical-surgical and pediatric nursing areas
7. When studying body systems and the associated diseases, remember to:
    a. Define the disease in terms of the pathophysiological process that is occurring
    b. Identify the client's early and late manifestations
    c. Identify the most important or life-threatening complications
    d. Define the medical treatment
    e. Identify and prioritize the nursing interventions associated with early and late manifestations
    f. Identify what the nurse teaches the client/family to prevent or adapt to disease
8. To schedule your study time:
    a. List the areas you need to review
    b. Count the number of days you have available to study
    c. Estimate the amount of time needed for each area
    d. On your calendar, write the area to review, the number of questions to answer, and the amount of time needed for each study day

C. Answer Many Questions

1. Answering questions will develop your test-taking skills
2. Use questions similar to those on the NCLEX exam
3. Answer a minimum of 3,000 test questions
4. Include answering test questions in your study plan. For example, answer 100 questions each day for a month.
5. If you are at high risk, answer 5,000 test questions
6. Use at least three different question-and-answer books, including MEDS Publishing's *Complete Q&A for the NCLEX-PN Exam* with CD-ROM
7. Using a variety of books provides a more comprehensive preparation
8. An online question and answer program which mimics the NCLEX exam such as MEDS StarNurse Exam-A-Day™ Gold will give you more realistic ex-

perience with answering alternative item format questions

D. Assess Your Progress
1. Each time you answer questions, check the number of questions you answered correctly
   a. If you answer less than 65% correctly, this is a warning signal! Spend lots of time reviewing content and answering more questions in this area of nursing.
   b. If you answer 65 to 75% correctly, your performance is average. Success in this area is uncertain. Continue working with this content until your score is above 75%. Work on building your confidence by answering more questions in this area.
   c. If you answer 75 to 85% correctly, your performance is very good. Only return to this area after you have at least 75% in all other areas. Feel confident.
   d. If you answer 85 to 95% correctly, your performance is superior. Don't waste time on this. Feel very confident.
2. For each wrong answer, identify why you answered wrong
   a. You may have answered a question wrong because you did not know the facts or got confused about the information
      1) Identify this as a content weakness
      2) Review the content again
   b. You may have answered a question wrong because you misread the question, did not understand what it was asking, or did not know how to select the best answer
      1) Identify this as a test-taking deficiency
      2) For further assistance with test-taking deficiencies, we recommend MEDS test-taking book, *Successful Problem Solving & Test Taking for Nursing and NCLEX-PN Exams*.
3. Check the number of questions that you identified as difficult and went back to answer later. See how many of them you answered correctly.

SECTION II

ANSWERING QUESTIONS

A. Identify the Critical Elements in the Question
1. Identify the issue in the question
   a. The issue is the problem about which the question is asking
   b. The issue may be a:
      1) Drug: for example, digoxin (*Lanoxin*), furosemide (*Lasix*)
      2) Nursing problem: for example, alteration in comfort, potential for infection

      3) Behavior: for example, restlessness, agitation
      4) Disorder: for example, diabetes mellitus, ulcerative colitis
      5) Procedure: for example, glucose tolerance test, cardiac catheterization
2. Identify the client in the question
   a. The client in the question is usually the person with the health problem
   b. The client in a test question may also be a relative or significant other or another member of the health care team with whom the nurse is interacting
   c. The correct answer to the question must relate to the client in the question
3. Look for the key words
   a. Key words focus attention on what is important
   b. Key words may appear in bold print
   c. Examples:
      1) During the early postoperative period, which nursing procedures would be **best**?
      2) The nurse would expect to find which characteristic in an **adult** diabetic?
      3) Which nursing action is **vital**?
      4) Which nursing action would be best **initially**?
4. Identify what the stem is asking and determine whether the question has a true response stem, a false response stem or a priority stem
   a. Be clear about what the stem is asking before you look at the options
   b. If the question is not clear to you, rephrase it using your own words
   c. Determine whether the question has a true response stem, a false response stem or a priority stem
      1) True response stem
         a) Definition: A true response stem requires an answer that is a true statement
         b) Examples:
            (1) The nurse would assign the nursing assistant to:
            (2) Which manifestation would the nurse expect to assess?
            (3) The therapeutic response by the nurse would be:
            (4) The nurse evaluates that the client has a positive response to the medication when the client has:
      2) False response stem
         a) Definition: A false response stem requires an answer that is a false statement

    b) Examples:
       (1) Which nursing action would be inappropriate?
       (2) Which statement by the client would indicate a need for further instruction?
       (3) Which describes incorrect placement of the hands during CPR?
       (4) Which action would place the client at risk?

   3) Priority response stem
    a) Definition: A priority response stem requires the candidate to select the best answer from four plausible responses
    b) Examples:
       (1) Which client would the nurse assess first?
       (2) The nurse's initial action would be to:
       (3) The nurse should give immediate consideration to:
       (4) The task that the nurse has the nursing assistant complete first would be:

B. Use a Selection Procedure to Eliminate Incorrect Options

1. Most NCLEX questions are standard multiple choice questions which have four options. The correct answer is the BEST answer. The other three options are "distractors."
2. Distractors are options made to look like correct answers. They are intended to distract you from answering correctly.
3. As you read each of the four options, make a decision about it.
   a. This option is true (+)
   b. This option is false (−)
   c. I am not sure about this option (?)
4. If the stem is a true response stem:
   a. An option that is true (+) might be the correct answer
   b. An option that is false (−) is a distractor. Eliminate this option
   c. An option that you are not sure about (?) is possibly the correct answer
5. If the stem is a false response stem:
   a. An option that is true (+) is a distractor. Eliminate this option.
   b. An option that is false (−) may be the correct answer
   c. An option that you are not sure about (?) is possibly the correct answer
6. Do not return to options you have eliminated
7. If you are left with one option, that is your answer
8. If you are left with one (+) option and one (?) op-

tion, select the (+) option as your answer
9. If you are left with two (+) options, use strategies to select the best answer

C. Use Test-Taking Strategies When You Are Unable to Select the Best Option

1. The Global Response Strategy
   a. A global response is a general statement that may include ideas of other options within it
   b. Look for a global response when more than one option appears to be correct
   c. The global response option will probably be the correct answer
2. The Similar Distractors Strategy
   a. Similar distractors say basically the same thing using different words
   b. Since there is only one correct answer in a question, similar distractors must be wrong
   c. Eliminate similar distractors. Select for your answer an option that is different.
3. The Similar Word or Phrase Strategy
   a. When more than one option appears to be correct, look for a similar word or phrase in the stem of the question and in one of the four options
   b. The option that contains the similar word or phrase may be the correct answer
   c. Use this strategy after you have tried to identify a global response option and eliminated similar distractors
4. The Absolute Word Strategy
   a. Absolute words include words such as "only", "every", "always", and "never"
   b. When a response includes an absolute word it is unlikely to be the correct answer

D. Answering Communication Questions

1. The NCLEX exam includes many communication questions because the ability to communicate therapeutically is essential for safe practice
2. Identify the critical elements as in all questions. Pay particular attention to identification of the client in the question. Remember that the answer must relate to the client.
3. Learn to identify communication tools that enhance communication.
   a. Being silent: Nonverbal communication
   b. Offering self: "Let me sit with you."
   c. Showing empathy: "You are upset."
   d. Focusing: "You say that . . ."
   e. Restatement: "You feel anxious?"
   f. Validation/clarification: "What you are saying is . . .?"
   g. Giving information: "Your room is 423."
   h. Dealing with the here and now: "At this time, the problem is . . ."
4. Learn to identify non-therapeutic communication

blocks.
  a. Giving advice: "If I were you, I would . . ."
  b. Showing approval/disapproval: "You did the right thing."
  c. Using clichés and false reassurances: "Don't worry. It will be all right."
  d. Requesting an explanation: "Why did you do that?"
  e. Devaluing client feelings: "Don't be concerned. It's not a problem."
  f. Being defensive: "Every nurse on this unit is exceptional."
  g. Focusing on inappropriate issues or persons: "Have I said something wrong?"
  h. Placing the client's issues "on hold": "Talk to your doctor about that."
5. When answering communication questions, select an option that illustrates a therapeutic communication tool. Eliminate options that illustrate non-therapeutic communication blocks.

E. Answering Questions that Focus on Setting Priorities
1. Priority-setting questions ask the test taker to identify either what comes first, is most important, or gets the highest priority
2. Examples:
  a. What is the nurse's initial response?
  b. The nurse should give immediate consideration to:
  c. Which nursing action receives the highest priority?
  d. What should the nurse do first?
3. Use guidelines to help you to answer priority setting questions
  a. Maslow's Hierarchy of Needs indicates that physiological needs come first
  b. Maslow's Hierarchy of Needs indicates that when no physiological need is identified, safety needs come first
  c. Nursing Process indicates that assessment comes first
  d. Communication Theory indicates focusing on feelings first
  e. Teaching/Learning Theory indicates focusing on motivation first

PREPARING FOR EXAM TIME

A. Plan for Everything
1. Assemble everything you will need for the exam the night before:
  a. Identification: two IDs with signatures, including one with recent photograph
  b. Watch
  c. Several sharpened pencils (with erasers) for calculations
2. Plan to arrive at the test site early:
  a. Know the route to the exam site
  b. Know how long it will take to get there
  c. Know where you will park and if you will need coins for a parking meter
3. Pay close attention to your own physiological needs:
  a. Dress in layers
  b. Get a good night's sleep the night before the exam
  c. Eat a good breakfast
  d. Avoid stimulants and depressants
  e. Use the bathroom just before the exam
4. During the exam:
  a. Listen to the instructions
  b. Pace yourself; don't spend too long on any one question
  c. Don't let yourself become distracted. Focus your attention on answering the questions.
  d. Go with your first choice. Use test-taking strategies only when you cannot decide between close options.
  e. Keep your thoughts positive!

B. Manage Your Anxiety Level
1. Moderate levels of anxiety increase your effectiveness
2. Don't cram the night before the exam
3. Do something enjoyable and relaxing the night before the exam
4. Learn and practice measures to manage your anxiety level during the exam as needed
  a. Take a few deep breaths
  b. Tense and relax muscles
  c. Tell yourself positive affirmations
  d. Visualize a peaceful scene
  e. Visualize your success

C. Test-Taking Tips

1. Prepare comprehensively and be sure to be well rested for the exam
2. Read each question carefully, identifying the critical elements. Each question must be answered in sequence, and you may not skip or go back to change your answers to any questions.
3. Don't panic if the computer stops after a short time! It does not mean that you failed. The computer stops when the exam is able to determine with at least 95% certainty that you have demonstrated the ability, or inability, to practice safely at the minimal level of nursing competency.
4. It is helpful to know that most students pass by answering a maximum of 119 questions. However, you can still pass the exam even if you answered all 205 questions.
5. If you are having difficulty choosing between the best two options, use the test taking strategies you have learned in this review.
6. You should anticipate that the test questions will increase in difficulty
7. Use your scratch paper wisely. Since you cannot review earlier questions to help recall previous facts, use the scratch paper provided for calculations to remember facts from previous questions. Sometimes, information from one question is helpful in answering another question.
8. Don't panic if someone finishes before you! The test adapts to each candidate's level of ability, and it means that you may take longer to prove that you are capable of practicing competently at the beginning level of nursing.
9. Keep a positive attitude! Remember that you have learned a great amount of nursing knowledge, and the exam is only designed to determine whether you are able to practice safely at the entry level.

NOTES

UNIT ONE

MEDICAL-SURGICAL NURSING

UNIT CONTENT

SECTION I. Review of Fluids and Electrolytes, Acid-Base Balance 11
SECTION II. Review of Respiratory System Disorders 15
SECTION III. Review of General Preoperative and Postoperative Care 23
SECTION IV. Review of Gastrointestinal, Hepatic, and Pancreatic Disorders 24
SECTION V. Review of Musculoskeletal Disorders 34
SECTION VI. Review of Endocrine System Functions and Disorders 38
SECTION VII. Review of Blood Disorders 46
SECTION VIII. Review of Cardiovascular System Disorders 48
SECTION IX. Review of Genitourinary System Disorders 56
SECTION X. Review of Neurological System Disorders 63
SECTION XI. Review of Oncology Nursing 70
SECTION XII. Review of Immunological Disorders 72
SECTION XIII. Review of Burns 73

SYMBOLS

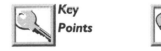 Key Points

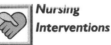 Nursing Interventions

 Points to Remember

REVIEW OF FLUIDS AND ELECTROLYTES, ACID-BASE BALANCE

Fluids and Electrolytes

A. Body Fluids
1. Adults
   a. Women: 50–55% body weight is water
   b. Men: 60–70% body weight is water
   c. Elderly: 47% body weight is water
2. Infant: 75-80% body weight is water
3. Intracellular: 80% of total body water
4. Extracellular: 20% of total body water
   a. Interstitial *between the cells*
   b. Intravascular (plasma)
   c. Other: cerebrospinal fluid, intraocular fluid, bone water, gastrointestinal secretions

B. Electrolytes (normal values may vary slightly between institutions and laboratories)
1. Extracellular
   a. Na^+ 135–145 mEq/L
   b. Ca^{++} 8-10 mg/dL
   c. Cl^- 85–115 mEq/L
   d. HCO_3^- 22–29 mEq/L
2. Intracellular
   a. K^+ 3.5-5.5 mEq/L
   b. PO_4 2.5-4.5 mg/dL
   c. Mg^+ 1.3-2.0 mEq/L
3. Function
   a. Promote neuromuscular excitability
   b. Maintain fluid volume
   c. Distribute water between fluid compartments
   d. Regulate acid-base balance

C. Movement of Fluids and Electrolytes
1. Diffusion: molecules move from an area of higher concentration to an area of lower concentration
2. Osmosis: water moves from an area of lower concentration of particles to an area of higher concentration
3. Filtration: water and dissolved substances move from an area of greater hydrostatic pressure to an area of lower hydrostatic pressure
4. Types of solution
   a. Isotonic 0.9% NaCl
      1) Same osmolarity as plasma
      2) Example: D_5W: To replace fluid volume or increase ADH activity
   b. Hypertonic 3.0% NaCl
   c. Hypotonic 0.45% NaCl
5. Types of pressures
   a. Osmotic
   b. Hydrostatic

D. Mechanisms of Fluid Balance
1. Kidneys: regulate fluids and electrolytes, secrete renin
2. Lungs: regulate CO_2 levels, water vapor
3. Skin: regulate fluid losses (sweat)
4. Hormonal control
   a. ADH (antidiuretic hormone)
   b. Aldosterone *to regulate Na & electrolyte balance*

E. Assessment of Fluid and Electrolyte Balance/Imbalance
1. Fluid volume deficit: water and electrolytes lost in same proportion (blood and urine become concentrated)
   a. Causes
      1) Fever
      2) Vomiting
      3) Diarrhea or ostomy losses
      4) Increased urine output
      5) Increased respirations
      6) Use of diuretics
      7) Insufficient IV fluid replacement
      8) Draining fistulas
      9) Third spacing (burns, ascites)
   b. Manifestations
      1) Weight loss
      2) Poor skin turgor
      3) Urine: decrease in volume, dark, odorous, increased specific gravity
      4) Increased respirations
      5) Dry mucous membrane
      6) Increased heart rate
      7) Increased hematocrit (hemoconcentration)
      8) Decreased central venous pressure (CVP)
   c. **NURSING INTERVENTIONS**
      1) Weigh client daily
      2) Monitor intake and output
      3) Replace fluid-P.O. or IV (Lactated Ringers, 0.9% NS) per order
      4) Measure urine specific gravity
      5) Correct underlying cause
2. Fluid volume excess
   a. Causes
      1) Excessive IV fluids
      2) Decreased kidney function, congestive heart failure (CHF), cirrhosis
      3) Excessive ingestion of table salt
   b. Manifestations (same as CHF)
      1) Cough, dyspnea, crackles, tachypnea
      2) Increased blood pressure, pulse
      3) Decreased hematocrit (hemodilution)
      4) Headache
      5) Weight gain (1 liter of water = 1 kg of

weight gain)

    6)   Increased CVP

    7)   Flushed skin

    8)   Late Signs

       a)   Neck vein distention

       b)   Tachycardia

       c)   Pitting edema

c. **NURSING INTERVENTIONS**

    1)   Administer diuretics - furosemide (*Lasix*) as per order

    2)   Restrict fluids, monitor intake and output

    3)   Weigh client daily

    4)   Provide skin care

    5)   Use Semi-Fowler's position

    6)   Maintain low-sodium diet

3. Electrolyte imbalances: (see table I-1. Major Electrolytes: Imbalance/Interventions)

F. Regulation of Body pH

1. Normal value is 7.35–7.45

2. Mechanisms regulating pH

  a. Chemical buffers: protein molecules, phosphate

  b. Lungs: control carbon dioxide levels

  c. Kidneys: bicarbonate

Metabolic/Respiratory Imbalance-Acidosis/Alkalosis

A. Acid-Base Imbalance

1. Metabolic acidosis

  a. Definition: base bicarbonate deficit; increase in hydrogen ion concentration

  b. Causes

    1)   Diarrhea

    2)   Renal failure

    3)   Systemic infections

    4)   Diabetic acidosis

    5)   Starvation, malnutrition, ketogenic (high-fat) diet

    6)   Excessive exercise

  c. Manifestations

    1)   Headache

    2)   Confusion, stupor

    3)   Loss of consciousness

    4)   pH below 7.35

    5) HCO_3^- below 22

    6)   Tachypnea (increased respirations) or Kussmaul's respirations

  d. **NURSING INTERVENTIONS**

    1)   Promote good air exchange

    2)   Monitor K^+ level

    3)   Give sodium bicarbonate as ordered

2. Metabolic alkalosis

  a. Definition: base bicarbonate excess; decrease in hydrogen ion concentration

  b. Causes

    1)   Vomiting (excessive loss of chloride)

    2)   Gastric suction

    3)   Alkali ingestion (excessive bicarbonate)

    4)   Long-term diuretic therapy

  c. Manifestations

    1)   CNS symptoms: confusion, irritability, agitation, coma

    2)   Shallow respirations

    3)   Tetany

    4)   pH above 7.45

    5) HCO_3^- above 26

  d. **NURSING INTERVENTIONS**

    1)   Restore fluid volume

    2)   Prevent metabolic alkalosis

       a)   Monitor K+ level

       b)   Evaluate need for intravenous K+ replacement for clients on gastric suction

       c)   Promote intake of K+ rich foods or oral replacement for clients on long term diuretic therapy

3. Respiratory acidosis

  a. Definition: excess carbonic acid; increase in hydrogen ion concentration

  b. Causes

    1)   Acute: respiratory suppression or obstruction due to pulmonary edema, oversedation, pneumonia

    2)   Chronic: chronic airflow limitation (CAL) or COPD

  c. Manifestations

    1)   Acute

       a)   Confusion

       b)   Restlessness

       c)   Weakness

       d)   Headache

       e)   Coma

       f)   pH below 7.35

       g) pCO_2 above 45 mm Hg

    2)   Chronic (These symptoms are classic signs of COPD)

       a) pCO_2 above 45 mm Hg

       b)   Tachypnea

       c)   Dyspnea

       d)   Weight loss

  d. **NURSING INTERVENTIONS**

    1)   Administer sodium bicarbonate per order

    2)   Promote good respiratory exchange

    3)   Administer bronchodilators per order

    4)   Monitor arterial blood gases (ABGs)

4. Respiratory alkalosis

  a. Definition: carbonic acid deficit; decrease in hydrogen ion concentration

  b. Causes

    1)   Hyperventilation - secondary to pain,

READ!!!

TABLE I-1.
MAJOR ELECTROLYTES: IMBALANCE/INTERVENTIONS

ELECTROLYTE	NORM. VALUE	SOURCES	LOW CAUSES	MANIFES-TATIONS	NURSING INTERVEN.	EXCESS CAUSES	MANIFES-TATIONS	NURSING INVERVEN.
1. Potassium: (K$^+$)	3.5 mEq/L 5.5 mEq/L	Fruits: bananas, figs, peaches, melons, prunes, raisins, apricots. Juices: tomato, orange, grape. Nuts & Veg.	Hypokalemia associated with renal loss, diuretics, burns, massive trauma, colitis, uncontrolled diabetes, diarrhea, excessive perspiration, decreased intake, vomiting, gastric suction	Muscle cramping, muscle weakness, weak pulse, dyspnea, mental changes, loquacious, hallucinations, depression, EKG changes (sensitivity to digitalis), respiratory arrest	- Keep I&O - Observe for ECG changes - Potassium supplements: Never give bolus injection IV or P.O - Check renal function before giving - Dilute and mix well before adm. Not greater than 40 mEq/L.	Hyperkalemia, renal failure, cell damage, Addison's disease, acidosis	CNS stimulation, listlessness, weakness, flaccid paralysis, abdominal cramps, arrhythmias, muscle weakness	- Monitor IV glucose and insulin (promote entry of K into cells), - Give fluids to increase urinary output, Kayexalate exchanges Na+ for K+ ion
2. Sodium: (Na$^+$)	135–145 mEq/L	Common Table Salt	Hyponatremia, increased perspiration, drinking water, gastrointestinal suction, irrigation of tube with plain water, adrenal insufficiency, potent diuretics	Lethargy, hypotension, cramps, vomiting, oliguria, apprehension, muscular weakness, headache, convulsions	- Use normal saline (not distilled water) for irrigation - Avoid tap water enemas - Drink juices and bouillon	Hypernatremia, decreased water intake, diarrhea, impaired renal function, acute tracheo bronchitis, unconsciousness, base bicarbonate deficit	Edema, hypertonicity, dry sticky mucous membranes, elevated temperature, flushed skin, thirst	- D$_5$W - Give water between tube feedings - Elderly clients to drink 8-10 glasses - Check humidifier water level
3. Calcium: (Ca^{++})	8.5–10.5 mg/dL or 4.5–5.5 mEq/L	Milk, cheese, sardines, salmon	Hypokalemia, massive infection, burns, administration of citrated blood, hypoparathyroidism, surgical removal of parathyroids	Tetany cramps, tingling, numbness hyperactive reflexes, cardiac arrhythmias	- Teach proper use of antacids/laxatives, Importance of adequate milk intake - Keep 10% calcium gluconate on hand for use, start after thyroid surgery	Hypercalcemia, excessive Vit. D milk ingestion, hyperparathyroid, multiple myeloma, prolonged bed rest, renal disease	Renal calculi, nausea, anorexia, weight loss, deep bone pain, flank pain, lethargy, anorexia, muscle weakness, pathological fractures	- Increase mobility - Avoid large doses of Vit. D supplementation - Adequate hydration
4. Magnesium: (mg^{++})	1.7 mEq/L 2.3 mEq/L or 2–7mg/ 100 mL	Fruit, peas, beans, nuts	Hypomagnesemia, vomiting, diarrhea, chronic alcoholism, impaired GI absorption, unterostomy drainage. Use of diuretics	Disorientation, convulsion, hyperactive deep reflexes, tremors, positive response to magnesium		- Hypermagnesemia, hypotension, respiratory, paralysis - Associated with renal failure, DM, dehydration		

MEDICAL-SURGICAL NURSING - **UNIT ONE** ❖ 13

anxiety, thyroid toxicosis
2) Decreased O_2 (pneumonia, pulmonary edema)
3) Elevated body temperature
4) Salicylate intoxication
c. Manifestations
1) Unconsciousness
2) Circumoral numbness
3) pCO_2 below 35 mm Hg
d. **NURSING INTERVENTIONS**
1) Have client breathe into paper bag
2) Have client breathe into cupped hands
3) Provide oxygen if hypoxic

B. Blood Gases

1. Arterial Blood Gases (ABG)s
   a. Most accurate means of assessing respiratory function
   b. Must be sterile, anaerobic
   c. Drawn into heparinized syringe
   d. Keep on ice and transport to lab immediately
   e. Document amount of oxygen delivered
   f. Document client's body temperature
   g. Apply pressure to site for 5-10 minutes
2. Components

   pH   measure of acidity or alkalinity of blood
           N = 7.35-7.45

   pCO_2 partial pressure of carbon dioxide respiratory parameter influenced by lungs only
           N = 35-45, remember this by taking the seven away from pH

   Hypoventilation results in hypercapnia ($\uparrow CO_2$)

   Hyperventilation results in hypocapnia ($\downarrow CO_2$)

   pO_2 partial pressure of oxygen measure of amount of oxygen delivered to the lungs
           N = 80-100

   HCO_3- bicarbonate, metabolic parameter influenced only by metabolic factors
           N = 22-26

POINTS TO REMEMBER:

1. Regardless of the pO_2, delivery of oxygen to the tissues is affected by the pH and temperature.
2. Ratio which dictates pH level: $H_2CO_3 : HCO_3$ 1 : 20
3. Remember: pCO_2 is inversely associated to pH if respiratory origin; HCO_3^- is directly associated to pH if metabolic origin

3. Examples:

TABLE I-2.
ACIDOSIS/ALKALOSIS

			ACIDOSIS	ALKALOSIS
Respiratory:	pCO_2		(52) (high)	(32) (low)
	pH		(7.32) (low)	(7.51) (high)
	HCO_3		(18) (low)	(29) (high)
Metabolic:	HCO_3		(16) (low)	(38) (high)
	pH		(7.3) (low)	(7.56) (high)
	CO_2		(30) (low)	(50) (high)
Norms:	pCO_2	: 35–45 mmHg		
	HCO_3	: 22–26 meql		
	pH	: 7.35–7.45		
	H_2CO_3	: HCO_3 1:20		

	pH	pCO_2	HCO_3^-
Respiratory Acidosis	$\downarrow$	$\uparrow$	Normal or $\uparrow$
Respiratory Alkalosis	$\uparrow$	$\downarrow$	Normal or $\downarrow$
Metabolic Acidosis	$\downarrow$	$\downarrow$	$\downarrow$
Metabolic Alkalosis	$\uparrow$	$\uparrow$	$\uparrow$

RESPIRATORY ACIDOSIS		RESPIRATORY ALKALOSIS	
pH	7.32	pH	7.48
pCO_2	48	pCO_2	33
HCO_3^-	20	HCO_3^-	28
pO_2	90	pO_2	90
METABOLIC ACIDOSIS		**METABOLIC ALKALOSIS**	
pH	7.32	pH	7.48
pCO_2	30	pCO_2	38
HCO_3^-	20	HCO_3^-	28
pO_2	90	pO_2	90

POINTS TO REMEMBER:

1. Clients with low sodium will present with acute onset of confusion.
2. Never give K^+ to a client who is not voiding: no "P," no "K"
3. When a client has a high calcium level, phosphorus levels will be low and vise versa; works like a see-saw

SECTION II

REVIEW OF RESPIRATORY SYSTEM DISORDERS

Anatomy and Physiology

A. Function of the Lungs
1. Respiration: overall process by which exchange takes place between the atmosphere and the cells of the body. Normal adult respiratory rate: 12–20 breaths per minute.
2. Ventilation: movement of air in and out of the airways, intermittently replenishing the oxygen and removing the carbon dioxide from the lungs
3. Dead space: the 150 mL area where there is no air exchange; anatomically from the nose and mouth to the alveoli. Therefore, 150 mL of the tidal volume is not used in any air exchange.

B. Thoracic Cavity-Lined by Visceral and Parietal Pleura
1. Right pulmonary space
2. Left pulmonary space
3. Pericardial space
4. Mediastinal space contains the esophagus, trachea, great vessels, and heart

C. Subdivisions of the Lungs
1. Right: 3 lobes, 10 segments
2. Left: 2 lobes, 8 segments
3. Alveoli: tiny distal air sacs where gas exchange takes place; produce surfactant, a phospholipid secretion of the alveoli (Type II cells) that reduces the surface tension of fluid lining the alveoli allowing expansion to take place. Without surfactant, the lungs would collapse; oxygen is required for surfactant production.
4. Diffusion: exchange of gases (oxygen and carbon dioxide) at the alveolar/capillary membrane

D. Factors Affecting Airflow
1. Normally airways are open, moist, intact, and not inflamed. Cilia clear foreign substances.
2. Objective of care is to keep the airways healthy by the nursing interventions:
   a. Promote adequate fluid intake
   b. Prevent exposure to infections
   c. Decrease exposure to tobacco smoke
   d. Decrease environmental pollutants
   e. Avoid triggers which cause inflammation of airways, such as allergens
3. If airways are affected, the diameter of the airways narrows causing an increase in airway resistance.

E. General Causes of Airway Illnesses Are:
1. Infections which cause mucus and swelling
2. Allergens which cause swelling and bronchospasm
3. Foreign bodies which cause obstruction
4. Obstructive disorders: COPD, bronchiectasis
5. Restrictive disorders: kyphoscoliosis, abdominal distension, edema
6. Trauma: stab wound, surgery

Diagnostic Tests

A. Chest X-ray: noninvasive procedure with no special preparation; lead shield for women of childbearing age

B. Mantoux Test: positive result only indicates client was exposed to Tuberculosis (TB); it is not diagnostic for active TB
1. Upper 1/3 inner surface forearm
2. Needle bevel up
3. 0.1 mL of purified protein derivative (PPD) subdermal
4. Read in 48-72 hours
5. Measure induration: if 10 mm or greater, it is a positive reading

C. Sputum Examination: first morning specimen preferable, approximately 15 mL required; always obtain before initiating antibiotics

D. Thoracentesis: aspiration of pleural fluid and/or air from the pleural space
1. Preparation
   a. Consent and explanation
   b. Position: sitting on side of bed with feet on chair, leaning over bedside table
   c. No more than 1,200 mL should be removed at one time
2. Post-procedure
   a. Apply pressure to puncture site
   b. Use Semi-Fowler's position or puncture site up
   c. Monitor for shock, pneumothorax, respiratory arrest, subcutaneous emphysema
   d. Assess breath sounds

E. Bronchoscopy: examination of tracheobronchial tree using a bronchoscope
1. Preparation
   a. Consent and explanation
   b. NPO after midnight
   c. ABG, oxygen administration
2. Post-procedure
   a. Keep client NPO until return of gag reflex is confirmed
   b. Monitor vital signs until stable

c. Assess for respiratory distress
d. Administer warm saline gargles after gag reflex returns
e. Use Semi-Fowler's position
f. Give water as first fluid
g. Inform client that it is possible to expectorate some blood tinged mucus secretions, especially when a biopsy was performed.

Management of Clients with Respiratory System Disorders

A. **Chronic Airflow Limitation** (CAL); also called **Chronic Obstructive Pulmonary Disease** (COPD)
1. Definition: a group of chronic lung diseases including pulmonary emphysema, chronic bronchitis, and bronchial asthma
2. Major diseases
   a. Pulmonary emphysema ("pink puffer")
      1) Definition: destruction of alveoli, narrowing of small airways (bronchioles) and the trapping of air resulting in loss of lung elasticity
      2) Etiology: cigarette smoking (#1 preventable cause of respiratory problems), deficiency of alpha anti-trypsin (enzyme that blocks the action of proteolytic enzymes that are destructive to elastin and other substances in the alveolar walls)
      3) Manifestations
         a) Shortness of breath
         b) Difficult exhalation
         c) Pursed-lip breathing
         d) Wheezing, crackles
         e) Shallow rapid respirations
         f) Hypoxia
         g) Productive cough
         h) Respiratory acidosis
         i) Barrel chest
         j) Anorexia, weight loss
         k) Finger clubbing
      4) **NURSING INTERVENTIONS**
         a) Position sitting up, leaning forward
         b) Provide pulmonary toilet
            (1) Bronchodilator medications via nebulization as ordered
            (2) Chest physiotherapy/pulmonary drainage (CPT/PD)
            (3) Assess if effective by checking the breath sounds and the pulse oximetry on a routine basis.
         c) Encourage frequent rest periods
         d) Use intermittent positive pressure breathing (IPPB)
         e) Administer oxygen at low flow (under most circumstances, limited to 1 liter, but may go no higher than a maximum 3 liters or less): to prevent CO_2 narcosis
         f) Encourage fluids: 3000 mL per day if not contraindicated
         g) Administer prophylactic antibiotics, as ordered
         h) Provide appropriate nutrition: decrease carbohydrates in order to decrease carbon dioxide. Increase calories and protein to meet increased energy requirements. Lower intake of gas forming foods to decrease dyspnea and SOB.
         i) Promote deep breathing exercises
         j) Promote energy conservation exercises to enhance rest
         k) Provide emotional support to decrease anxiety
         l) Address sexual concerns
         m) Provide teaching
            (1) Avoid crowds
            (2) Diaphragmatic breathing
            (3) Pursed-lip breathing
            (4) Report first sign of upper respiratory infection (URI)
            (5) Avoid allergens (examples: dust, odors, dander, etc.)
   b. Chronic bronchitis (blue bloater)
      1) Definition: excessive mucus secretions within the airways and recurrent cough
      2) Etiology: heavy cigarette smoking, pollution, infection
      3) Manifestations
         a) Cough (copious sputum)
         b) Dyspnea on exertion, later at rest
         c) Hypoxemia resulting in polycythemia: ruddy look to skin, compensation
         d) Crackles, rhonchi
         e) Pulmonary hypertension leading to cor pulmonale and signs of right heart failure such as peripheral dependent edema
      4) **NURSING INTERVENTIONS**
         a) Prevent exposure to irritants
         b) Reduce irritants
         c) Increase humidity: 70% is best
         d) Relieve bronchospasm through deep breathing and medications
         e) Provide chest physiotherapy (CPT)
         f) Provide postural drainage (PD)
         g) Promote breathing techniques; same as COPD
   c. Asthma
      1) Definition: condition of abnormal bronchial hyperreactivity to certain

substances
2) Etiology
   a) Extrinsic: antigen-antibody reaction triggered by food, drugs, or inhaled particles
   b) Intrinsic: pathophysiological conditions within the respiratory tract, non-allergic form
3) Manifestations: acute attack
   a) Severe, sudden dyspnea
   b) Use of accessory muscles; for adults neck muscles; child will get retractions
   c) Sitting up
   d) Diaphoresis
   e) Anxiety, apprehension
   f) Wheezing
   g) Cyanosis: very late sign
   h) Remember, an improvement in wheezes with no improvement in the client's condition may actually indicate worsening of the condition and tightening of airways to the point where air flow is diminishing
   i) Decrease in tidal volume is measured by a spirometer
4) **NURSING INTERVENTIONS**
   a) Remain with client
   b) Use High-Fowler's position
   c) Provide emotional support
   d) Monitor respiratory status: ABGs, lung sounds, and pulse oximetry
   e) Promote hydration with fluids
   f) Administer epinephrine hydrochloride (*Adrenalin*) subcutaneously and monitor its effectiveness
   g) Administer aminophylline, theophylline and ethylenediamine (*Phyllocontin*) IV
      (1) Monitor for side effects such as GI upsets (nausea and vomiting) and seizures
      (2) Monitor theophylline level to assure therapeutic action and eliminate toxic effects: therapeutic serum level is 10-20 mcg/mL
   h) Provide bronchodilators via nebulization and metered dose inhalers (MDI)
   i) Monitor oxygen therapy
   j) Administer corticosteroids: to decrease airway inflammation and open airways
5) Status Asthmaticus: attack lasting more than 24 hours; medical emergency
   a) Use High-Fowler's position
   b) Monitor vital signs for signs of

hypoxia
   c) Monitor respiratory status
   d) Administer aminophylline (*Phyllocontin*) IV as ordered
   e) Administer bronchodilator therapy as ordered
   f) Provide emotional support

B. **Complications of CAL** (COPD)
   1. Cor pulmonale (form of heart failure)
      a. Definition: right ventricular hypertrophy or failure secondary to disease of the lungs, pulmonary vessels or chest wall
      b. Etiology: causes increased pressure and pulmonary hypertension
         1) Decrease in the size of the pulmonary vascular bed from destruction of the pulmonary capillaries
         2) Increased resistance of pulmonary capillary bed
         3) Shunting of unaerated blood across the collapsed alveoli
      c. Manifestations: signs of heart failure; initially the right heart fails, then the left heart fails because of decreased cardiac output
         1) Right heart failure
            a) Peripheral edema (dependent)
            b) Jugular vein distension
         2) Left heart failure
            a) Dyspnea
            b) Cyanosis
            c) Cough
            d) Substernal pain
            e) Syncope on exertion
            f) Paroxysmal nocturnal dyspnea (PND) and orthopnea
      d. **NURSING INTERVENTIONS**
         1) Promote bed rest
         2) Monitor oxygen therapy
         3) Maintain low-sodium diet
         4) Monitor for side effects of digitalis (*Digoxin*) and diuretics
   2. Carbon dioxide narcosis/oxygen toxicity
      a. Definition: near comatose state secondary to increased CO_2 due to chronic retention
      b. Etiology: carbon dioxide retention and secondary to excessive oxygen delivery
      c. Manifestations: signs of hypoxia
         1) Drowsy
         2) Irritable
         3) Hallucinations
         4) Coma
         5) Paralysis
         6) Convulsions
         7) Tachycardia
         8) Arrythmias
         9) Poor ventilation

d. **NURSING INTERVENTIONS**
1) Avoid high concentrations of oxygen – keep below 3 L. per minute, no more than 70% oxygen delivered. Make sure you know the approximate concentration delivered by the oxygen delivery method you are using. Cannula: 40%; mask: 60%; rebreather mask: 100%.
2) Monitor response to oxygen therapy; monitor blood gases. If pCO_2 level is above normal, it is not preferable to have the oxygen at normal level because it will shut off the hypoxic drive which is triggered by a low O_2 level. This will cause client to go into respiratory arrest.

3. Pneumothorax
   a. Definition: collection of air or fluid in the pleural space. Can come from outside chest wall or inside the lung.
   b. Etiology
      1) Trauma: gunshot, stabbing
      2) Thoracic surgery: open thoracotomy
      3) Positive pressure ventilation: causes segment of the lung to rip open, expose pleural space.
      4) Iatrogenic, adverse effects of
         a) Thoracentesis
         b) Central venous pressure line insertion
         c) Unknown cause
   c. Types
      1) Spontaneous
      2) Tension: due to build up of pressure. Results in a shift of the major organs and vessels in the chest cavity.
      3) Open: from trauma such as a gunshot or stab wound
   d. Manifestations: depend on severity
      1) Spontaneous
         a) Sudden, sharp chest pain
         b) Sudden shortness of breath with violent attempts to breathe
         c) Hypotension
         d) Tachycardia
         e) Hyperresonance and decreased breath sounds over the affected lung
         f) Anxiety, diaphoresis, restlessness
      2) Tension
         a) Subcutaneous emphysema (crepitus), dyspnea
         b) Cyanosis
         c) Acute chest pain
         d) Tympany on percussion
      3) Mediastinal shift: contents of mediastinum pushed to unaffected side
         a) Cyanosis
         b) Tracheal deviation–away from injured side

c) Cardiovascular compromise: may have signs and symptoms depending on degree of deviation
e. **NURSING INTERVENTIONS**
1) Remain with client and remain calm
2) Position in High-Fowler's
3) Assess vital signs and breath sounds
4) Provide oxygen therapy as ordered
5) Prepare for chest x-ray
6) Provide thoracentesis tray to reestablish negative pressure or relieve pressure with tension pneumothorax
7) Monitor ABGs
8) Monitor for shock
9) Assist with insertion of chest tubes
   a) At the bedside or in operating room by physician
   b) Aseptic technique
   c) Local anesthetic, stab wound
      (1) Upper for evacuation of air
      (2) Lower for evacuation of fluid
   d) Occlusive dressing

C. **Closed Chest Drainage**
1. Purposes
   a. Remove fluid and/or air from the pleural space
   b. Reestablish normal negative pressure in the pleural space
   c. Promote re-expansion of the lung
   d. Prevent reflux of air/fluid into pleural space from the drainage apparatus
   e. Used commonly after thoracic surgery or pneumothorax
2. General Principles: the nurse must ask the following when confronted with any chest drainage system:
   a. Where is the water seal? How can it be maintained?
   b. What controls the suction in the system? Is it gravity or is it a negative pressure? What is the setting?
   c. Where does the drainage collect, and how can I maintain the patency of this system? How can I measure the drainage?
3. Usage: the most commonly used today are disposable chest tube systems (Pleur-Evac, Thora-seal)
   a. Replacing two and three-bottle systems, these are made of molded plastic to form three chambers.
      1) Suction control chamber (closest to suction): when on should be continuously bubbling. Amount is usually determined by a water level in the suction control chamber.
      2) Water seal chamber is middle seal; intermittent bubbling occurs if there is air in

the chest. In this area, you will observe the rise and fall of fluid in the system with respirations This is called tidaling.

    3) Drainage collection (closest to chest tube)

b. Suction is controlled by the amount of water in the suction control chamber. Make sure evaporation does not change the amount of suction by lowering the water level.

4. **NURSING INTERVENTIONS**
   a. Check for bubbling and fluctuation
   b. Assess respiratory status
   c. Turn client; ask client to cough, deep breathe
   d. Mark the amount of drainage at the beginning of each shift. Should see a decrease in the amount over time.
   e. Note character of drainage
   f. Be sure tubing is without kinks, coiled on the bed
   g. Keep bottles below level of heart
   h. Maintain water seal
   i. Maintain dry, sterile, occlusive dressing
   j. Do not strip tubes, avoid milking
   k. Obtain STAT Chest x-ray (CXR)

5. Removal of chest tubes: done by physician
   a. Provide equipment: suture removal kit, sterile gauze, petroleum gauze, adhesive tape
   b. Use Semi-Fowler's or High-Fowler's position
   c. Instruct client on that removal of tubes will be done during expiration or at end of full inspiration
   d. Apply air-occlusive dressing immediately
   e. Obtain STAT Chest x-ray
   f. Assess for complications: subcutaneous emphysema, respiratory distress. Major complication is pneumothorax.

POINTS TO REMEMBER:

1. Problem: Continuous, rapid bubbling in water-seal bottle/chamber
   Solution: Locate leak in the system; repair or replace. Start at chest and move down the tubing to see where the leak is.

2. Problem: No fluctuation in water-seal chamber with respirations
   Solution: Check for kinks in the tubing. Listen for breath sounds. Assess for respiratory distress. Lung may have re-expanded.

3. Problem: No bubbling in suction-control bottle/chamber
   Solution: Turn up suction until gentle continuous suctioning; check fluid level

4. Problem: Damaged system or chest tube disconnected from water seal
   Solution: Insert end of chest tube into sterile water until the system can be replaced

5. Problem: Tube pulled out
   Solution: Cover wound site with petroleum (*Vaseline*) air occlusive dressing and call primary healthcare provider immediately

D. Infectious Pulmonary Diseases

1. Tuberculosis
   a. Reportable, communicable, infectious, inflammatory disease that can occur in any part of the body
   b. Etiology: mycobacterium tuberculosis (nonmotile, aerobic, killed by heat and ultraviolet light); droplet nuclei spread by laughing, sneezing, coughing. Can spread to other areas of the body and is called miliary TB. Causes caseation in the lungs and Ghon tubercles which can stay with the client for years, lay dormant then open again and reinfect the client.
   c. Risk factors
      1) Overcrowded, poor living conditions
      2) Poor nutritional status
      3) Previous infection
      4) Inadequate treatment of primary infection leads to multi-drug resistant organisms
      5) Close contact with infected person
      6) Immune dysfunction or HIV
      7) Long-term care facilities, prisons
      8) Elderly
      9) Substance abuse
   d. Manifestations: same as other pulmonary inflammations and infections
      1) Productive cough
      2) Night sweats, low-grade fever
      3) Hemoptysis
      4) Dyspnea
      5) Malaise
      6) Weight loss
      7) Anorexia, vomiting, indigestion
      8) Pallor
   e. Diagnostic tests
      1) Mantoux test
      2) Sputum for acid-fast bacillus, x3
      3) Chest x-ray
      4) History and physical exam
   f. Treatment
      1) Chemotherapy (all are hepatotoxic)
         a) Ethambutol (*Myambutol*): impairs RNA synthesis; side effects: optic neuritis, skin rash

b) Rifampicin (*Rifadin*): impairs RNA synthesis; side effects: red-orange color to urine and feces; negates birth control pill; nausea, vomiting, thrombocytopenia

c) Isoniazid (*INH*): interferes with DNA synthesis used in prophylactic treatment; side effects: peripheral neuritis, hepatotoxicity, GI upset; must take vitamin B$_6$ (*pyridoxine*) (*Beesix*) in conjunction with this therapy to prevent peripheral neuritis

d) Streptomycin; side effects: 8th nerve damage, use with caution in renal disease. Should have hearing tests done routinely.

2) **NURSING INTERVENTIONS**

a) Teaching plan includes:
(1) Preventive measures to avoid catching viral infections (infection control)
(2) Drugs must be taken in combination to avoid bacterial resistance
(3) Drugs should be taken either once each day or 2-3 times per week, but always at the same time of day and on an empty stomach
(4) Drugs must be taken for 6–12 months
(5) Maintaining adequate nutritional status
(6) Promoting yearly checkups
(7) Make sure the client knows to have liver function tests.

b) Hospital care
(1) Teaching: hand washing, cover nose and mouth when sneezing, coughing
(2) Wear special particulate respirator mask when in the client's room
(3) Isolation room ventilated to outside (negative pressure room); discontinued when client no longer considered infectious
(4) Psychological support: reinforcement of the need to take medications. Many clients choose to stop drug therapy.

POINTS TO REMEMBER:
1. Obtain sputum specimens before drug therapy is initiated
2. Multiple drug therapy is necessary to prevent the development of resistant organisms
3. Give drugs in a single daily dose

4. Drug therapy must be continued for 6–12 months even though the x-ray, sputum specimens, and manifestations are within normal limits
5. Client is generally considered noninfectious after 1–2 weeks of continuous drug therapy
6. Avoid use of alcohol during drug therapy to reduce risk of hepatotoxicity

2. Pneumonia
a. Definition: inflammation of the lung parenchyma caused by infectious agents
b. Etiology: classified as community acquired or hospital acquired (nosocomial)
1) Community acquired
a) Streptococcus pneumoniae or pneumococcal
b) Haemophilus influenzae
c) Legionella pneumonia
d) Atypical pneumonia: most commonly seen in children; usual organism is mycoplasma pneumoniae; differs from the others in that minimal mucus is produced
2) Hospital acquired
a) Staphylococcus aureus
b) Klebsiella pneumoniae
c) Pseudomonas pneumoniae
d) Fungi (various types, i.e., histoplasmosis)

c. Persons at risk
1) Elderly
2) Infants
3) Substance abusers
4) Cigarette smokers
5) Postoperative clients or those on prolonged bed rest
6) Clients with chronic illnesses such as COPD; CAL
7) Clients with AIDS - Pneumocystis carinii pneumonia (PCP)
8) Other immunosuppressed clients

d. Common manifestations
1) Sudden onset of chills, fever
2) Cough: dry and painful at first, later produces rusty colored sputum
3) Dyspnea
4) Flushed cheeks
5) Pallor, cyanosis
6) Pleuritic pain that increases with respiration
7) Tachypnea, tachycardia

e. **NURSING INTERVENTIONS**
1) Administer drug therapy as ordered
a) Cough suppressants (be careful giving to children and clients who have chest congestion; generally only

given to them for sleep), expectorants
- b) Bronchodilators; teach use of metered dose inhaler
- c) Antibiotics as ordered
- d) Mild analgesic – to decrease pain and enable client to deep breathe
2) Encourage ambulation as tolerated
3) Provide pulmonary toilet
4) Assess for sputum thickness, color
5) Administer oxygen to maintain oxygen saturations >95%
6) Provide small frequent meals, increase fluid intake
7) Maintain fluid and electrolyte balance
8) Isolate as indicated
9) Provide oral hygiene

POINTS TO REMEMBER:

1. Most pneumonias have a sudden onset
2. Penicillin remains the drug of choice for pneumococcal pneumonias (unless allergic to PCN)
3. Antibiotics must be given on time to maintain blood levels
4. Watch for side effects of penicillin therapy – especially allergies

E. Cancer of the Lungs (see also under oncology)

1. Definition: primary or secondary (metastatic from a primary site) malignant tumor located in the lung or bronchi
2. Etiology: cigarette smoking, exposure to asbestos and other carcinogens (coal dust, uranium, nickel)
3. Manifestations:
   a. Asymptomatic in the early stages
   b. Later stages:
      1) Coughing
      2) Wheezing
      3) Dyspnea
      4) Hemoptysis
      5) Weight loss
      6) Anorexia
      7) Fever
   c. NURSING INTERVENTIONS
      1) Support cessation of smoking
      2) Postoperative care for lung excision
         a) Pneumonectomy: removal of an entire lung (reasons: cancer, abscess); postop: dorsal recumbent or Semi-Fowler's position on affected side; range of motion to affected shoulder; no chest tube. Make sure nursing interventions are instituted to prevent infection in the other lung.
         b) Lobectomy: removal of a lobe for TB or abscess; postop: chest tube
         c) Segmentectomy: removal of a lobe

(reason: infection in localized area); postop: chest tube
- d) Wedge resection: removal of a small portion of lung tissue (reason: small localized area of disease near the surface of the lung); postop: chest tube
3) Encourage turn, cough, deep breathe
4) Administer oxygen
5) Provide pain interventions so that client will be able to move and deep breathe
6) Promote fluids to maintain thin respiratory tract secretions
7) Instruct client to splint chest incision when coughing
8) Teach client exercises for arm on affected side to prevent frozen shoulder
9) Place needed articles on side of surgery so client will move arm to get them
10) Assess wound for infection

F. Disorders of the Pleural Space

1. Pleural effusion (secondary to other disorders)
   a. Definition: accumulation of nonpurulent fluid in the pleural cavity
   b. Etiology
      1) Blood vessels exudate
      2) Tissue surfaces transudate, associated with leukemia, lymphomas, pneumonia, pulmonary edema, cirrhosis of the liver, following cardiac (coronary artery bypass graft; CABG) and pulmonary surgery
2. Empyema
   a. Definition: accumulation of pus in the pleural cavity
   b. Etiology: spread of infection from lungs, chest wall; complication of pneumonia, TB, abscess, bronchiectasis
   c. Treatment: antibiotics, possible chest tube
   d. Interventions
      1) Follow care of the client with a chest tube. Drainage will depend on what is present in the pleural space. If only a limited amount of effusion or pus is present, may be able to remove with a thoracentesis.
      2) Assess respiratory status
      3) Maintain infection control measures

Pulmonary Therapies

A. Chest Physiotherapy (CPT) (using cupped hands)

1. Definition: percussion and vibration over the thorax to loosen secretions in the affected areas of the lung
2. Procedure

     a. Keep a layer of material (gown or pajamas) between your hands and the client's skin

     b. Stop if pain occurs

     c. Best time to do is in the morning upon rising, 1 hour before meals or 2–3 hours after meals

     d. Client must be instructed to deep breathe and cough during the procedure

     e. Should be followed with oral hygiene

3. Contraindications

     a. When bronchospasm is increased by its use

     b. History of pathological fractures, rib fractures, or osteoporosis

     c. Obesity

     d. New incisions in the chest area or upper abdominal area

     e. Pain in the chest

B. Postural Drainage

1. Definition: use of gravity to drain secretions from segments of the lung; may be combined with chest PT

2. **NURSING INTERVENTIONS**

     a. Proper positioning (lung segment to be drained is uppermost)

     b. Stop if cyanosis or exhaustion increases

     c. Provide mouth care after procedure; best time is in the morning upon rising, 1 hour before meals or 2–3 hours after meals

     d. Maintain position 5–20 minutes or as tolerated

3. Contraindications

     a. Unstable vital signs

     b. Increased intracranial pressure

C. Pulmonary Toilet

1. Cough
2. Breathe deeply
3. Chest PT
4. Turn and position

D. Intermittent Positive Pressure Breathing (IPPB)

1. Definition: delivery of aerosolized medications to the bronchial tree by positive pressure

2. Adverse effects

     a. Dizziness

     b. Headache

     c. Anxiety

     d. Cardiac arrhythmias

     e. Pneumothorax

E. Inhalers and Nebulizer Treatments

1. Inhaler Therapy:

     a. Doses may vary per order. Generally, 2 puffs are a standard for metered dose inhalers, with no more than 12 puffs administered in 24 hours.

     b. For maximum effectiveness, administer ordered bronchodilators and nebulizer treatments prior to CPT/PD

     c. Types of Inhalers

TABLE I-3.
INHALER THERAPY

Drug	Nebulization Dose	Inhaler Dose	Side Effects
albuterol (*Proventil*)	2.5mg, 3–4/daily	2 puffs q 4–6h	tachycardia
isoetharine (*Bronkosol*)	0.25 mL of 1% solution diluted into 2.5 mL NS q4h	1–2 puffs q 4h	- headache - tachycardia
isoproterenol (*Isuprel*)	0.25 mL of 1% solution diluted into 2.5 mL NS q4h	1–2 puffs q 4h	- tachycardia - arrhythmias
terbutaline (*Brethine*)		2 puffs q 4–6h	tachycardia

1) Bronchodilators

     a) Relax airways and open diameter thereby decreasing airway resistance

     b) Common side effects include tachycardia and headache

     c) Types:

        (1) Albuterol (*Proventil*)

        (2) Isoetharine (*Bronkosol*)

        (3) Terbutaline (*Brethine*)

        (4) Salmeterol xinafoate (*Serevent*)

           (a) Used for long-term maintenance therapy of asthma

           (b) Prevents bronchospasm

           (c) Cannot be used to treat acute symptoms

2) Steroids

     a) Decrease inflammation and open airways thereby decreasing airway resistance

     b) May cause oral superinfection therefore always follow with oral hygiene

     c) May mask the signs of infection

     d) When administering inhalers, always give the steroid last

     e) Types:

        (1) Triamcinolone acetonide (*Azmacort*)

        (2) Fluticasone propionate (*Flovent*)

3) Mast cell inhibitors

     a) Prevents allergic response in airways

     b) Used for prophylaxis only

     c) Never use at onset of attack

     d) Types:

        (1) Cromolyn (*Intal*)

2. Using inhalers (metered dose inhalers); teach client procedure
   a. Shake the inhaler
   b. Remove the cap from the inhaler
   c. Breathe deeply in and out through the mouth (breathe out as much as possible)
   d. Hold the mouthpiece 1-2 inches away from the lips and open the mouth.
   e. With the index finger on top of the canister, depress the top while inhaling deeply and consistently
   f. Close mouth and hold breath for as long as possible
   g. Exhale
   h. Wait 2-5 minutes before the next puff
   i. If possible, follow with mouth care. Must do after steroid inhalers.
3. Use of Spacer devices:
   a. Used to deliver inhalant medications
   b. Increase the amount of medication delivered to the lungs significantly over standard inhalers and should be used whenever possible.

F. Suctioning

1. Indications: client is unable to raise secretions after coughing or chest PT; to obtain a sputum sample; airway filled with secretions.
2. Can be oral or via endotracheal tube/tracheostomy
   a. Oral is not sterile
   b. Endotracheal tube/tracheostomy is sterile
3. Procedure: Tracheostomy
   a. Pre-lubricate catheter before insertion with normal saline
   b. Pre-oxygenate client
   c. Advance catheter during inspiration without suction
   d. Pull catheter back 2–3 cm after reaching the bronchial bifurcation
   e. Withdraw catheter while applying intermittent suction and rotating catheter between thumb and index finger maximum 10-15 seconds
   f. Oxygenate client
   g. Rinse catheter and discard with gloves
   h. Document client response, character and volume of sputum
   i. Maintain standard precautions including mask, goggles, and gloves
   j. Listen to breath sounds to determine effectiveness of intervention
3. Adverse effects
   a. Hypoxia
   b. Dysrhythmia
   c. Bronchospasm
   d. Infection

REVIEW OF GENERAL PREOPERATIVE AND POSTOPERATIVE CARE

Preoperative Care

A. Purposes

1. Ensure the client is in the best physical and psychological condition for surgery
2. Eliminate or reduce postoperative discomfort and complications
3. Preop teaching
   a. Enhances client participation
   b. Decreases anxiety
   c. Helps to ensure good postop recovery

B. General Preoperative Care

1. Psychological support: stress experience, consider the effects here
2. Client teaching specific to scheduled procedure
   a. Coughing and deep breathing
   b. Supporting the wound: use of pillow, splinting
   c. Leg exercises
   d. Turning, positioning, and ambulation
   e. Analgesics and pain control: discuss the option of patient controlled analgesia (PCA)
   f. Recovery room procedures
   g. Other postoperative expectations: type of dressing, Nasogastric tube (NG), drains, IV
3. Informed consent: nurse only witnesses permit, surgeon must explain procedure to client
4. Latex allergies: assess for and identify clients at risk (multiple surgeries or procedures)
5. Preoperative checklist must be complete
6. Physical care
   a. Baseline vital signs: client must be afebrile
   b. Nutritional support for wound healing
   c. Skin preparation as indicated
   d. Oral hygiene: check loose teeth
   e. Enema if ordered. (Not routine except for bowel surgery)
7. Preoperative drugs
   a. Purpose
      1) Reduce anxiety
      2) Decrease secretions
      3) Reduce amount of general anesthesia required
      4) Control nausea and vomiting
   b. Common preoperative drugs: Medication is rarely given IM, usually IV when the client gets to the OR
      1) Meperidine (*Demerol*), morphine sulfate
      2) Hydroxyzine (*Vistaril*), promethazine

(*Phenergan*) synergistic to narcotics

    3) Atropine, scopolamine to dry oral secretions during anesthesia

    4) Pentobarbital sodium (*Nembutal*), secobarbital sodium (*Seconal*) night before to help to sleep

    5) Midazolam (*Versed*) causes conscious sedation and is very popular; client will get amnesia post procedure so will not remember what happened

C. Anesthetics

1. General: Causes the most effects postoperatively
   a. Inhalation
   b. Intravenous
2. Local
   a. Topical
   b. Spinal
      1) Side effects: hypotension, nausea, vomiting, headache

      2) **NURSING INTERVENTIONS**
         a) Increase fluids per order
         b) Increase caffeine per order
         c) Flat for six to eight hours postop

General Postoperative Care

A. Immediate "Head-to-Toe" Assessment

1. Pulmonary
   a. Airway (check gag reflex)
   b. Bilateral breath sounds
   c. Encourage coughing, deep breathing
2. Neurological
   a. Level of consciousness
   b. Reflexes/pattern of movement
3. Circulatory
   a. Vital signs
   b. Peripheral perfusion
4. Gastrointestinal
   a. Bowel sounds
   b. Distention
5. Genitourinary
   a. Urinary output
   b. Intake and output
6. Equipment
   a. Intravenous line (IV)
   b. Dressings: expect mostly serosanguineous drainage
   c. Drainage tubes: expect some sanguineous drainage postop but monitor amount and evaluate in light of vital signs
   d. Nasogastric tube: evaluate need for KCL in IV to prevent metabolic alkalosis

B. NURSING INTERVENTIONS

1. Assess for complications
   a. Take vital signs routinely according to policy
   b. NPO until alert & gag reflex returns
   c. Suction oral cavity prn
   d. Monitor intake and output
2. Pain Interventions
   a. Pharmacologic interventions
      1) PRN scheduling: pain medication is given, as ordered, to the client on a demand basis when pain occurs. Is least effective strategy.
      2) Fixed scheduling: pain medication is given around the clock (usually every 4 hours). Not only treats, but prevents pain.
      3) Patient Controlled Analgesia (PCA): pain medication is self administered by client via an infusion system. Client must be able to participate in this intervention.
      4) Most pharmacologic interventions use narcotic drugs; therefore client must be carefully assessed for the complication of respiratory depression
   b. Non-pharmacologic interventions
      1) Distraction
      2) Relaxation techniques
      3) Back rubs
      4) Acupuncture, acupressure
3. Positioning
   a. Head to side, chin forward if unconscious
   b. Lateral Sims, semiprone
   c. Turn and position the client; have the client cough and deep breathe

REVIEW OF GASTROINTESTINAL, HEPATIC, AND PANCREATIC DISORDERS

Nursing Assessment

A. History of Problem

B. General Appearance:
1. Thin, emaciated
2. Obese
3. Skin turgor

C. GI System:
1. Nausea and vomiting: what precipitates it, what relieves it, appearance, characteristics

TABLE I-4.
COMMON POSTOPERATIVE COMPLICATIONS

COMPLICATION	PREVENTION	COMMON CAUSES	OCCURRENCE	MANIFESTATIONS
Atelectasis	Cough and deep breathe	Shallow respirations	First 48 hours	Fever, increased pulse and respiration
Hypostatic pneumonia	Cough and deep breathe	Shallow respirations	After 48 hours	-Fever, increased pulse and respiration -Crackles and rhonchi
Hypoxia	-Cough and deep breathe -Ambulation and turning	Anesthesia causing depressed respirations	48 hours	Confusion, increased BP and pulse, SOB
Nausea	Slowly progress with diet	Reaction to anesthesia or narcotics	48 hours	Nausea
Shock	-Assess routinely for signs of shock -Identify populations at risk -Monitor for bleeding	-Loss of fluids and electrolytes -Bleeding from wound or surgical site	48 hours	-Decreased BP, pulse, urinary output -Cold, clammy, pale skin -Change in level of consciousness
Urinary retention	-Upright to void (male) -Monitor I and O	-Medications (narcotic) -Local edema	2-3 days or later	Inability to void, restlessness, bladder distention
Wound hemorrhage	Monitor site for healing	Slipping of suture, wound evisceration	Immediately or later	-Signs of shock -Bleeding (sanguinous drainage) from tubes or site of surgery
Thrombophlebitis	-Leg exercises, elastic stockings, pneumatic stockings -Identify at-risk populations for intervention	Venous stasis, IV irritation, pressure to legs	7-14 days	Redness, warmth, pain and swelling at the site
Wound infection	-Maintain nutritional status -Maintain aseptic technique with manipulations of dressings	Poor aseptic technique, debilitated, obesity	3-5 days	Wound area red and edematous, increased pain in incisional area, increase in the amount and/or change in the character of the drainage: common for drainage to be purulent
Wound dehiscence and evisceration	-Identify those at risk -Maintain nutritional status in high-risk populations	Debilitated, obese, elderly	4-15 days	Wound opens and contents may come out onto abdominal area. Intervention: place sterile saline soaked gauze over site and place in recumbent position.
Urinary tract infection	-Maintain sterility of catheter, increase fluids -Remove catheter as soon as possible	Indwelling catheter, urinary retention post anesthesia	5-8 days	Dysuria, hematuria, urgency, frequency

2. Pain: location, what precipitates it, what relieves it, radiation how long, characteristics, quality
3. Elimination pattern: pattern and consistency of stools, laxative use
4. Nutrition: intake and output; difficulties in swallowing; likes and dislikes (consider cultural diversity here), normal intake per day

D. Examination of Abdomen: inspection, auscultation, percussion, palpation

E. Associated Symptoms: flatus, eructation, heartburn, pain

Diagnostic Procedures

A. Upper GI
1. Method: barium swallow
2. Purpose: assessment of esophagus and stomach
3. NPO 6–8 hours before procedure
4. Laxative after procedure
5. Follow-up x-ray 6 hours after procedure

B. Lower GI
1. Method: barium enema
2. Purpose: assessment of large colon
3. Liquid diet before procedure
4. Laxative before and after procedure
5. Initially, feces will be white. Should be normal color within 72 hours.

C. Endoscopy (Gastroscopy, Esophagogastric Duodenoscopy)
1. Method: visualization of the inside of the body by means of a lighted tube
2. Purpose: assessment of esophagus, stomach
3. Gag reflex inactivated
4. NPO 6–8 hours before procedure
5. Resume diet only after gag reflex returns
6. Complications: perforation, bleeding, bloating

D. Sigmoidoscopy/Colonoscopy
1. Method: endoscope inserted through the anus
2. Purpose: assessment of sigmoid colon
3. Administer enema before
4. Monitor for complications: perforation, bleeding, bloating, flatus

E. Analysis of Gastrointestinal Secretions
1. Stool Analysis:
   a. Method: culture, fat analysis, guaiac - no aspirin (*ASA*), NSAID, red meat, Vitamin C for 3 days before
   b. Purpose: assessment for bacteria, virus, ova & parasites, malabsorption, blood
   c. Do not refrigerate stool samples
2. Gastric Secretion Analysis

   a. Method: contents of stomach analyzed
   b. Purpose: assessment of ulcers, rule out pernicious anemia
   c. NPO for 8-10 hours prior to procedure, no smoking, no anticholinergics

F. Evaluation of the Gallbladder and Liver
1. Cholecystogram (Gallbladder Series)
   a. Method: dye conjugated in the liver and excreted into the bile that outlines the gallbladder
   b. Purpose: assessment of gallstones, proper gallbladder function
   c. Check for allergy to iodine or seafood
   d. Telepaque tablets 12 hours before test
   e. NPO after midnight
   f. Less commonly performed than ultrasound
2. Cholangiogram
   a. Method: bile ducts visualized
   b. Check for allergy to iodine or seafood
3. Ultrasound of Gallbladder and Liver
   a. Strict NPO after midnight prior to procedure
   b. Able to visualize if stones are present

G. Flat Plate of the Abdomen
1. No preparation
2. Gives a good overall impression of the abdominal cavity

H. Liver Biopsy
1. Method: removal of liver tissue to rule out liver disease
2. Obtain consent and results of hemostasis tests before the biopsy
3. Usually performed under fluoroscopic guidance
4. Two weeks prior, client must discontinue aspirin, NSAIDS and anticoagulants
5. NPO after midnight
6. Position on left side during biopsy
7. Position on right side after biopsy for two hours
8. Bed rest for prescribed time after biopsy
9. Observe for complications (bleeding, pneumothorax)

I. Paracentesis
1. Removal of fluid accumulated in the peritoneum
2. Indicated when ventilation is impaired, abdominal discomfort
   a. Therapeutic: to relieve shortness of breath when ventilation is impaired
   b. Diagnostic: to examine contents of peritoneal fluid
3. Void immediately prior to procedure
4. During procedure: sitting up with feet resting on stool
5. Fluid should be removed slowly over 30–90 minutes, generally <1500 mL

6. Bed rest after the procedure
7. Observe for complications-for example, hypovolemia; shock secondary to fluid shift, tachycardia, oliguria, infection, peritonitis

J. Liver Function Tests
1. Alkaline phosphatase
   a. Elevated in cardiac disorder, bone disease, biliary obstruction
   b. Enzyme found in liver tissue
   c. Released during liver damage
2. Prothrombin time
   a. Value is prolonged with liver damage
   b. Assess extrinsic clotting process
3. Blood ammonia: assess liver's ability to deaminate protein by products
4. Serum transaminase studies
   a. Elevated in liver disease
   b. SGOT, SGPT, LDH, AST, ALT
5 Cholesterol
   a. Increased in bile duct obstruction
   b. Decreased with liver damage
   c. Produced by liver
6. Bilirubin
   a. Direct: indicative of pre-hepatic causes
   b. Indirect: indicative of post-hepatic causes

Gastrointestinal Intubation

A. Types
1. Nasogastric tube: decompression of stomach
2. Salem sump: for continuous or intermittent suction, prevents trauma to stomach lining
3. Miller-Abbot/Anderson: intestinal suction – Reposition client hourly for insertion of the tube and movement into the intestines
4. Ewald: removal of secretions through the mouth
5. Sengstaken-Blakemore: for treatment of esophageal varices, requires intensive care. Not used much because of the trauma and potential complications it causes for the client. Major complications are rebleeding, pneumonia and respiratory obstruction.

B. Nasogastric Tube Feeding/Suction
1. Feeding Tube **NURSING INTERVENTIONS**
   a) Assess placement before each feeding and every 4 hours with continuous feeding
   b) Semi-Fowler's position
   c) Check for residual: always refeed unless amount increases
   d) Nose and mouth care
   e) Hold for aspirates of >100 mL, recheck in one hour
   f) Replace aspirated contents to prevent metabolic alkalosis

2. Suction Tube **NURSING INTERVENTIONS**
   a) Should drain stomach contents
   b) Over time should see a decrease in volume of drainage
   c) Always irrigate with normal saline

C. Gastrostomy Tube
1. Anterior wall of the stomach is sutured to the abdominal wall and the tube is sutured in place; skin care is important
2. Primarily placed for long term feeding needs

D. Percutaneous Endoscopic Gastrostomy (PEG)
1. No need to check placement
2. Primarily placed for long term feeding needs
3. Preferred over gastrostomy tube because of ease of insertion and care
4. Make sure tube is anchored continuously with ring at same number point on tube. This assures that the stomach is clearly anchored to the abdominal wall and decreases the chance of complications.

E. Total Parenteral Nutrition (TPN)
1. Definition: intravenous administration of a hypertonic solution of glucose, nitrogen and other nutrients to achieve tissue synthesis and anabolism; lipids may be given as a supplement; provides 3,000–4,000 calories per day Note: Any concentration of glucose greater than 10% must be given through a central intravenous line.
2. Indications for use
   a. Inability of the gastrointestinal tract to absorb nutrients adequately (e.g., malabsorption syndrome, gastrointestinal obstruction, paralytic ileus, bowel resection, ulcerative colitis, "gut rest")
   b. Inability to take food by mouth (e.g., neurosurgical problems (coma), anorexia nervosa)
   c. Excessive nutritional needs that cannot be met by the usual methods (e.g., burns, multiple fractures, carcinoma being treated with chemotherapy or radiation therapy, severe infections)
3. **NURSING INTERVENTIONS**
   a. Chest x-ray immediately after subclavian line insertion for proper placement
   b. Assess weight, baseline electrolytes, blood glucose, zinc and copper levels before treatment begins
   c. Maintain aseptic (sterile) technique during dressing changes
   d. Maintain infusion rate, do not increase or decrease rate without order; may cause hyper or hypoglycemia
   e. Assess weight daily: should maintain or increase weight while receiving TPN

f. Monitor for complications
   1) Infection-filters and tubing changed with every bottle
   2) Hypoglycemia
   3) Hyperglycemia
   4) Air embolism: Never open central line to air. Chance of air embolism is decreased with multiple lumen set-ups. When central line is inserted or opened, have client perform Valsalva maneuver and place in Trendelenburg position.
   5) Pneumothorax, especially during insertion
   6) Zinc deficiency
   7) Fluid overload
   8) Hyperglycemic, hyperosmolar nonketotic coma

g. Gradual decrease in rate of solution when discontinuing therapy thereby avoiding hypoglycemia

h. Continually evaluate effectiveness of therapy. Seek consultation if it is not effective.

TABLE I-5.
COMPARISON OF CHRONIC DUODENAL AND CHRONIC GASTRIC ULCERS

	CHRONIC DUODENAL	CHRONIC GASTRIC
Age:	Usually 25–50 yrs	Usually 50 yrs or more
Sex:	M:F–3:1	M:F–2:1
Incidence:	80%	20%
General nourishment:	Well-nourished	Malnourished
Etiology factors:	Most result from Helicobacter pylori infection, smoking, 0 blood type	Excessive ingestion of salicylates, smoking
Acid production in stomach:	Hypersecretion	Normal to hyposecretion
- Location: - Pain:	- Within 3 cm. of pylorus - 2–3 hours after meal; night, early morning. Ingestion of food relieves pain. Pain is a gnawing sensation sharply localized in mid-epigastrium or in back.	- Lesser curvature - 1/2–1 hour after meal; rarely at night. Relieved by vomiting. Ingestion of food does not help; sometimes causes pain.
Vomiting:	Uncommon	Common: caused by pyloric obstruction either by muscular spasm of pylorus or by mechanical obstruction from scarring.
Hemorrhage:	Melena more common than hematemesis	Hematemesis more common than melena
Malignancy possibility:	None	Usually less than 10%
Complications:	Hemorrhage, perforation and obstruction	Hemorrhage and perforation
Ulcerogenic drugs:	Salicylates, Butazolidin, steroids	Same

Duodenal and Gastric Ulcer

A. Types of Ulcers

1. Chronic duodenal and gastric ulcers (see table I-5.)
2. Stress ulcers
   a. May be caused by physical as well as psychological stress
   b. Burns cause Curling's ulcer
   c. Steroid therapy
      1) Usually occurs at least one to two weeks after stress
      2) No pain
      3) May be diagnosed due to gastric bleeding and resulting low hemoglobin and hematocrit

B. NURSING INTERVENTIONS

1. Major goal is to prevent complications and allow ulcer to heal
   a. Rest: physical and mental; lower stress
   b. Eliminate stimulants: caffeine, alcohol, spicy foods, cigarette smoking
   c. Diet has no therapeutic effect; milk may be used but is not recommended
   d. Antacid: aluminum hydroxide (*Amphojel*); magnesium carbonate (*Maalox*)
   e. Cimetidine (*Tagamet*): decreases acid production
   f. Ranitidine (*Zantac*): decreases acid production
   g. Sucralfate (*Carafate*): protects lining of stomach
   h. Omeprazole (*Prilosec*): heals ulcer

TABLE I-6.
COMPARISON OF CROHN'S DISEASE AND ULCERATIVE COLITIS

	CROHN'S DISEASE Small Bowel	ULCERATIVE COLITIS Large Bowel
Pathology:	Transmural: primarily involving ileum and right colon	Mucosal ulceration of lower colon and rectum
Age:	20–30, 40–50	20–40
Etiology factors:	Unknown genetic, Jewish	Unknown familial, Jewish
Bleeding:	Usually not	Common, severe
Perianal involvement:	Common	Rare, mild
Fistulas:	Common	Rare
Rectal involvement:	20%	100%
Diarrhea:	Less severe	Severe
Abdominal pain after eating:	Yes	Yes
Weight loss:	Yes	Yes
Treatment:	Steroids: sulfasalazine (*Azulfidine*) hyperalimentation; partial or complete colostomy & ileostomy or anastomosis	Steroids: sulfasalazine (*Azulfidine*) partial or complete colostomy and proctocolectomy & ileostomy
History:	Deteriorating, progressive	Exacerbations, remissions
Complications:	Scarring, obstruction	Perforation; susceptible to cancer; toxic megacolon; fistulas obstruction, abscess

i. For H. pylori ulcers: antibiotics

C. Gastric Resection
1. Types
   a. Billroth I (gastroduodenostomy)
   b. Billroth II (gastrojejunostomy)
   c. Total gastrectomy: will cause pernicious anemia

 2. **NURSING INTERVENTIONS**
   a. NG tube in place: do not move as it may stimulate bleeding at surgical site
   b. Evaluate need for KCL in IV to prevent metabolic alkalosis
   c. NPO until suture line is totally healed
   d. Assess drainage: will initially be sanguinous but should change to greenish in 2-3 days
3. Complications
   a. Hemorrhage
   b. Pulmonary
   c. "Dumping syndrome": due to rapid entry of ingested food into the jejunum without proper mixing and normal digestive process of the duodenum
      1) Early: 5–30 minutes after eating, vertigo, sweating, diarrhea, nausea; due to fluid shifts
      2) Late: 2–3 hours after meals, hypoglycemia occurs due to excess insulin secretion
      3) Intervention: avoid salty, high-carbohydrate meals; eat small, frequent meals; avoid liquids with meals; lie down after meals (30 – 60 minutes); avoid antispasmodics; eat high-protein, high-fat, low-carbohydrate meals. No fluids for 1 hour before, with, or 2 hours after meals.
   d. Major complication: Peritonitis

Diverticulitis and Diverticulosis

A. Definition:
1. Outpouching of colon is diverticulosis
2. When the outpouching becomes infected, it is called diverticulitis
3. Problem: the pouch gets filled with feces, becomes inflamed, can obstruct and perforate leading to peritonitis

B. NURSING INTERVENTIONS
1. Prevent by increasing fiber in diet
2. Avoiding all seeds
3. Preventing constipation by using bulk agents and increased water

Crohn's Disease and Ulcerative Colitis

See Table I-6. for Comparisons

Hernia

A. Definition:
1. Protrusion of bowel through the muscles of the abdominal cavity
2. Problem: strangulation and gangrene of the bowel

TABLE I-7.
COMPARISON OF COLOSTOMY AND ILEOSTOMY

	COLOSTOMY	ILEOSTOMY
Defined:	Portion of the colon brought through the abdominal wall, creating a temporary or permanent opening for exit of waste products	Portion of the ileum brought through the abdominal wall creating a permanent opening for exit of waste products
Areas:	Involves large bowel	Involves small bowel
Indications:	Inflammatory or obstructive process of the lower intestinal tract; trauma to intestinal tract; cancer of the rectum or sigmoid where anastomosis is not possible	-Crohn's disease -Ulcerative colitis
Stool:	Semiformed to formed	Liquid
Control:	May be controlled by diet and/or irrigation depending on location in colon, may be able to control evacuation	No control, must wear appliance at all times

B. **Types**
1. Umbilical
2. Ventral
3. Inguinal

C. **NURSING INTERVENTIONS**
1. Prevent pressure in the abdominal area
2. Support the area with binder, for example
3. Prevent constipation
4. Surgical repair

Hiatal Hernia

A. **Definition:** portion of the stomach is herniated through the esophageal hiatus of the diaphragm

B. **Manifestations**
1. Heartburn
2. Dysphagia

C. **NURSING INTERVENTIONS**
1. Small, frequent meals
2. Upright position during and after meals
3. Head of bed elevated
4. Antacids
5. Avoid anticholinergic drugs
6. Avoid coughing
7. Reduce intra-abdominal pressure by avoiding lifting and tight clothes around waist area
8. Reduce spicy food intake

Bowel Obstruction

A. **Definition:** anything that obstructs the colon; inflammation, tumor

B. **Manifestations:**
1. Increased bowel sounds proximal to the obstruction
2. No stool
3. Pain
4. Distention
5. Vomiting (projectile from reverse peristalsis)
6. Hypovolemia and shock

C. **NURSING INTERVENTIONS**
1. Intestinal tube: refer to care in preceding section
2. Ambulation
3. Treat cause and relieve
4. Surgical intervention; colon resection

General Bowel Surgery

A. **Preoperative NURSING INTERVENTIONS:**
1. Oral antibiotics as ordered to sterile bowel

2. Laxatives and enemas until clear to evacuate intestines

B. **Postoperative NURSING INTERVENTIONS:**
1. Nasogastric tube
2. Evaluate need for KCL in intravenous line
3. TPN may be needed
4. Pain control because of location of surgery
5. Aseptic wound care to prevent infection
6. Early ambulation decreases risks of complications: increased peristalsis, decreased risk of thrombophlebitis, decreased risk of atelectasis

Colostomy and Ileostomy

A. **Types of Intestinal Ostomies** (see table I-8: Types of Intestinal Ostomies)

B. **NURSING INTERVENTIONS**
1. Preoperative care
   a. Emotional support (anticipatory grieving)
   b. Client teaching concerning impending surgery (ileostomy/colostomy)
2. Postoperative care
   a. General postoperative care
   b. Psychological support
   c. NG tube
   d. Observe stoma, surrounding tissues, and type of excretion (should be pink; above skin level; may have bloody discharge at first)
   e. Teach self-care to client
      1) Type of equipment to use and how
      2) Skin care
      3) Diet: decrease fat and odor forming foods

Hepatitis A; Hepatitis B; Hepatitis Non-A, Non-B; Hepatitis C

See Table I-9. for Comparisons

Cirrhosis

A. **Definition:** liver cells destroyed and replaced by scar tissue; cause not clear; frequently seen in alcoholics, but also occurs in non-alcoholics; associated with nutritional deficiency with decreased protein intake

B. **Functions of the Liver**
1. Synthesis of clotting factors (fibrinogen, prothrombin, factors VII, IX, X)
2. Metabolism of hormones (aldosterone, antidiuretic hormone, estrogen, testosterone)
3. Synthesis of albumin
4. Carbohydrate metabolism
5. Protein metabolism

TABLE I-8.
TYPES OF INTESTINAL OSTOMIES

	ILEOSTOMY	ILEAL LOOP (Urinary Conduit)	TRANSVERSE COLOSTOMY	DESCENDING OR SIGMOID COLOSTOMY
Intestinal segment involved	End of ileum	Pouch is made from loop of ileum into which ureters are transplanted for urine drainage	Transverse colon	Descending or sigmoid colon
Consistency of excretion	Liquid	Urine only	Semiformed to soft	Formed
Appliance worn	Open-ended pouch, no appliance if Kock's (continent) ileostomy	Open-ended pouch	Open-ended pouch	If controlled, no appliance

TABLE I-9.
COMPARISON OF HEPATITIS A; HEPATITIS B; HEPATITIS NON-A, NON-B; HEPATITIS C

	HEPATITIS A (Infectious Hepatitis)	HEPATITIS B (Serum Hepatitis)	HEPATITIS Non-A, Non-B	HEPATITIS C
Cause	-Virus transmitted by fecal-oral contact; often seen during floods, earthquakes -Transmitted by the 4 F's: food, fingers, feces, and floods	Virus transmitted through percutaneous or oral exposure to the blood of person with Hepatitis B	Thought similar to type B	-Transmitted via blood, by personal contact & possibly fecal-oral route -Hepatitis C causes 4% of hepatitis cases; causes 90% of post transfusion hepatitis -Risk factors are the same as Hepatitis B
Manifestations	Flu-like, upper-respiratory infection, headache, malaise, jaundice, dark urine, liver tenderness	Similar to type A without respiratory symptoms	Same as type B	Same as Type B; may lead to need for liver transplantation (30%)
Nursing	Enteric precautions, bed rest, low fat diet, fluids, drug therapy, reduced to minimum vitamins B_{12}	Same as type A except "blood precaution" instead of enteric precautions	Same as type B	Same as Type B
Prevention	Good sanitation; if in contact with infected client, administer immune serum globulin within 2–7 days; Hepatitis A vaccine is available	Mandatory screening of blood donors-use of disposable needles and syringes; administer Hepatitis B immune globulin 2–7 days after exposure. Hepatitis B vaccine: series of 3 injections over 6 months	Same as type B	No sharing of needles by drug users; care to avoid accidental needlesticks (health care workers); safe sexual practices

6. Fat metabolism through bile production
7. Filter action, especially drugs
8. Blood storage

C. **Manifestations:** these would be the same for a client with liver failure from other causes also, except for the enlargement of the liver and the alcohol related psychosis
1. Early stage (same as those for Hepatitis)
   a. Enlarged liver with fatty infiltration
   b. Jaundice
   c. GI disturbances
   d. Abdominal discomfort
2. Late stage
   a. Liver becomes smaller and nodular
   b. Spleen enlarges: anemia
   c. Ascites, distended abdominal veins; back-up of pressure in the portal system
   d. Bleeding tendencies; decreased vitamin K and prothrombin
   e. Wernicke-Korsakoff psychosis: alcohol related
   f. Esophageal varices, internal hemorrhoids; back-up of pressure in portal area
   g. Dyspnea from ascites and anemia
   h. Pruritus from dry skin
   i. Clay colored stools: no bile
   j. Tea-colored urine: bile in urine
3. End stage
   a. Hepatic encephalopathy stages
      1) Prodromal: slurred speech, vacant stare, restless; involves neuro deterioration
      2) Impending: asterixis, apraxia, lethargy, confusion
      3) Stuporous: noisy, abusive, somnolence
      4) Coma: positive Babinski, fetor hepaticas, decorticate/decerebrate posturing
   b. Convulsions
   c. Death

D. **NURSING INTERVENTIONS:** goal is treating the manifestations and maximizing liver functions
1. Encourage client to rest
2. Avoid hepatotoxic drugs and alcohol
3. High-calorie, low-protein (20 – 40 g/day), low-fat, low-sodium diet (Maintain protein restriction during stages I & II of encephalopathy; no protein allowed during stages III & IV)
4. Fat-soluble vitamin supplements, folic acid may need to be given intravenously
5. Restrict fluids
6. Albumin IV
7. Weigh client daily
8. Measure abdominal girth
9. Skin care: cool temperature, Aveeno baths, lubricate
10. Monitor intake and output
11. Assess for bleeding, hemorrhoids also

12. Diuretics: spironolactone (*Aldactone*), furosemide (*Lasix*)
13. Neomycin: reduces intestinal bacteria, thereby decreases breakdown of protein reducing ammonia levels
14. Lactulose (*Heptalac*): decreases ammonia levels
15. Thiamine daily

Bleeding Esophageal Varices

A. **Definition:** esophageal varices are dilated veins found in the lower esophagus that occur secondary to portal hypertension; bleeding may result because of coughing, trauma, or vomiting; bleeding esophageal varices is a medical emergency

NURSING INTERVENTIONS
1. Maintain client airway before insertion of Sengstaken-Blakemore tube
2. Care of client with Sengstaken-Blakemore tube
   a. Maintain traction and manometer pressure: 40 mm HG
   b. Keep scissors by bedside
   c. Oral suctioning, mouth care; cannot swallow saliva or will aspirate
   d. Deflate gastric balloon every 24–36 hours; usually deflate esophageal balloon every 12 hours as ordered
3. Semi-Fowler's position
4. Take vital signs
5. Monitor intake and output
6. Vitamin K
7. Vasopressin (*Pitressin*): vasoconstrictor
8. Endoscopic sclerotherapy
   a. Sclerosing agent introduced via endoscope
   b. Thromboses and obliterates the distended veins

C. **Surgical Interventions**
1. Portosystemic shunts: splenorenal, portocaval
2. Transesophageal ligation
3. TIPS: transjugular intrahepatic portosystemic shunt (angiographic method of creating shunt) to relieve pressure

Gallbladder Disease

A. **Definitions**
1. Cholecystitis: inflammation of the gallbladder
2. Cholelithiasis: stones in the gallbladder
3. At-risk: fair, fat, forty, oral contraceptive users

B. **Manifestations**
1. Right upper-quadrant or epigastric pain, shoulder pain
2. Nausea and vomiting
3. Fat intolerance

4. Murphy's sign: Have client take deep breath and palpate the right subcostal area. If the client has extreme pain and stops breathing on inspiration, this is a positive Murphy's sign and indicative of acute cholecystitis.
5. Jaundice: indicates obstruction

C. **NURSING INTERVENTIONS**
1. Relieve pain - meperidine (*Demerol*). Do not use morphine.
2. Maintain fluid and electrolytes balance
3. Administer antiemetic prn
4. Maintain low-fat diet

D. **Cholecystectomy:** postoperative
1. Nursing care same as any abdominal surgery
2. Penrose drain in gallbladder area
3. T-tube to gravity after cholecystostomy and choledochostomy: to prevent total loss of bile drainage, tube may be elevated above level of abdomen
4. Resume regular diet as tolerated

E. **Laparoscopic Cholecystectomy**
1. One-day surgery
2. Very popular because it requires short hospitalization
3. Postop problem: pain in shoulder from gas in abdominal area needed to visualize organs. Post-op instructions are important as client needs to assess self at home.

Pancreatitis

A. **Definition:** inflammation brought about by the digestion of this organ by the very enzymes it produces. Clients at greatest risk are those suffering from alcohol abuse, clients with other liver and gallbladder diseases.

B. **Manifestations**
1. Extreme upper-abdominal pain radiating into back
2. Persistent vomiting
3. Abdominal distention
4. Weight loss
5. Steatorrhea: bulky, pale, foul smelling stools
6. Elevated serum amylase and lipase
7. Pleural effusion

C. **NURSING INTERVENTIONS:** rest the organ
1. Administer anticholinergics, antacids, pancreatic extracts: pancrelipase (*Viokase*)
2. NPO with nasogastric tube in place: no ice chips or hard candies as these will stimulate the pancreas
3. IV fluids; may require TPN in moderate or severe cases
4. Provide meperidine (*Demerol*) for pain relief

5. Administer fat soluble vitamins
6. Home care management/teaching
   a. NO alcohol or caffeine
   b. Infusion of IV fluids
   c. Signs and symptoms of complications to report (fever, nausea, vomiting, respiratory distress)

SECTION V

REVIEW OF MUSCULOSKELETAL DISORDERS

Rheumatoid Arthritis and Osteoarthritis

See Table I-10. for Comparisons

Fractures

A. **Definition:** break in the continuity of bone
1. Prevention through safety measures
2. Identify populations at risk and intervene through teaching

B. **First Aid**
1. Maintain airway
2. Prevent shock
3. Splint limb
4. The "five P's"
   a. Pain
   b. Pallor
   c. Pulselessness
   d. Paresthesia
   e. Paralysis
5. Monitor for fat embolism up to 2 weeks following long bone fractures
   a. Signs and symptoms of fat embolism; synonymous with a pulmonary embolus
      1) Restlessness
      2) Altered mental status
      3) Tachypnea
      4) Tachycardia
      5) Fever
      6) Petechiae

C. **Traction**
1. Types (must be maintained continuously to be effective)
   a. Skin
      1) Buck's extension (5–10 lbs maximum)
      2) Pelvic (up to 20 lbs maximum)
   b. Skeletal

l)   Thomas splint with Pearson attachment

2)   Crutchfield tongs

 2. **NURSING INTERVENTIONS**

   a. General

     1)   Maintain positioning

     2)   Maintain weights hanging freely

     3)   Maintain alignment

     4)   Prevent complications of prolonged bed rest

     5)   Monitor for vascular occlusion; CMS checks:

        a)   Circulation

        b)   Motion/movement

        c)   Sensation

   b. Skin

     1)   General care as above

     2)   Detection of pressure points

     3)   Provide daily rewrapping

     4)   Maintain countertraction; usually bed on shock blocks

   c. Skeletal

     1)   Inspection

     2)   Skin/pin care

   d. Muscles

     1)   Strengthening exercises for uninvolved extremities

     2)   Preparation for crutch walking

D. Casts

1. Applied to maintain immobilization while the fracture heals

 2. **NURSING INTERVENTIONS**

   a. Handle wet cast with palms of hands, not fingers

   b. Cast should be allowed to air dry

   c. Elevate the cast on one to two pillows during drying

   d. Adhesive tape petals reduce irritation at cast edges

   e. Assess for vascular occlusion; CMS checks

   f. Prevent complications of immobility

   g. Compartment syndrome (serious complication of fractures)

     1)   Ischemic pain, especially with elevation of extremity

     2)   Change in sensation; "pins & needles;" weak movement

     3)   Pallor and coolness

     4)   Pulselessness (late sign)

     5)   If untreated, results in paralysis in about 6 hours; may require amputation of extremity

E. Hip Fractures

1. Classification

   a. Fracture of the neck of femur (intracapsular)

   b. Fracture of trochanteric region of femur (extra-capsular)

   c. Subtrochanteric fracture

2. Treatment

   a. Skin traction for immobilization (preop); decrease pain and muscle spasms

   b. Trochanter roll (prevents external rotation)

   c. Open reduction and internal fixation

   d. Total hip replacement (THR)

 3. **NURSING INTERVENTIONS**

   a. Preoperative care

     1)   Immobilization (if pin is placed, client can get out of bed right immediately postop)

     2)   Anticoagulation therapy

     3)   Assess for complications, because of client age and the immobility imposed; that is why intervention is aimed at ambulating ASAP after surgery

        a)   Skin breakdown

        b)   Thromboembolism

        c)   Fat embolism

        d)   Respiratory congestion

        e)   Senile dementia

   b. Postoperative care

     1)   Turning and positioning (if total hip, may use an abductor device)

     2)   Exercise

     3)   Observation for complications

        a)   Thromboembolism

        b)   Pneumonia

        c)   Fat embolism

        d)   Neurovascular checks; CMS checks

     4)   Crutch walking (may need a walker depending on upper body strength)

        a)   Measure for crutches in walking shoes

        b)   Avoid leaning on crutches (will cause nerve damage)

        c)   Good leg first going upstairs, "bad" leg first when going down

     5)   Total Hip Replacement (THR) postoperative care

        a)   Avoid adduction, flexion, and external rotation

        b)   Abductor device (care when turning)

        c)   Drain/dressing care

        d)   Teaching: no crossing of the legs; no hip flexion greater than 90°; no leaning over forward, may dislocate the hip

F. Osteoporosis

1. Definition: demineralization of the bones; the leading cause in crippling hip fractures in women

2. Risk factors:

   a. Immobility

b. Decreased calcium diet
c. Menopause, men older than 65, amenorrhea at any age
d. Thin and light-haired women
e. Smoking
f. Steroid use

3. Prevent by:
a. Weight-bearing exercises
b. Adequate calcium intake - 1200 mg pre-menopause; 1500 mg post-menopause

4. **NURSING INTERVENTIONS**
a. Weight-bearing exercises
b. Care with activities to prevent falls
c. Medical checkups and bone density testing
d. Adequate calcium intake
e. 5 lbs weight-bearing limit
f. Administer alendronate (*Fosamax*) to increase bone density
   1) Administer first thing in the morning with a full glass of water
   2) Be sure client does not lie down or eat for 30 minutes after its administration

g. Hormone Replacement therapy
   1) Contraindicated with history of ovarian cancer and phlebitis
   2) Evista: non-estrogen hormone that increases bone mass

G. Pelvic Fractures
1. **NURSING INTERVENTIONS**
a. Major assessments
   1) Bladder injuries: watch for hematuria
   2) Bowel injuries: watch for signs of peritonitis
   3) Bleeding
b. Immobilization
   1) Bed rest
   2) Pelvic sling (may be removed intermittently)

Amputation

A. Preoperative Care
1. Psychological adjustment; "anticipatory grieving"

TABLE I-10.
COMPARISON OF RHEUMATOID ARTHRITIS AND OSTEOARTHRITIS

	RHEUMATOID ARTHRITIS (systemic)	OSTEOARTHRITIS (local and unilateral - wear and tear)
Onset:	20–50 years	Middle to older age
Sex:	Women 3:1	Women 20:1
Defined:	Chronic systemic disease of unknown cause, with recurrent inflammation involving the synovium or lining of the joints	Degeneration of the articular cartilage in the joints caused by prolonged wear and tear of joint surfaces
Joints involved:	Any finger joint, cervical, spine; systemic disease can involve heart, lung, etc.	Distal interphalangeal joints (Heberden's nodes); weight bearing joints: hips, knees, spine
Joints appearance:	Bilateral involvement; tenderness, swelling, warm, redness, subcutaneous nodules; every bone prominence; remission and exacerbation; increased symptoms in morning, decreasing with moderate activity	Normal on exam; grating (crepitus) during movement; pain and stiffness worsen after inactivity or after exercise
Other symptoms:	Low-grade temperature, malaise, fatigue stiffness	
Treatment:	Rest with joints extended; emotional support, heat: warm baths, paraffin baths; daily exercise program; drugs: ASA, NSAIDs, Phenylbutazone (*Butazolidin*), gold salts (*Myochrysine*), steroids (P.O. or into joints); other rheumatoid drugs not effective	Normal amount of rest; rest affected joint; avoid over-activity, emotional support; heat: hot packs, warm soaks, paraffin baths exercise: ROM; drugs: ASA, steroids in joints only; phenylbutazone (*Butazolidin*), indomethacin (*Indocin*)
Nursing interventions:	Position joints in extension; maintain body alignment; balance rest with exercise; nutritious diet	

2. Teaching
3. Increase upper-body strength
4. Trapeze on bed

B. Surgical Approaches
1. Closed
2. Opened
3. Immediate post-surgical prosthesis
   a. Improved position sense
   b. Early ambulation

C. Postoperative Care
1. Positioning
   a. Extended position (to prevent flexion deformity)
   b. Elevated (only for the first 24 hours)
2. Complications
   a. Hemorrhage
   b. Infection: very common in clients who required amputation because of poor circulation in extremity
   c. Phantom limb/phantom pain

D. Rehabilitation
1. Exercise
   a. Stretching of flexor muscles and upper extremities
   b. ROM
   c. No prolonged sitting in bed or chair; will enhance flexion deformities
   d. Maintain proper alignment of extremity
2. Stump conditioning
   a. Stump shrinking with wrapping
   b. Stump "toughening"
   c. Compression dressing

Gout

A. Definition: inflammatory type of arthritis caused by deposits of urate crystals in and around the joints; there is an hereditary error in purine metabolism that results in excessive uric acid production; risk factors are alcoholism, chemotherapy, heredity

B. Manifestations
1. Severe pain, usually in great toe
2. Joints are red, warm, painful, and swollen
3. Large accumulations of crystals in the joints (tophi) and connective tissue
4. Joint damage and deformity increase with each attack
5. Monarticular or polyarticular
6. Hyperuricemia - greater than 7 ng/dL
7. Sporadic and usually diet related

C. Treatment
1. Nonsteroidal Anti-inflammatories (NSAID)

a. Can cause bone marrow suppression and liver damage
   b. Indomethacin (*Indocin*)
   c. Probenecid (*Benemid*)
2. Allopurinol (*Zyloprim*)
3. Colchicine (*Colchicine*)
   a. Reduces uric acid
   b. Can use during acute phase
 4. **NURSING INTERVENTIONS**
   a. Bed rest during acute attacks
   b. Keep covers away from affected joints
   c. Applications of heat or cold
   d. Fluid intake
   e. Limit intake of high purine foods (organ and red meats), wine
   f. Limit alcohol intake
   g. Increase fluid intake
   h. Weight loss strategies

Systemic Lupus Erythematosus

A. Definition: chronic inflammatory disease that involves the vascular and connective tissue of multiple organs; cause is unknown, may be autoimmune

B. Manifestations
1. Insidious onset
2. Characterized by remissions and exacerbations
3. Erythematous "butterfly rash" on both cheeks and across the bridge of the nose; rash worsens on exposure to sunlight (most common sign)
4. Polyarthralgia
5. Normochromic, normocytic anemia
6. Fever, malaise, weight loss
7. Positive for antinuclear antibodies (ANA); LE Cell prep
8. Raynaud's phenomenon

C. NURSING INTERVENTIONS
1. Supportive (depends on organs involved)
2. Teaching
   a. Avoid the sun (wear large-brimmed hats, sunscreen)
   b. Avoid stressful situations
   c. Adequate rest, exercise
   d. Regular, nutritious meals
   e. Follow medical treatment regimen (salicylates, NSAIDS, steroids)
   f. Oral contraceptives and/or pregnancy can precipitate an acute exacerbation
   g. No intrauterine devices

KEY INFORMATION
Lupus nephritis occurs early in the disease
   1) Manifestations

a) Microscopic hematuria
b) Proteinuria
c) Red cell casts
2) Treatment
a) Symptomatic
b) Salicylates, steroids
c) Dialysis
3) Prognosis: variable

SECTION VI

REVIEW OF ENDOCRINE SYSTEM FUNCTIONS AND DISORDERS

Pituitary Gland

See Table I-11. for Hormones Produced and Functions

Endocrine System Disorders

A. Disorders of Anterior Pituitary
1. Acromegaly
   a. Definition: hypersecretion of GH that occurs in adulthood; commonly associated with benign pituitary tumors
   b. Manifestations
      1) Enlargement of skeletal extremities (e.g., nose, jaw, hands, feet)
      2) Protrusion of the jaw and orbital ridges
      3) Course features
      4) Visual problems, blindness
      5) Hyperglycemia, insulin resistance
      6) Hypercalcemia
   c. Treatment
      1) Irradiation of pituitary
      2) Transphenoidal hypophysectomy: removal of pituitary gland
         a) Assess for signs of increased cranial pressure-signs of adrenal insufficiency, hypothyroidism, and temporary diabetes insipidus
         b) Elevate head of bed 30 degrees
         c) Avoid coughing, sneezing, blowing nose
         d) Check for CSF in nasal packing
      3) Bromocriptine (*Parlodel*) with surgery or radiation
    d. **NURSING INTERVENTIONS**
      1) Provide emotional support
      2) Directed toward symptomatic care
2. Gigantism
   a. Definition: hypersecretion of GH that occurs in childhood
   b. Manifestations
      1) Proportional overgrowth in all body tissue
      2) Overgrowth of long bones: height in childhood may reach 8 or 9 feet
   c. Treatment (see acromegaly)
   d. Nursing responsibilities (see acromegaly)
3. Dwarfism
   a. Definition: hyposecretion of GH during childhood
   b. Manifestations
      1) Retarded symmetrical physical growth
      2) Premature body aging processes
      3) Slow intellectual development
   c. Treatment
      1) Removal of the causative factor (for example: tumors)
      2) Human growth hormone injections (HGH)
   d. Nursing responsibilities (see acromegaly)

B. Disorder of Posterior Pituitary
1. Diabetes insipidus
   a. Definition: hyposecretion of ADH, due to a tumor or damage of the posterior lobe of the pituitary; may be idiopathic; may be genetic; very common following neurosurgery or head trauma
   b. Manifestations
      1) Polyuria
      2) Polydipsia
      3) Hypernatremia
      4) Weight loss
      5) Dehydration/dry skin
   c. Treatment
      1) Desmopressin acetate (*DDAVP*) nasal spray
      2) Vasopressin tannate (*Pitressin Tannate*) in Oil (IM for chronic severe cases)
      3) Lypressin (*Diapid*) nasal spray
   d. **NURSING INTERVENTIONS**
      1) Maintain adequate fluids
      2) Avoid foods with diuretic-type action
      3) Monitor intake and output: report any changes; can sometimes have 800 mL output per hour
      4) Teach self-injection techniques
      5) Daily weights (very important)
      6) Specific gravity (should be greater than 1.004)
2. Syndrome of inappropriate secretion of antidiuretic hormone (SIADH)
   a. Definition: inappropriate, continued release of antidiuretic hormone resulting in water intoxication; caused by neoplastic tumors, respiratory disorders, drugs
   b. Manifestations

1) Mental confusion/irritability
2) Lethargy/seizures
3) Dilutional hyponatremia
4) Weight gain
5) Anorexia, nausea and vomiting
6) Weakness

c. Treatment
1) Fluid restriction (less than 500 mL/24 hours) with hypertonic solutions to treat the hyponatremia
2) Strict intake and output
3) Treat underlying cause (surgery, radiation, chemotherapy)
4) Demeclocycline HCL (*Declomycin*) to facilitate free water clearance
5) Daily weight

Adrenal Gland

See Table I-12. for Hormones Produced and Functions

A. Disorders of Adrenal Cortex
1. Addison's disease
   a. Definition: hyposecretion of adrenal cortex hormones, (insufficiency of cortisol, aldosterone and androgens); discontinuing steroid medications abruptly without weaning off of them
   b. Manifestations
      1) Slow, insidious onset
      2) Malaise and generalized weakness from increased potassium retention
      3) Hypotension, hypovolemia from increased sodium excretion
      4) Increase pigmentation of the skin: "eternal tan"

TABLE I-11.
PITUITARY GLAND: HORMONES PRODUCED AND FUNCTIONS

ENDOCRINE GLAND	HORMONES PRODUCES	FUNCTION
Pituitary gland		Controlled primarily by the hypothalamus; termed "master gland" as it directly affects the function of other endocrine glands
Anterior lobe	-Adrenocorticotropic hormone (ACTH)	-Concerned with growth and secretory activity of adrenal cortex, which produces steroids
	-Thyrotropic hormone (TSH)	-For growth and secretory activity of thyroid; controls release rate of thyroxine, which controls rate of most chemical reactions in the body; target is thyroid gland
	-Somatotropic hormones (STH or GH)	-Promote growth of body tissue
	-Gonadotropic hormones and estrogen secretion; follicle stimulating hormone (FSH)	-Stimulate development of ovarian follicles, seminiferous tubules, and sperm maturation
	-Luteinizing hormone (LH)	-Works with FSH in final maturation of follicles; promotes ovulation and progesterone secretion
	-Prolactin	-Maintains corpus luteum and progesterone secretion
	-Melanocyte stimulating hormone (MSH)	-Produces the characteristic skin darkening
Posterior lobe	-Vasopressin (ADH)	-Influences water absorption by kidney
	-Oxytocin	-Influences the menstrual cycle, labor, and lactation

5) Anorexia, nausea, vomiting
6) Electrolyte imbalance (hyponatremia, hyperkalemia)
7) Weight loss
8) Loss of libido
9) Hypoglycemia
10) Personality changes

c. Treatment
1) Lifelong steroid replacement: hydrocortisone (*Florinef*); complications of long-term steroid therapy include osteoporosis
2) High-protein, high-carbohydrate diet may increase Na$^+$ intake (low K+ intake)
3) Monitor fluid and electrolytes routinely
4) Decrease stress, emotional and physical

d. **NURSING INTERVENTIONS**
1) Observe for addisonian crisis (sudden extreme weakness; severe abdominal, back, and leg pain; hyperpyrexia; coma; death) secondary to stress caused by infection, trauma, surgery, pregnancy or stress
2) Observe for side effects of hormone replacement; this will be the same symptoms as hypersecretion of this gland
3) Provide emotional support
4) Teaching (lifelong medications, prompt treatment of infection, illness, stress management)
5) Monitor fluid and electrolyte balance regularly

2. Cushing's syndrome
a. Definition: hypersecretion of the glucocorticoids; overdose of steroid medications
b. Manifestations
1) Central-type obesity, moon face, buffalo hump and obese trunk with thin extremities
2) Mood swings (80% meet the criteria for a major affective disorder)
3) Malaise and muscular weakness (increase protein catabolism)
4) Masculine characteristics in females (hirsutism)
5) Hypokalemia (may cause arrhythmias)
6) Hyperglycemia (insulin resistant)
7) Hypertension (edema; may lead to CHF or CVAs)
8) Acne (striae on chest, abdomen, legs)
9) Amenorrhea
10) Osteoporosis; thin skin with ecchymosis
11) Increased susceptibility to infections
12) Peptic ulcer

c. Treatment
1) Adrenalectomy: unilateral or bilateral
2) Chemotherapy: bromocriptine (*Parlodel*); mitotane (*Lysodren*), or aminoglutethimide (*Cytadren*)

TABLE I-12.
ADRENAL GLAND: HORMONES PRODUCED AND FUNCTIONS

HORMONE PRODUCED	FUNCTION
Cortex:	- Cannot live without the secretions from this gland; therefore if missing, hormones must be replaced
- Glucocorticoids - Cortisol - Cortisone - Corticosterone	- Affect carbohydrate, fat, and protein metabolism; affect stress reactions and the inhibition of the inflammatory process
- Mineralocorticoids - Aldosterone - Corticosterone - Deoxycorticosterone	- Regulate sodium and electrolyte balance
- Sex Hormones - Androgens - Estrogens	- Influence the development of sexual characteristics
Medulla: - Catecholamines - Epinephrine - Norepinephrine	- Stimulate "fight or flight" response to danger, sympathetic nervous system response

3) High-protein, low-carbohydrate, low-sodium diet with potassium supplement
  d. **NURSING INTERVENTIONS**
     1) Protect from infection
     2) Protect from accidents and falls due to osteoporosis
     3) Client education concerning lifelong self-administration of hormone suppression therapy
  e. Steroid replacement (similar to Cushing's syndrome but in lesser effect)
     1) Purpose
        a) Anti-inflammatory and antiallergic reaction
        b) Enables one to tolerate high degree of stress
     2) Indications
        a) Crisis (for example: shock, bronchial obstruction)
        b) Long-term therapy (for example: post-adrenalectomy, arthritis, leukemia)
     3) Side effects due to prolonged use (refer to Cushing's manifestations)
     4) Dosage schedule
        a) Large dosages should be given at 8:00 a.m. (2/3 morning, 1/3 night) to simulate the normal excretion by the body
        b) Should be taken same time every day
        c) Withdraw steroids by tapered dosages or will get symptoms of Addison's disease
        d) Can be given with antacids to minimize GI upset and ulceration
  3. Aldosteronism (Conn's syndrome)
     a. Definition: hypersecretion of aldosterone from adrenal cortex (usually due to a tumor)
     b. Manifestations
        1) Hypokalemia and hypernatremia
        2) Hypertension from hypernatremia
        3) Muscle weakness and cardiac problems related to hypokaliemia
     c. Treatment
        1) Surgical removal of tumor/adrenal gland
        2) Potassium replacement
        3) Antihypertensive drugs: spironolactone (*Aldactone*)
  d. **NURSING INTERVENTIONS**
     1) Provide quiet environment
     2) Monitor BP and cardiac activity
     3) Monitor potassium level

B. Disorders of Adrenal Medulla
  1. Pheochromocytoma
     a. Definition: hypersecretion of the hormones of adrenal medulla (exact cause unknown)
     b. Manifestations (sudden onset): seen in young women and men
        1) Hypertension (principal manifestation): very high crisis
        2) Sudden attacks resemble manifestations of overstimulation of sympathetic nervous system
           a) Sweating
           b) Apprehension
           c) Palpitations
           d) Nausea
           e) Vomiting
           f) Orthostatic hypotension
           g) Headache
           h) Tachycardia
        3) Hyperglycemia
     c. Treatment
        1) Surgical excision of tumor or adrenal gland
        2) Symptomatic if surgery not feasible
  d. **NURSING INTERVENTIONS**
     1) Provide high-calorie, nutritious diet (avoid caffeine)
     2) Promote rest
     3) Preoperative: control hypertension (this is essential; high risk for hypertensive crisis)

Thyroid Gland

See Table I-13. for Hormones Produced and Functions

A. Disorders of Thyroid Gland
  1. Myxedema: highest incidence between ages 50 & 60; more often in women
     a. Definition: hyposecretion of thyroid hormone in adulthood
     b. Manifestations
        1) Slow rate of body metabolism
        2) Personality changes (depression)
        3) "Dull" appearance
        4) Anorexia and constipation
        5) Intolerance to cold
        6) Decreased sweating
        7) Hypersensitivity to barbiturates and narcotics
        8) Generalized interstitial edema
        9) Husky voice from swelling of vocal cords
        10) Coarse, dry skin
        11) Thin hair
        12) Generalized weakness
        13) Goiter
        14) Weight gain
        15) Puffy appearance (nonpitting)
        16) Anemia
        17) Increased cholesterol and lipids
        18) Menstrual disorders in women
     c. Treatment: drug therapy-Levothyroxine

(*Synthroid*)

1) Thyroid replacement hormones should be taken on an empty stomach
2) Monitor heart rate: fewer than 100 beats per minute is desirable; monitor for cardiac symptoms of angina at initiation of therapy

d. **NURSING INTERVENTIONS**

1) Directed toward manifestations of decreased metabolism
   a) Provide warm environment
   b) Low-calorie, low-cholesterol, low-saturated-fat diet
   c) Increase roughage
   d) Moderate fluids
   e) Avoid sedatives
   f) Plan rest periods
   g) Weigh client
2) Observe for overdosage manifestations of thyroid preparations (these will be the same as the manifestations of hyperthyroidism with the exception of exophthalmus; see below)

2. Cretinism
   a. Definition: hyposecretion of thyroid hormones in the fetus or neonate
   b. Diagnosed shortly after birth thru newborn screening; testing for thyroid hormones is mandated in all 50 states
   c. Can lead to severe, irreversible mental retardation if not treated
   d. Requires lifelong hormone replacement therapy

3. Hyperthyroidism (Graves' disease, diffuse toxic goiter)
   a. Definition: hypersecretion of thyroid hormone; over-treatment of hypothyroidism
   b. Manifestations
      1) Increased rate of body metabolism
      2) Personality changes
      3) Enlargement of the thyroid gland
      4) Exophthalmos (never goes away)
      5) Cardiac dysrhythmia and hypertension
      6) Increased appetite (but weight loss)
      7) Diarrhea
      8) Diaphoresis and heat intolerance
      9) Easy fatigability
      10) Anxiety/insomnia
      11) Nervous appearance
      12) Amenorrhea
   c. Treatment
      1) Drug therapy
         a) Methimazole (*Tapazole*): blocks thyroid hormone production
         b) Propylthiouracil (*Propyl-Thyracil*): blocks thyroid hormone production
            (1) Can cause agranulocytosis
            (2) Client must have frequent CBCs performed
         c) Iodides: decrease vascularity; inhibit release of thyroid hormones
            (1) Lugol's solution (use is decreasing because this medication is expensive and inactivates thyroid medications in the bowel)
            (2) Saturated solution of potassium iodide (*SSKI*); use prior to thyroidectomy
         d) Propranolol (*Inderal*): relief of tachycardia, new onset palpitations
      2) Radioiodine therapy: slowly destroys hyperfunctioning thyroid tissue (I 131; radioactive cocktail; client must be in isolation for about three days and care must be taken with wastes during this time)
      3) Thyroidectomy: subtotal or total
   d. **NURSING INTERVENTIONS**
      1) Provide adequate rest
      2) Provide cool, quiet environment
      3) Provide high-caloric (4000–5000 cal/day), high-protein, carbohydrate, vitamin diet without stimulants, extra fluids
      4) Weigh client daily
      5) Provide emotional support; activities; nothing repetitive
      6) Provide eye protection: ophthalmic medicine; tape eyes at night; decrease sodium and water

TABLE I-13.
THYROID GLAND: HORMONES PRODUCED AND FUNCTIONS

HORMONES PRODUCED	FUNCTION
Thyroxine (T4)	Acts as a catalyst; influences metabolic rate, growth, and development
Triiodothyronine (T3)	Controls rate of body metabolism, growth, and nutrition
Thyrocalcitonin	Assists in control of calcium levels; decreases reabsorption of bone

TABLE I-14.
PARATHYROID GLAND: HORMONES PRODUCED AND FUNCTIONS

HORMONES PRODUCED	FUNCTION
Parathyroid hormone (PTH)	Controls calcium and phosphate metabolism

7) Elevate head of bed
8) Be alert for complications
   a) Corneal abrasion
   b) Heart disease
   c) Thyroid storm (usually occurs after thyroid surgery)
e. Thyroidectomy
   1) Definition: removal of the thyroid gland, either total or partial
   2) Preoperative goals
      a) Thyroid function in normal range: saturated solution of potassium iodide (SSKI)
      b) Signs of thyrotoxicosis are diminished
      c) Weight and nutritional status normal

   3) **NURSING INTERVENTIONS** (postoperative care)
      a) Semi-Fowler's position
      b) Check dressing: especially back of neck
      c) Observe for respiratory distress: tracheostomy tray, oxygen, and suction apparatus at bedside
      d) Be alert for signs of hemorrhage
      e) Talking limited, note any hoarseness; may indicate injury to laryngeal nerve
      f) Observe for signs of tetany: Chvostek's sign and Trousseau's sign (parathyroid glands may accidentally be removed)
      g) Calcium gluconate IV at bedside
      h) Observe for thyroid storm (life-threatening); increase release of thyroid hormone
         (1) Fever
         (2) Tachycardia
         (3) Delirium
         (4) Irritability
         (5) Important to assess temperature routinely
      i) Gradually increase range of motion to neck; support when sitting up

Parathyroid Gland

See Table I-14. for Hormones Produced and Functions

A. **Disorders of Parathyroid Gland**
   1. Hypoparathyroidism
      a. Definition: hyposecretion of the parathyroid hormone; accidental removal during thyroid surgery
      b. Manifestations
         1) Hypocalcemia
         2) Acute: increased neuromuscular irritability tetany (positive Chvostek and positive Trousseau)
         3) Chronic
            a) Poor development of tooth enamel
            b) Lethargic
            c) Thin hair; brittle nails
            d) Mental retardation
            e) Circumoral paraesthesia with numbness and tingling of fingers
      c. Treatment
         1) Acute: IV calcium gluconate
         2) Chronic
            a) Oral calcium salts
            b) Vitamin D and aluminum hydroxide gel (*Amphojel*)
            c) High-calcium, low-phosphorous diet

      d. **NURSING INTERVENTIONS**
         1) Provide quiet room, no stimulus
         2) Assess for increased signs of neuromuscular irritability
   2. Hyperparathyroidism (causes are tumor or renal disease)
      a. Definition: hypersecretion of parathyroid hormone
      b. Manifestations (causes loss of calcium from the bones to the serum)
         1) Bone deformities, susceptible to fractures
         2) Calcium deposits in various body organs
         3) Hypercalcemia
         4) Gastric ulcers and GI disturbances
         5) Apathy, fatigue, weakness, depression
         6) Nausea, vomiting, anorexia
         7) Constipation, abdominal pain
         8) Joint and bone pain
         9) Polyuria
         10) Polydipsia
         11) Azotemia
         12) Hypertension
      c. Treatment

1) Subtotal surgical resection of parathyroid gland
2) Hydration and diuretics - furosemide (*Lasix*) excretes excess calcium
3) Plicamycin (*Mithracin*) or gallium nitrate (*Ganite*)

d. **NURSING INTERVENTIONS**
1) Force fluids
2) Provide a low-calcium, low vitamin D diet
3) Prevent constipation and fecal impaction
4) Strain all urine
5) Safety measures to prevent breaks
6) Calcitonin; binds phosphate; in renal failure

Pancreas

See Table I-15. for Hormones Produced and Functions

A. Disorder of the Pancreas

1. Diabetes mellitus
   a. Definition: chronic disorder of carbohydrate metabolism characterized by an imbalance between insulin supply and demand; either a subnormal amount of insulin is produced or the body requires abnormally high amounts
      1) Type 1: usually juvenile onset
      2) Type 2: usually adult onset
   b. Manifestations-"3 Polys"
      1) Polyuria
      2) Polydipsia
      3) Polyphagia
      4) Weight loss
   c. **NURSING INTERVENTIONS** (Balance of diet, insulin, and exercise; it is monitored by the capillary blood sugar levels)
      1) Administer insulin therapy (insulin is the hormone necessary to open the door for glucose to enter the cell and be used for energy)
      2) Administer hypoglycemics (increases the amount of insulin released by the pancreas for use by glucose in the body)
         a) Tolbutamide (*Orinase*)
         b) Chlorpropamide (*Diabinese)*
         c) Glyburide (*Micronase*)
         d) Metformin (*Glucophage*)
   3) Maintain diet therapy
      a) Goal is to provide the body with adequate nutrients for cell growth and function
      b) Maintain a balance between the amount of glucose in the body and the amount of insulin present to utilize that glucose
      c) Caloric requirements prescribed by physician in conjunction with the health care team
   4) Monitor for complications
      a) Hypoglycemia (occurs quickly; the most serious diabetic problem is no food for the brain)
         (1) Causes: decreased dietary intake, excess insulin, increased exercise
         (2) Manifestations
            (a) Tachycardia
            (b) Diaphoresis
            (c) Tremors
            (d) Weakness, fatigue
            (e) Irritability, anxiety
            (f) Confusion
         (3) **NURSING INTERVENTIONS**
            (a) Give hard candy (if conscious)
            (b) Apple juice/orange juice
            (c) Soft drinks
            (d) Follow with meal or carbohydrates within 1/2 hour
      b) Ketoacidosis (hyperglycemia); takes days to occur

TABLE I-15.
PANCREAS: HORMONES PRODUCED AND FUNCTIONS

HORMONES PRODUCED	FUNCTIONS
Insulin	Decreases blood sugar by: - Stimulating active transport of glucose into muscle and adipose tissue - Promoting the conversion of glucose to glycogen for storage - Promoting conversion of fatty acids into fat - Stimulating protein synthesis
Glucagon	Increases blood sugar by promoting conversion of glycogen to glucose

(1) Causes: lack of insulin, infection, stress
(2) Manifestations
    (a) Three Polys (polyuria, polydipsia, polyphagia)
    (b) Nausea
    (c) Vomiting
    (d) Dry mucous membranes
    (e) Kussmaul respirations
    (f) Coma
    (g) Ketone breathe
    (h) Flushed skin
    (i) Electrolyte shifts
    (j) Headache and decreased awareness
    (k) Vascular collapse
(3) **NURSING INTERVENTIONS**
    (a) Give regular insulin
    (b) Treat shock if present
    (c) Monitor electrolyte levels

c) Lipodystrophy: indurated areas of subcutaneous tissue secondary to injecting cold insulin or not rotating sites

d) Hyperglycemic hyperosmolar nonketotic coma (HHNK)
  (1) Extremely high glucose levels cause dehydration
  (2) No ketosis; elevated BUN
  (3) Treatment: replace fluids; give insulin and electrolytes

5) Insulin pump
  a) External device that provides a basal dose of regular insulin with a bolus dose before meals; does not read blood sugar
  b) Needles are inserted into subcutaneous abdominal tissue (changed every 24 to 48 hours)
  c) Complications
    (1) Insulin overdosage
    (2) Continued insulin injections during hypoglycemia

6) Health teaching
  a) Foot care: daily cleanse feet in warm soapy water; rinse and dry carefully; inspect, don't break blisters; trim nails to follow natural curve of toe; always wear breathable shoes such as leather; no crossing of the legs; no cream between toes; inspect visually daily
  b) Injection techniques (IntraSite rotation)
  c) Dietary management

d) Quit smoking
e) Stress management (stress increases blood sugar)
f) Complications
  (1) Neuropathy: causes pain in legs, then no feeling; safety issues ensue; causes impotence in men
  (2) Renal: affects microcirculation of kidneys and can cause renal failure
  (3) Cardiovascular: diabetics are 4 times more likely to have a myocardial infarction; unknown cause, but also increases occurrence of hypertension and decreased peripheral circulation
  (4) Eyes: number one cause of blindness and increases occurrence of cataracts
  (5) Infections: increased sugar in body fluids makes them an ideal medium for growth of microorganisms, urinary tract infections, cellulitis, etc.
  (6) **NURSING INTERVENTIONS:**
    (a) Assess for each complication early
    (b) Teach client to maintain control of the illness and to consistently keep blood sugar within normal ranges

TABLE I-16.
INSULIN

INSULIN	ONSET	PEAK	DURATION
Rapid acting Insulin analog (*Humalog*)	15 minutes	2-4 hrs	6-8 hrs
Short acting: Regular (*Semilente*)	1/2–1 hr	2-4 hrs	6–8 hrs
Intermediate: NPH (*Lente*)	1–2 hrs	7–12 hrs	24–30 hrs
Long acting: Protamine Zinc (*Ultralente*)	4–6 hrs	18+ hrs	30–36 hrs

Mixing insulin: draw up regular first, then NPH

SECTION VII

REVIEW OF BLOOD DISORDERS

Anemia

A. **Definition:** a deficiency of red blood cells that is characterized by a decreased red blood cell count and a below-normal hemoglobin (Hgb) and hematocrit (HCT); this results in a decrease in oxygen to the cells directly related to the degree of anemia present

TABLE I-17.
BLOOD VALUES

Normal values: RBC: female 4.2–5.4 mil/cu. mm, male 4.6-6.2 mil/cu. mm

Hgb: female 12–16 gm/dL, male 13–18

HCT: female 37%–48%, male 45%–52%

Note: 3 x Hgb = HCT

B. **Causes**
1. Acute or chronic blood loss (example: GI ulcers)
2. Greater than normal destruction of red blood cells (example: spleen diseases)
3. Abnormal bone marrow function (example: chemotherapy)
4. Decreased erythropoietin (example: renal failure)
5. Inadequate maturation of red blood cells (example: cancer)

C. **Manifestations**
1. Fatigue
2. Weakness
3. Dizziness
4. Pallor: first seen in conjunctival area (Caucasian) and oral area (dark and black-skinned population)
5. Cardiac, if decreased oxygen to heart
6. Decreased activity tolerance
7. Decreased Hgb, HCT, RBC levels
8. Shortness of breath and dyspnea

D. **NURSING INTERVENTIONS**
1. Activity as tolerated
2. Protect skin from breakdown; decrease pressure
3. Remove the cause or minimize as much as possible
4. Oxygen therapy as needed
5. Maximize rest and delivery of oxygen to tissues
6. Administer blood products as necessary

E. **Blood Transfusions**
1. Equipment
   a. Y-type tubing with filter
   b. Normal saline
   c. Blood

2. **NURSING INTERVENTIONS**
   a. Check ID, name, blood type; information verified by two nurses
   b. Take baseline vital signs including temperature
   c. Stay with the client for the first 15 minutes
   d. Infuse within 4 hours
   e. Monitor for transfusion reaction
      1) Allergic (pruritus, respiratory distress, urticaria), flushing; if expect a minor reaction to something in the blood, may give diphenhydramine (*Benadryl*) and continue to infuse
      2) Hemolytic: ABO incompatibility (flank pain, chest pain, fever, chills, tachycardia, tachypnea)
   f. Treat transfusion reaction
      1) Stop blood immediately
      2) Start saline
      3) Take vital signs
      4) Notify physician
      5) Follow facility policy (for example: send urine sample, CBC, send bag and tubing to lab for analysis)

F. **Classifications**
1. Hypoproliferation anemia; bone marrow is unable to produce adequate numbers of cells
   a. Anemia secondary to renal disease (lack of erythropoietin); treat by administering Epogen
   b. Iron deficiency anemia
      1) Due to chronic blood loss (for example: bleeding ulcer); treat the ulcer by methods discussed in GI section; if due to a tumor in GI tract, remove
      2) Due to nutritional deficiency; administer iron preparations
      3) Common in infants, young adult women, older adults
   c. Aplastic anemia (treat by eliminating the cause, administering steroid therapy, bone marrow transplantation, antibiotics, and splenectomy)
      1) Lack of precursor cells in the bone marrow with a decrease in all blood cell components (WBC: leukopenia; platelet: thrombocytopenia; RBC: anemia) due to drugs, virus, toxins, irradiation
      2) Manifestations

a) Hypoxia, fatigue, pallor (related to anemia)
b) Increased susceptibility to infection (related to leukopenia)
c) Hemorrhage, ecchymosis/leukopenia (related to thrombocytopenia)

3) **NURSING INTERVENTIONS**

a) General nursing interventions as previously listed
b) Protective isolation
c) Psychological support
d) Monitor for manifestations of infection

2. Megaloblastic anemia (deficiency of B_{12} and folic acid)
a. Pernicious anemia: a vitamin B_{12} deficiency due to a lack of the intrinsic factor in the gastric juice or deficiency in diet
b. Causes
1) Atrophy of the gastric mucosa/hypochlorhydria
2) Total gastrectomy
3) Malabsorption (secondary to Crohn's disease, pancreatitis)
4) Malnutrition
c. Manifestations (low Hgb and HCT)
1) Numbness, tingling of extremities
2) Paresthesia/hypoxemia
3) Gait disturbances
4) Behavioral problems
d. **NURSING INTERVENTIONS**
1) General interventions discussed
2) Assist with Schilling's test
3) B_{12} three times a week for two weeks; two times a week for two weeks; then once a month; must be given by injection if due to lack of intrinsic factor
4) Encourage client to have physical examination twice per year due to high risk potential of developing gastric carcinoma

KEY INFORMATION

B_{12} combines with intrinsic factor for absorption in the small intestine

B_{12} is important for RNA production, which is necessary for maintenance of CNS integrity

3. Hemolytic anemia, due to excessive RBC destruction
a. Causes
1) Trauma
2) Lead poisoning
3) TB
4) Infections

5) Transfusion reactions
6) Toxic agents
b. **NURSING INTERVENTIONS**
1) General interventions discussed
2) Steroids as needed
3) Treat underlying disease to remove the cause

4. Congenital anemia
a. Sickle cell anemia (see also Unit IV, Section VII): defective hemoglobin molecule that assumes a sickle shape when oxygen in venous blood is low; the sickle cells become lodged in the blood vessels, especially the brain and the kidneys as they have a constant need for oxygen
b. Manifestations
1) Severe pain
2) Swelling
3) Fever
4) Jaundice
5) Susceptibility to infection
6) Hypoxic damage to organs
c. Risk factors that will cause an attack by enhancing sickling in the cells
1) Stress
2) Dehydration
3) Hypoxia
4) High altitudes
d. **NURSING INTERVENTIONS** (symptomatic)
1) Refer for genetic counseling
a) Autosomal recessive inheritance
b) More common in African-American clients
2) Hydration (make sure adequate)
3) Oxygen
4) Analgesics (may need narcotics)
5) Rest
6) Eliminate risk factors

Administration of Iron Preparations

A. Oral
1. Dilute liquid preparations in juice or water and administer with a plastic straw to avoid staining teeth
2. Orange juice facilitates absorption
3. Monitor for constipation, GI upset

B. Intramuscular
1. Use large bore needle (19 gauge)
2. Use one needle to draw up iron; change needle before administering (to prevent staining)
3. Z-track (to buttocks only, never arm)
4. Do not massage

REVIEW OF CARDIOVASCULAR SYSTEM DISORDERS

Cardiovascular System in Failure

A. Deficits Present in at Least One Area:
1. Adequately pumps blood to all parts of the body, thus good working cardiac muscles and conduction system
2. Good circulating blood volume to meet body's needs
3. Peripheral vascular resistance must be sufficient to maintain adequate blood pressure
4. Normal heart rate 60–100 beats per minute

Diagnostic Procedures

A. Laboratory Tests
1. Blood electrolytes (see table I-1.)
2. Sedimentation rate (0–30); increased with myocardial infarction
3. Blood coagulation tests
   a. PTT (16–40 seconds); significant if client is on heparin therapy
   b. PT (9–12 seconds); significant if client is on warfarin sodium (*Coumadin*) therapy
   c. Clotting time (10 min.)
   d. INR (2–3.5); universal test not affected by variations in lab norms
4. BUN (6–20 mg/dL); reflects kidney function or increased muscle breakdown
5. Serum cholesterol (150–250 mg/dL); greater than 200, treatment required
   a. Low-density lipids (LDL): less than 130 mg/dL; "bad" cholesterol
   b. High-density lipids (HDL): greater than 35 mg/dL; "good" cholesterol
6. Blood cultures
7. Enzymes (indicates actual death of myocardial muscles; heart attack)
   a. CPK-MB: men: 55–170 units/mL; women: 30–135 units/mL; rises 2–5 hours after myocardial infarction (MI), (peaks in 24 hours)
   b. LDH: 150–450 units/mL; rises 14–24 hours after MI, (peaks in 48 hours)
   c. SGOT: 5–40 units/mL, rises 6–8 hours after MI, (peaks in 48 hours)
   d. MB Fraction: rises 4–6 hours after MI, (peaks by 18 hours)
   e. Troponin I and T: <1.0 ng/mL, rises 3–12 hours after MI, may remain elevated 1–2 weeks
      1) Highly specific for myocardial injury

2) Considered the new "gold standard" in diagnosis of MI

B. Central Venous Pressure (normal = 5–10 cm water)
1. Provides an indication of pressure in the right atrium
2. Trends are more important than values

C. Electrocardiogram (ECG)
1. Definition: a record showing the electrical activity of the heart
2. Interpretation
   a. P wave: atrial depolarization
   b. QRS complex: ventricular depolarization
   c. T wave: ventricular repolarization
   d. PR interval: 0.12–.20 seconds
   e. QRS: 0.08–.10 seconds

D. Arteriography/Angiography
1. Definition: injection of contrast medium into the vascular system to outline an area of the body; when it is done to the vessels around the heart, it is usually done with cardiac catheterization
2. Purpose: obtain information regarding coronary anatomy, structural abnormalities of the coronary artery
3. **NURSING INTERVENTIONS**
   a. Standard preop preparation
   b. General care following any type of angiogram
      1) Monitor vital signs q 15 minutes until stable
      2) Check routinely for bleeding at puncture site(s)
      3) Check distal extremity to puncture site for CMS checks
      4) Force fluids
      5) Maintain bed rest 8–12 hours

E. Cardiac Catheterization
1. Definition: a diagnostic procedure; catheter is introduced into the right or left side of the heart through either the femoral or brachial artery
2. Purpose
   a. Measure oxygen concentration, saturation, tension, and pressure in various chambers of the heart
   b. Detect shunts
   c. Obtain blood samples
   d. Determine cardiac output and pulmonary blood flow
   e. Determine need for cardiac bypass surgery
3. **NURSING INTERVENTIONS**
   a. Prior to catheterization
      1) Know approach: right (venous) or left (arterial)
      2) Keep client NPO for 6 hours
      3) Mark distal (baseline) pulses

4) Explain procedure to client and what to expect
   a) May have metallic taste in mouth
   b) May feel flushed when dye is injected
5) Assess client for history of allergy to dye, shellfish
6) Obtain consent form from client
b. After catheterization
1) Monitor blood pressure and apical pulse q 15 minutes for 2–4 hours
2) Check peripheral pulses q 15 minutes for 2–4 hours (CMS checks)
3) Check puncture sites for bleeding
4) Apply sandbag to area to maintain hemostasis
5) Assess for chest pain
6) Keep extremity extended 4–6 hours
7) Maintain bed rest; no hip flexion; no sitting up in bed
8) Increase fluid intake to flush body of dye

Disorders

A. Angina (syndrome)
1. Definition: insufficient coronary blood flow, thus inadequate oxygen supply causing intermittent chest pain
2. **NURSING INTERVENTIONS**
   a. Assess pain
      1) Location: jaw and/or arm as well as chest
      2) Character
      3) Duration: goes away with rest and/or nitroglycerine (*Nitro-bid*)
      4) Precipitating factors (once identified, eliminate or minimize to avoid attacks)
   b. Educate client to help client to adjust living style to prevent episode of angina
      1) Avoid excessive activity in cold weather
      2) Avoid overeating
      3) Stop smoking
      4) Avoid constipation
      5) Rest after meals
      6) Exercise
      7) Decrease stress
   c. Teach client that anything that decreases cardiac output or increases workload of heart can cause chest pain
   d. Teach client how to cope with an attack: use of nitroglycerin (*Nitro-bid*) - peripheral vasodilation decreases myocardial oxygen demand; coronary artery vasodilation increases supply of oxygen to myocardium
      1) When to take: daily to prevent and/or as needed at onset of chest pain; if client knows an activity can cause pain, should take before (for example: sexual intercourse)

2) How often: if at onset of attack, q 5 minutes x 3; if chest pain still not relieved, call 911
3) Storage (dark, dry; only good for 3 months; "no tingle—no good")
4) Side effects (headache; hypotension)
5) Types: tablets, ointment, patch, spray
   a) If given daily for prevention, client must be nitroglycerine free daily for 12 hours to prevent tolerance
   b) If patch user: "On" upon waking, "off" at bedtime
6) Never take nitroglycerin (*Nitro-stat*) without sitting down and stopping activity
7) Client on regular or intermittent nitroglycerines (*Nitro-bid, Nitro-stat*) must not take sildenafil citrate (*Viagra*) due to the increased risk of sudden cardiac death

B. Myocardial Infarction
1. Definition: process by which myocardium tissue is destroyed due to reduced coronary blood flow and lack of oxygen; actual necrosis of heart muscle occurs
2. Causes
   a. Atherosclerotic heart disease
   b. Coronary artery embolism
3. Manifestations
   a. Chest pain
      1) Heavy (viselike, crushing, squeezing) chest pain that may radiate down left arm, hand, jaw, neck
      2) Not relieved by rest, often lasts longer than 15 minutes
      3) Women have a slightly different presentation: back pain, indigestion with nausea, cold sweating, weakness, pallor
   b. Nausea, vomiting due to stress reaction
   c. Diaphoresis, dizziness due to sympathetic reaction
   d. Drop in blood pressure
   e. ECG changes: inverted T wave and depressed ST segment indicate ischemic changes, elevated ST segment and widened QRS indicate infarction
   f. Denial/anxiety
   g. Increased Troponin I and T, MB-CPK, LDH isoenzymes: done in serials of three to see trends
4. **NURSING INTERVENTIONS:** aimed at resting myocardium
   a. Early
      1) Treat dysrhythmia promptly: antiarrhythmics such as lidocaine (*Xylocaine*)
      2) Give analgesics: morphine

3) Maintain bed rest: Semi-Fowler's position to decrease venous return and rest myocardium
4) Administer oxygen via cannula
5) Monitor vital signs
6) Administer aspirin and heparin to decrease thrombosis
7) Administer propranolol HCl (*Inderal*): decreases heart rate and decreases work of myocardium
8) Administer calcium channel blockers: decrease afterload; vasodilators: increase oxygen to myocardium
9) Administer nitroglycerin IV: vasodilator; increases oxygen to myocardium; decreases preload and afterload
10) Provide emotional support
11) Administer streptokinase (*Kabikinase*) or TPA ("clot busters"): if client arrives within first 6 hours; major side effect is bleeding

b. Later
1) Administer stool softeners to decrease myocardial workload
2) Provide low-fat, low-cholesterol, low-sodium diet, soft food
3) Utilize bedside commode: causes less energy expenditure than using a bedpan
4) Promote self-care to tolerance; stop at the onset of pain
5) Plan for cardiac rehabilitation
   a) Exercise program: stop if fatigue or chest pain occurs
   b) Stress management
   c) Teach modifiable risk factors reduction
      (1) Obesity
      (2) Stress
      (3) Diet
      (4) Hypertension
      (5) Smoking
      (6) Lack of exercise
   d) Recognize nonmodifiable risk factors
      (1) Heredity
      (2) Race
      (3) Age
      (4) Sex
      (5) "Type A" personality
   e) Psychological support
   f) Long-term drug therapy
      (1) Antiarrhythmics: quinidine (*Quinora*), lidocaine (*Xylocaine*)
      (2) Anticoagulants: heparin (*Hep-Lock*), aspirin, warfarin (*Coumadin*), enoxaparin (*Lovenox*)

(3) Antihypertensives: propranolol (*Inderal*), chlorothiazide (*Diuril*), and calcium channel blockers
(4) Vasodilators - nitroglycerin (*Nitro-bid*) and calcium channel blockers

C. Cardiac Surgery
1. Percutaneous transthoracic cardiac angioplasty (PTCA)
   a. Done through a left cardiac catheterization
   b. Dilates the blocked coronary artery and often places a stent in the vessel to hold it open
   c. **NURSING INTERVENTIONS**
      1) Same as post-angioplasty care
      2) Monitor for complications: vasospasm, dysrhythmia, rupture of coronary vessel leading to a myocardial infarction
2. Coronary artery bypass graft (CABG)
   a. Done to replace damaged coronary arteries and reestablish perfusion in areas of myocardium
   b. Most procedures in use require open chest/heart approach with bypass machine
      1) Preoperative care; general care
      2) Psychological support: may need to be done on an emergency basis
      3) Postoperative care
         a) Chest tubes
         b) General postoperative care including pain management and care of wound
         c) Will have endotracheal tube for a day postop; prepare client about and provide sterile technique when caring for tube and suctioning
         d) Assess all systems since they all can be affected by decreased cardiac output; for example: vital signs, urine output, circulation in legs, chest pain
         e) Assess for complications: myocardial infarction, pleural effusion, dysrhythmia

D. Congestive Heart Failure
1. Definition: inability of the heart to meet tissue requirements for oxygen (not pumping effectively); usually the body tries to compensate by increasing the rate (tachycardia), increasing the size of the muscle and increasing the length of the heart fibers; all these changes are aimed at increasing cardiac output
2. Left ventricular failure: inadequate ejection of blood into the systemic circulation, usually associated with MI, hypertension
   a. Manifestations (primarily respiratory symptoms)

1) Dyspnea and PND
2) Moist cough
3) Crackles, wheezing
4) Orthopnea
b. Pulmonary edema results, causing excessive quantity of fluid in pulmonary interstitial spaces or alveoli evidenced by:
1) Moist crackles, frothy sputum
2) Severe anxiety
3) Marked dyspnea and cyanosis
4) Edema in pulmonary system
c. NURSING INTERVENTIONS
1) Administer morphine sulfate for pain: decreases rate and increases effective breathing; causes pooling of blood in the peripheral vessels, thus decreasing cardiac return and decreasing the work of the heart
2) Administer furosemide (*Lasix*) for diuretic
3) Deliver high-flow oxygen therapy
4) Monitor client for possible intubation
5) Maintain bed rest in Semi-Fowler's position
6) Administer digitalis (*Digoxin*) to increase efficiency of the myocardium as a pump
3. Right ventricular failure: congestion due to blood not adequately pumped from systemic system to the lungs; also related to COPD/CAL;
a. Manifestations (primarily systemic symptoms)
1) Peripheral edema (dependent in nature)
2) Distended neck veins
3) Weight gain (greater than 2 lbs in one day)
4) Enlarged liver
5) Elevated central venous pressure (CVP)
6) Hypotension (from decreased cardiac output)
7) Tachycardia ← *trying to compensate*
b. NURSING INTERVENTIONS
1) Provide psychological support for relief of anxiety and stress
2) Deliver oxygen
3) Decrease fluid intake to decrease preload
4) Improve myocardial contraction with digitalis (*Digoxin*), dobutamine hydrochloride (*Dobutrex*)
c. Digitalis (*Digoxin*) therapy
1) Purpose: decrease heart rate, improve ventricular filling, stroke volume and coronary artery perfusion; improve strength of contraction
2) Manifestations of toxicity - check digitalis (*Digoxin*) level in serum; 0.5 – 2.0 is normal
a) Halo around lights
b) Anorexia, diarrhea

c) Nausea and vomiting
d) Bradycardia, frequent premature ventricular contractions (PVCs)

3) NURSING INTERVENTIONS   *S/E green*
a) Monitor K$^+$ levels; decreased potassium levels enhance digitalis (*Digoxin*) toxicity
b) Monitor apical heart rate: verify if >60 BPM before each dose
c) Teach client: live within cardiac reserve; report symptoms of CHF
d) Weigh daily: report weight gain of greater than 2 lbs in one day of 3 lbs in one week
e) Administer diuretics: decrease preload
f) Implement cardiac diet: decreased sodium, decreased fluid intake

E. **Dysrhythmia**
1. Atrial dysrhythmia (significance is how they are affecting ventricular functioning and pulse rate)
a. Atrial fibrillation
1) Irregular, rapid rate   *organic*
2) Usually due to organic cause
3) Treated with medication such as beta blockers   *LA pooling from atrium*
4) May require cardioversion
5) Can cause mural thrombi which can lead to a stroke, so clients with this dysrhythmia should be taking warfarin (*Coumadin*)
b. Atrial tachycardia
1) Regular rate greater than 100 BPM
2) Examples of causes: anxiety, caffeine, medications, exercise
3) Treated by removing the cause
c. Atrial bradycardia
1) Rate below 60 BPM
2) Normal in athletes
3) Significance relates to how it affects cardiac output
4) Treated by administering anticholinergic medication (example: Atropine)   *↓ speeds up!*
2. Ventricular dysrhythmia
a. Ventricular tachycardia
1) Pulse rate above 150   *side parking of a pacing*
2) Severely affects cardiac output
3) Treatment: cardioversion   *hook the paddle or medication*
b. Ventricular ectopic beats
1) Indicates irritability of the ventricles
2) Could lead to cardiac arrest or ventricular tachycardia so must treat   *arrythmia*
3) Treatment: antiarrhythmic medications
a) Procainamide hydrochloride (*Pronestyl*)
b) Lidocaine (*Xylocaine*)
4) Side effects: slowing of the heart rate,

decreased blood pressure
  c. Ventricular fibrillation
    1) Most serious dysrhythmia
    2) Synonymous with cardiac arrest; treatment CPR and defibrillation

F. AV Heart Block
  1. Definition: altered transmission of impulse from SA node through AV node; impulse blocked from getting to the ventricles; therefore the pulse rate drops and the cardiac output drops
    a. First degree
      1) Delayed transmission of impulse through the AV node
      2) Prolonged PR interval (> 0.20)
      3) No treatment necessary
    b. Second degree
      1) Some impulses pass through AV node, some do not
      2) May be: 2:1, 3:1, or 4:1 block
      3) May progress to more lethal heartblock
      4) Pacemaker may be necessary
    c. Third degree
      1) No impulses pass through AV node
      2) Atria and ventricles essentially beat independently of each other
      3) Ventricular pacemaker takes over and the ventricles are a very slow and unreliable source to generate cardiac heart rate
      4) Indication for a pacemaker
    d. Pacemaker
      1) Definition: electronic device that provides repetitive electrical stimuli to the heart muscle to control heart rate
      2) Types
        a) Permanent pacemakers
          (1) Ventricular demand: fires at preset rate when client's heart rate drops below a predetermined/preprogrammed rate
          (2) Ventricular fixed: fires constantly at preset/preprogrammed rate, regardless of the client's own heart rate
          (3) Dual chamber: stimulates both the atria and the ventricles
          (4) Atrial Demand: fires as needed when the atria do not originate a rhythm
          (5) Variable rate: senses oxygen demands and increases firing rate to meet the client's needs
        b) Temporary pacemakers
          (1) Transcutaneous (skin); external, for use in emergency pacing situations
          (2) Transvenous

    3) Lower limit: All permanent pacemakers are set at a definitive lowest rate whereby the pacemaker will fire and stimulate the heart if the pulse rate drops below this predetermined/preprogrammed rate. The nurse must know this rate to assess and teach the client. If the pulse ever drops below this rate, it must be reported.
    4) **NURSING INTERVENTIONS**
      a) Teach client preoperatively
      b) Postoperative care
        (1) Monitor EKG and pulse rate
        (2) Check wound for hematoma, infection
        (3) Administer analgesics as necessary
        (4) Maintain electrically safe environment; client will need to avoid large generators, magnets, MRI machines
        (5) Observe for hiccoughs; indicates pacemaker is malpositioned and is pacing the diaphragm
        (6) Maintain sterile technique at insertions site for wound care
      c) Monitor for complications after pacemaker insertion
        (1) Observe for local infection (will have to remove pacemaker)
        (2) Monitor for hematoma
        (3) Monitor for dysrhythmia
        (4) Prevent accidental dislodging of the electrode; client must be careful using arm on the affected side until site is completely healed: no raising the arm high over the head
        (5) Observe for signs of pacemaker malfunction (failure to capture, sense or pace)
      d) Teach client
        (1) Carry ID information at all times
        (2) Battery change intervals (3–15 years for lithium batteries)
        (3) How to transmit data via telephone from pacemaker to healthcare provider
        (4) Wear loose fitting clothes
        (5) No contact sports

G. Valvular Disorders
  1. Definition: results in narrowing of valve that prevents or impedes blood flow (stenosis) or impaired closure that allows backward leakage of blood (regurgitation); affects mitral, aortic, or tricuspid: stenosis or insufficiency; rheumatic fever

history frequent causative factor (or infection such as endocarditis)

2. Manifestations
   a. Right heart failure (mitral stenosis, mitral regurgitation, tricuspid stenosis)
   b. Left heart failure (aortic stenosis, insufficiency)
   c. Murmurs → *little pound*
   d. Decreased cardiac output

3. **NURSING INTERVENTIONS**

   a. Same as CHF
   b. Administer antibiotic therapy for damage due to infection
   c. Administer prophylactic antibiotics prior to any invasive procedure, dental work

4. Surgical management
   a. Heart valve replacement (can actually hear the click)
   b. Mitral commissurotomy (valvulotomy)
      1) **NURSING INTERVENTIONS**
         a) Routine post-operative care
         b) See post-operative care for client after cardiac surgery
      2) **NURSING INTERVENTIONS** (rehabilitation)
         a) Allow activities as tolerated
         b) Implement cardiac diet: low-sodium, low-cholesterol
         c) Administer medications (anticoagulant therapy) for lifetime
         d) Instruct client in life long need for antibiotics prior to any invasive procedures and dental work

H. **Arterial Disorders of the Peripheral Vascular System**
1. Causes
   a. Arteriosclerosis - *plaque*
   b. Atherosclerosis - *hardening*
2. Classic manifestations
   a. Intermittent claudication; increases the more you use the extremity, like angina but in the leg
   b. Tingling and numbness of toes
   c. Cool extremities
   d. Trophic changes to extremity: thick toenails, dry skin, hairless
   e. Difficulty in assessing peripheral pulses; grade pulses so can compare for assessment of changes
3. Client teaching
   a. Stop smoking
   b. Avoid stressful situations
   c. Avoid constricting garments
   d. Keep legs in straight plane or dependent; do not cross legs
   e. Buerger-Allen exercises
4. Arteriosclerosis obliterans (ASO): usually affects aorta or the arteries of the lower extremities

   a. Characteristics
      1) Commonly associated with diabetes
      2) Occlusion usually proximal to pain zone
      3) Advanced manifestations: pain at rest, commonly at night
   b. Surgical management
      1) Vascular grafts
      2) Patch grafts
      3) Endarterectomy
   c. **NURSING INTERVENTIONS**
      1) Frequently check extremities for pulses, color and temperature
      2) Observe for paralysis of lower extremities after operation upon thoracic aorta
      3) Ensure adequate circulating blood volume through arterial repair: intake and output; central venous pressure
      4) Teach client: avoid dependent positions, elevate extremities, use of support hose/ anti-embolism stockings
      5) Administer heparin

5. Buerger's disease (thromboangiitis obliterans)
   a. Definition: recurring inflammation of the arteries and veins of lower and upper extremities resulting in thrombus and occlusion (cause unknown)
   upper & lower extremities
   b. Characteristics
      1) Occurs in men ages 20–40 years
      2) Most common manifestations: pain in legs relieved by inactivity, numbness and tingling of toes and fingers in cold weather/ intermittent claudication
      3) Cessation of smoking important; client teaching is same as arteriosclerosis
      4) Ulcerations and gangrene with amputation are common

6. Raynaud's syndrome *hands*
   a. Definition: vasospastic or obstructive condition of arteries that occurs with exposure to cold or stress and primarily affects the hands
   b. Characteristics
      1) Arteriolar vasoconstriction results in coldness, pallor, and pain
      2) Occasional ulceration of the fingertips
      3) Color changes from white to blue to red (can be bilateral or symmetrical)
   c. **NURSING INTERVENTIONS**
      1) Teach client to avoid cold (keep extremities warm); gloves
      2) Educate client to stop smoking; limit caffeine
      3) Administer nifedipine (*Procardia*); drug of choice → *dilator*
      4) Sympathectomy

I. **Vascular Disorders** → *cut the nerves*
1. Aortic aneurysm

a. Definition: local distention of the artery wall, usually thoracic or abdominal (four times more common); watch until it gets above 5 cm, then rate of rupture increases so surgery is required

b. Cause
1) Infections (mycotic)
2) Congenital
3) Atherosclerosis or hypertension

c. Manifestations (frequently asymptomatic)
1) Thoracic: pain, dyspnea, hoarseness, cough, dysphagia
2) Abdominal: abdominal pain, persistent or intermittent low back or flank pain; may be asymptomatic; pulsating abdominal mass; shock

d. Treatment: usually surgery
1) Preoperative: careful monitoring because of a possible rupture; prepare for abdominal surgery
2) Postoperative: same as abdominal surgery, careful monitoring of peripheral circulation below level of aneurysms
3) Postoperative complications
   a) Myocardial infarction
   b) Emboli
   c) Renal failure → no perfusion
   d) Spinal cord ischemia

2. Hypertension
a. Definition: persistent BP above 140/systolic and 90/diastolic; called "silent killer"

128/80
90-140/60-90

b. Primary hypertension
1) 90% have this kind
2) Hereditary disease
3) More common among African-Americans
4) Cause unknown
5) Late manifestations: headaches, fatigue, dyspnea, edema, nocturia, blackouts
6) Usually no signs or symptoms are displayed until end-organ involvement occurs

c. Secondary hypertension
1) Due to identifiable problem
2) Pheochromocytoma → from blood
3) Renal pathology

d. **NURSING INTERVENTIONS**
1) Counsel client on weight control methods
2) Teach client to stop smoking
3) Educate client to avoid stimulants (decrease alcohol and caffeine intake); moderate amount of alcohol is actually good: less than 1 ounce of alcohol OR 24 ounces of beer a day
4) Promote a program of regular physical exercise
5) Promote lifestyle with reduced stress
6) Maintain salt-restricted diet
7) Teach risk factors

KIKOMAN NAPPA!

e. Antihypertensive drugs
1) Potassium depleting diuretics
   a) Loop diuretics: bumetanide (*Bumex*) and furosemide (*Lasix*)
   b) Chlorothiazide (*Diuril*)
   c) Hydrochlorothiazide (*HydroDIURIL*)
   d) Ethacrynic acid (*Edecrin*)
   e) **NURSING INTERVENTIONS**
      (1) Administer potassium supplements as ordered
      (2) Teach dietary sources of potassium
      (3) Be aware of possible interaction of low K^+ and digitalis (*Digoxin*) preparations
2) Potassium sparing diuretics
   a) Spironolactone (*Aldactone*)
   b) Triamterene (*Dyrenium*)
   c) Watch for increased potassium level
3) Central acting adrenergic inhibitors (Beta blockers)
   a) Propranolol HCl (*Inderal*)
   b) Atenolol (*Tenormin*)
   c) Metoprolol (*Lopressor*)
   d) **NURSING INTERVENTIONS**
      (1) Watch for major side effect of bradycardia
      (2) Monitor daily pulse
      (3) Monitor for signs and symptoms of CHF
      (4) Contraindicated in asthmatics
      (5) Watch for reflex tachycardia due to decreased cardiac output and hypotension
4) Central acting anti-adrenergic agents
   a) Clonidine (*Catapres*)
   b) Side effects: drowsiness, sexual dysfunction, dry mouth
   c) Methyldopa (*Aldomet*); major side effect is postural hypotension
5) Vasodilators
   a) Hydralazine (*Apresoline*); major side effects are headache, flushing/palpitations
   b) Minoxidil (*Loniten*)
6) Calcium agonist
   a) Nifedipine (*Procardia*): Major side effects-headache/dizziness, bradycardia, peripheral edema
   b) Verapamil (*Calan*) and diltiazem (*Cardizem*): Major side effects-flushing, arrhythmias, constipation
7) Angiotensin-converting enzyme (ACE) inhibitors
   a) Captopril (*Capoten*)
   b) Enalapril (*Vasotec*)

c) Lisinopril (*Zestril*)
d) Major side effects: cough, headache, angioedema of face and limbs

Venous Disorders

A. **Thrombophlebitis**
1. Definition: clot in the vein with inflammation of the wall
2. Precipitating factors
   a. Stasis
   b. Hypercoagulability
   c. Damage to intima of blood vessels/trauma
   d. Pregnancy or estrogen (oral contraceptives)
   e. Malignancy or obesity
3. Manifestations
   a. Edema of affected limb
   b. Local swelling, bumpy, knotty
   c. Red, tender, local induration
   d. Positive Homans' sign (not very reliable sign)
4. **NURSING INTERVENTIONS**
   a. Maintain bed rest
   b. Elevate leg and apply moist warm compresses
   c. Administer anticoagulant therapy
   d. Initiate anti-embolism stockings/support hose
   e. Administer pain medication
   f. Increase fluids
   g. Encourage deep breathing
   h. Assist client with ROM
   i. Teach client
      1) Avoid green leafy vegetables while on warfarin (*Coumadin*)
      2) Care to area of phlebitis
      3) Watch for bleeding

B. **Varicose Veins**
1. Precipitating factors
   a. Prolonged standing
   b. Pregnancy
   c. Obesity
   d. Heredity
2. Manifestations (accentuated by gravity)
   a. Enlarged, tortuous veins in lower extremities
   b. Pain
   c. Edema (after upright)
3. **NURSING INTERVENTIONS** (teaching)
   a. Elevate legs frequently
   b. TEDS (below the knee except immediately after surgery)
   c. Avoid constrictive clothing, prolonged sitting or standing
   d. Avoid crossing legs at knee
   e. Postop care for vein stripping and ligation
      1) Monitor circulation (elastic stockings to entire leg postop only)
      2) Elevate feet

3) Stand, lie down
4. Ulcers
   a. Arterial: looks punched-out; no edema present
   b. Venous: around ankle usually, reddened and bluish, edema present many times

Shock

A. **Definition:** Lack of oxygen and nutrients at the cellular level (due to impaired tissue perfusion) for cellular metabolism, regardless of the etiology

B. **Types**
1. Cardiogenic: failure of the heart to pump adequately
2. Hypovolemic: decreased blood volume
3. Distributive (vasogenic)
   a. Neurogenic: increased size of vascular bed due to loss of vascular tone
   b. Anaphylactic: hypersensitivity reaction
   c. Septic: systemic reaction vasodilation due to infection

C. **General Manifestations** (related to decreased tissue perfusion)
1. Tachycardia
2. Tachypnea
3. Oliguria
4. Cold, moist skin
5. Color ashen: pallor
6. Hypotension
7. Metabolic acidosis
8. Decreased LOC

D. **NURSING INTERVENTIONS**
1. Elevate feet
2. Secure client IV
3. Administer oxygen
   a. Record vital signs q 5 minutes
   b. Promote rest; decrease movement
   c. Monitor urine output
4. Treat underlying cause

E. **Emergency Drugs**
1. Atropine: increases heart rate
2. Dopamine (*Intropin*): vasoconstrictor; increases BP and tissue and renal perfusion
3. Epinephrine HCl (*Adrenalin*): increases body reaction to stress
4. Isoproterenol (*Isuprel*): increases heart rate and cardiac output
5. Dobutamine (*Dobutrex*): inotropic; increases force of myocardial contraction in cardiogenic shock
6. Norepinephrine levarterenol (*Levophed*): vasoconstrictor; increases tissue perfusion
7. Sodium bicarbonate: decreases acidosis

Cardiopulmonary Resuscitation (CPR)

A. **Indications**
1. Absence of palpable carotid pulse
2. Absence of breath sounds

B. **Purpose**
1. Establish effective circulation and respiration
2. Prevent irreversible cerebral anoxic damage

C. **Procedure**
1. Determine unresponsiveness
2. Airway (head tilt/chin lift)
3. Breathing (two breaths)
4. Circulation
5. American Heart Association 2001 recommendations:
   a. Ratio of 15 compressions to 2 ventilations for either single or two rescuer *[handwritten: for everybody]*
   b. Compression rate of 100 per minute for all age groups

D. **Complications**
1. Fractured ribs
2. Punctured lungs
3. Lacerated liver
4. Abdominal distension

E. **Stop CPR When:**
1. Physician pronounces client dead
2. Exhausted
3. Help arrives
4. Heartbeat returns

F. **Automated External Defibrillator** (AED)
1. Computerized defibrillator analyzes cardiac rhythm once pads are placed on client's chest
2. Mechanical voice tells rescuer if/when to deliver shock to client
3. Do not have to be a professional rescuer but must be trained in use of machine

G. **Obstructed Airway**
1. Conscious
   a. Establish that victim is choking
   b. Heimlich maneuver until successful or client becomes unconscious
2. Unconscious
   a. Establish unresponsiveness
   b. Attempt to ventilate
   c. Reposition and reventilate
   d. Tongue-jaw lift, finger-sweep
   e. Reattempt ventilation
   f. Abdominal thrusts

g. Repeat steps d through f until successful or EMS arrives

REVIEW OF GENITOURINARY SYSTEM DISORDERS

Assessment of the Client

A. **Functions of the Kidney**
1. Regulates acid-base balance
2. Excretes metabolic wastes (creatinine, urea)
3. Regulates blood pressure: renin (stimulated by decreased blood pressure or blood volume) stimulates production of angiotensin I, which is converted to angiotensin II in the lungs; angiotensin II is a strong vasoconstrictor and also stimulates aldosterone secretion; vasoconstriction and sodium reabsorption result in increased blood volume and increased blood pressure *[handwritten: cardiac + renal work together]*
4. Secretes erythropoietin
5. Converts vitamin D to its active form for absorption of calcium
6. Excretes water soluble drugs and drug metabolites *[handwritten: ADEK → fat soluble]*

B. **History**
1. Has there been renal disease in the past?
2. Is there a family history of renal disease?
3. Age: developmental issues; incontinence and prostatic problems
4. Gender: incontinence increased in women; benign prostate hypertrophy (BPH): older men

C. **Manifestations**
1. Pain (usually in acute conditions): flank radiating to upper thigh, testis, or labium
2. Changes in voiding: hematuria, proteinuria, dysuria, frequency, urgency, burning, nocturia, incontinence, polyuria, oliguria, anuria
3. Thirst, fatigue, edema (generalized)

Diagnostic Tests

KEY INFORMATION

A. **Urinalysis**
1. Specific gravity: 1.010–1.030
2. Color: yellow/amber
3. Negative glucose, protein, red blood cells and white blood cells
4. pH: 5–8
5. First voided morning sample preferred; 15 mL
6. Send to lab immediately or refrigerate *[handwritten: used for cultures]*

7. If clean catch, get urine for culture prior to starting antibiotics
   a. Cleanse labia, glans penis
   b. Obtain midstream sample

B. **Renal Function Tests** (several tests over a period of time are necessary)
   1. BUN (blood urea nitrogen): 10–20 mg/100 mL
   2. Serum creatinine: 0–1 mg/dL
   3. Creatinine clearance: 100–120 mL/minute; collect 24 hour urine (refrigerate); blood drawn at start (measures glomerular filtration rate)
   4. Uric acid (serum): 3.5–7.8 mg/dL
   5. Uric acid (urine): 250–750 mg/24 hour; 24 hour urine
   6. Prostate-specific antigen (PSA): 0.85 ng/mL

C. **Radiologic Test**
   1. KUB (x-ray): shows size, shape and position of kidneys, ureters, bladder; no preparation
   2. Intravenous pyelography (IVP): visualization of urinary tract

      a. **NURSING INTERVENTIONS**
         1) Obtain consent
         2) Keep client NPO for 8–10 hours
         3) Administer laxatives to clear bowel
         4) Restrict fluids
         5) Check for allergies to iodine or shellfish
         6) Inform client that flushing, warmth, nausea, salty taste may accompany injection of dye
         7) Have emergency equipment available during procedure
         8) Push fluids after procedure to flush out dye
   3. Renal angiography: visualization of renal arterial supply; contrast material injected through a catheter
      a. **NURSING INTERVENTIONS:** same as IVP plus
         1) Shave proposed injection sites: groin or ankle
         2) Locate and mark peripheral pulses
         3) Have client void before procedure
         4) Teach client: procedure takes 1/2 hour to 2 hour; client will feel heat along vessel
      b. **NURSING INTERVENTIONS** (after procedure)
         1) Maintain bed rest 4–12 hrs
         2) Monitor vital signs until stable
         3) Apply cold compresses to puncture site
         4) Observe for swelling and hematoma
         5) Palpate peripheral pulses/vascular checks
         6) Monitor urinary output

D. **Cystoscopy**
   1. Diagnostic uses: inspect bladder and urethra;

insert catheters into ureters; see configuration and position of urethral orifices
   2. Treatment uses: remove calculi from urethra, bladder and ureter; treat lesions of bladder, urethra, prostate

   3. **NURSING INTERVENTIONS** (general preop care)
      a. Maintain NPO if general anesthesia; liquids if local anesthesia
      b. Administer preop cathartics/enemas
      c. Teach client deep breathing exercises to relieve bladder spasms
      d. Monitor for postural hypotension
      e. Inform client that pink-tinged or tea-colored urine is common following the procedure; bright red urine or clots should be reported to physician
      f. Inform client that post-procedural pain may be present
         1) Leg cramps due to lithotomy position
         2) Back pain and/or abdominal pain
         3) Warm sitz baths comforting
      g. Push fluids/analgesics
      h. Monitor intake and output; make sure no obstruction

E. **Needle Biopsy of Kidney**
   1. **NURSING INTERVENTIONS** (pre-biopsy)
      a. Obtain bleeding, clotting and prothrombin times
      b. Obtain results of pre-biopsy x-rays of kidney, IVP
      c. Inform pregnant client that ultrasound may be used
      d. Keep client NPO 6–8 hours
      e. Position client prone with pillow under abdomen, shoulders on bed
   2. **NURSING INTERVENTIONS** (post biopsy)
      a. Keep client supine, bed rest for 24 hours
      b. Monitor vital signs q 5–15 minutes for 4 hours, then decrease if stable
      c. Maintain pressure to puncture site 20 minutes
      d. Observe for pain, nausea, vomiting, BP changes
      e. Push fluids to 3,000 mL
      f. Assess HCT and Hgb 8 hours after procedure
      g. Measure output
      h. Educate client to avoid strenuous activity, sports, and heavy lifting for at least 2 weeks

F. **Catheterization**
   1. Purpose: to empty contents of bladder, obtain a sterile specimen, determine residual urine, allow irrigation of bladder, bypass an obstruction; procedure is sterile

   2. **NURSING INTERVENTIONS**
      a. Maintain closed system
      b. Measure output each shift

c. Keep drainage bag below bladder

d. Have client increase fluid intake

e. Ensure that there are no dependent loops

f. Discontinue as soon as possible due to risk for urinary tract infection

Specific Disorders and Nursing Interventions

A. Cystitis

1. Definition: inflammation of the urinary bladder

2. Etiology: ascending infection after entry via the urinary meatus; acute infections usually E. coli

   a. More common in females

   b. Benign prostate hypertrophy in men

3. Manifestations

   a. Frequency and urgency

   b. Dysuria

   c. Suprapubic tenderness; pain in region of bladder or flank pain

   d. Hematuria

   e. Fever/malaise/chills

   f. Cloudy, foul-smelling urine

4. **NURSING INTERVENTIONS**

   a. Obtain urine for culture and sensitivity (before initiating antibiotic therapy)

   b. Give antimicrobial medications - sulfonamides are the drugs of choice unless allergic; for example co-trimoxazole, sulfamethoxazole-trimethoprim (*Bactrim*) and nitrofurantoin microcrystal (*Macrodantin*)

   c. Maintain acidic urine pH

   d. Force fluids (greater than 3,000 mL per day)

   e. Give analgesics - phenazopyridine (*Pyridium*)

   f. Apply heat to perineum

   g. Teach client: good perineal care, cotton underwear, avoid bubble baths, high fluid intake

B. Glomerulonephritis

1. Definition: inflammatory disease involving the renal glomeruli of both kidneys; thought to be an antigen-antibody reaction that damages the glomeruli of the kidney (usually in children); good prognosis if treated

2. Etiology: group A beta-hemolytic streptococcal infection; usually a history of pharyngitis or tonsillitis 2–3 weeks prior to manifestations

3. Manifestations

   a. Hematuria, proteinuria fever, chills, weakness, pallor, nausea, vomiting

   b. Edema (especially facial and periorbital/ascites)

   c. Oliguria or anuria

   d. Hypertension

   e. Headache

   f. Increased blood urea nitrogen (BUN); elevated

BUN is azotemia

   g. Flank pain/abdominal pain

   h. Anemia

4. **NURSING INTERVENTIONS**

   a. Goal: protect kidney; recognize and treat infection

   b. Maintain bed rest

   c. Administer penicillin for streptococcal infection (substitute other antibiotics for clients with penicillin allergy)

   d. Reduce dietary protein and sodium; increase calories

   e. Restrict fluids

C. Nephrotic Syndrome

1. Definition: clinical disorder associated with protein-wasting secondary to diffuse glomerular damage

2. Etiology: unknown; kidneys become more permeable to protein

3. Manifestations

   a. Insidious onset of pitting edema (generalized edema is anasarca)

   b. Proteinuria; hypoalbuminemia and hyperlipidemia

   c. Anemia

   d. Anorexia and malaise

   e. Nausea

   f. Oliguria

   g. Ascites

4. **NURSING INTERVENTIONS**

   a. Goal: preserve renal function

   b. Maintain bed rest (during severe edema only)

   c. Maintain low-sodium, low-potassium, moderate-protein, high-calorie diet

   d. Protect client from infection

   e. Monitor intake and output

   f. Weigh client daily

   g. Measure abdominal girth

5. Drug therapy

   a. Loop diuretics: furosemide (*Lasix*)

   b. Steroids: prednisone (*Deltasone*)

   c. Immunosuppressive agents: cyclophosphamide (*Cytoxan*)

D. Urolithiasis (Urinary calculi)

1. Definition: stones in the urinary system

2. Etiology

   a. Obstruction and urinary stasis

   b. Proteus infection

   c. Dehydration

   d. Immobilization

   e. Hypercalcemia

   f. More common in men 30–50

   g. Tends to recur

   h. Most stones are calcium or magnesium with phosphate or oxalate, although type of stone is commonly based on alkalinity or acidity of urine

3. Manifestations (based on location, size of stone)
   a. Pain: severe renal colic (ureter); dull, aching (kidney); radiates to the groin
   b. Nausea, vomiting, diarrhea, or constipation
   c. Hematuria
   d. Manifestations of urinary tract infection

4. **NURSING INTERVENTIONS**
   a. Goals: to eradicate the stone, determine stone type and prevent nephron destruction
   b. Force fluids: at least 3,000 mL/day (IV or PO)
   c. Strain all urine
   d. Give drugs as ordered (depends on type of stone)
   e. Maintain proper urine pH (depends on stone type):
   f. Implement diet therapy if stone type is known (see Appendix B: Therapeutic Diets)
      1) Antibiotics
      2) Lithotripsy (crush stone through sound waves)
         a) No surgery required but pain occurs because of shock waves
         b) Measure intake and output and strain all urine post-procedure

E. Acute Renal Failure

1. Definition: abrupt reversible cessation of renal function; may be result of trauma, allergic reactions, kidney stones
2. Etiology: any condition that obstructs renal blood flow
   a. Pre-renal: hemorrhage, dehydration, burns, anaphylaxis, pulmonary emboli
   b. Renal: acute tubular necrosis, trauma, hypokaliemia, transfusion reaction
   c. Post-renal: BPH, tumors, strictures, calculi, infection
   d. Hemolytic uremic syndrome (HUS): acute renal failure following an acute gastroenteritis with bloody diarrhea; usually related to ingestion of undercooked beef; causative organism is E. coli 0.57
3. Manifestations: three phases
   a. Oliguric phase (8th–14th day): sudden onset, less than 400 mL/24 hours, edema, elevated BUN, creatinine and potassium; decreased specific gravity
   b. Period of diuresis (14th–24th day): dilute urine, 1,000 mL/24 hours, BUN and creatinine rise in early stage; decrease in specific gravity
      1) Recovery period: up to one year
      2) Fluid and electrolyte imbalances

4. **NURSING INTERVENTIONS**
   a. Treat, eliminate or prevent cause
   b. Prevent acidosis by maintaining fluid and

electrolyte balance
   c. Monitor and treat increased potassium level
      1) Kayexalate (an ion exchange resin given orally or by enema)
      2) IV glucose and insulin or calcium carbonate (causes K^+ to enter cells)
   d. Implement diet
      1) Oliguric phase: low-protein, high-carbohydrate, restrict K^+ intake to reverse glucogenesis
      2) Diuresis phase: low-protein, high-calorie, restrict fluids as indicated
   e. Administer phosphate binding gels to increase calcium levels; aluminum hydroxide (*Amphojel*)
   f. Prevent infection
   g. Weigh client daily
   h. Monitor intake and output; replacement is usually based on previous output
   i. Maintain dialysis; care for catheter
   j. Assess for pericarditis; friction rub

F. Chronic Renal Failure

1. Definition: a slower or progressive failure of the kidneys to function that results in death unless hemodialysis or transplant is performed; irreversible
2. Etiology
   a. Chronic glomerulonephritis
   b. Pyelonephritis → pus in the kidney
   c. Uncontrolled hypertension
   d. Diabetes mellitus
   e. Congenital kidney disease
   f. Renal vascular disease
3. Stages of renal failure
   a. Diminished renal reserve (creatinine 1.6–2.0)
   b. Renal insufficiency (creatinine 2.1–5.0)
   c. Renal failure (creatinine >8.0)
   d. Uremia: end stage (creatinine >12.0)
4. Manifestations (progressively worsen)
   a. Fatigue
   b. Headache
   c. Nausea, vomiting, diarrhea
   d. Hypertension
   e. Irritability
   f. Convulsions/coma
   g. Anemia
   h. Edema
   i. Hypocalcemia/hyperkalemia
   j. Pruritus, uremic frost
   k. Pallid, gray-yellow complexion
   l. Metabolic acidosis/elevated BUN and creatinine
5. **NURSING INTERVENTIONS**
   a. Goal: help the kidneys maintain homeostasis
   b. Maintain bed rest
   c. Implement renal diet: low-protein, low-potassium, high-carbohydrate, vitamin and

calcium supplements, low-sodium, low-phosphate

d. Treat hypertension/give diuretics
e. Maintain strict I & O; fluid replacement: 500–600 mL more than 24-hour urine output
f. Monitor electrolytes
g. Administer aluminum hydroxide gel (*Amphojel*); binds phosphate to increase calcium
h. Do not administer any magnesium or phosphorus (for example: M.O.M., Fleets Phospho-Soda)
i. Maintain dialysis
j. Administer diuretics
k. Provide skin care (collects kidney wastes)
l. Provide emotional support to client and family
m. Assess for and prevent bleeding tendencies
n. Evaluate need for Kayexalate orally to keep potassium levels down
o. Care for anemia: administer epoetin alfa, erythropoietin (*Epogen*) to stimulate red blood cell formation and transfuse as necessary

G. Dialysis
1. Goals
   a. Remove end products of metabolism (urea and creatinine) from the blood
   b. Maintain a safe concentration of the serum electrolytes
   c. Correction of acidosis and restoration of blood buffer system
   d. Removal of excess fluid from the blood
2. Hemodialysis:
   a. Definition: process of cleansing the blood of accumulated waste products; used for end-stage renal failure and those clients who are acutely ill and require short-term treatment; uses diffusion, osmosis, and filtration
   b. **NURSING INTERVENTIONS**
      1) Weigh client before and after procedure
      2) Monitor client continuously during procedure; BP may "bottom out"
      3) Provide care to access site to prevent clotting and infection
      4) Assess bruit and thrill; feel for patency
      5) Provide adequate nutrition
      6) Monitor for hypotension
      7) Maintain fluid restrictions
      8) Withhold regular morning medications prior to dialysis
      9) Observe for psychological and physiological complications
3. Peritoneal dialysis
   a. Definition: substitute for kidney function during failure that uses the peritoneum as a dialyzing membrane; usually short term; peritoneal catheter inserted by physician

b. **NURSING INTERVENTIONS**
   1) Have client void (if applicable) prior to procedure
   2) Weigh client daily
   3) Monitor vital signs, baseline electrolytes
   4) Maintain asepsis
   5) Keep accurate record of fluid balance
   6) Procedure
      a) Warm dialysate (1–2 liters of 1.5%, 2.5%, or 4.25% glucose solution)
      b) Allow to flow in by gravity
      c) 5–10 minutes inflow time; close clamp immediately
      d) 30 minutes of equilibration (dwell time)
      e) 10–30 minutes of drainage (clear yellow)
   7) Continue for 24–48 exchanges
   8) Monitor for complications: peritonitis, bleeding, respiratory difficulty, abdominal pain; bowel, or bladder perforation
4. Continuous Ambulatory Peritoneal Dialysis (CAPD)
   a. Definition: dialyzing method involving almost continuous peritoneal contact with a dialysis solution for clients with end-stage renal disease
   b. Procedure (slightly different from peritoneal dialysis)
      1) Permanent indwelling catheter into peritoneum
      2) Fluid infused by gravity (1.5 – 3 liters)
      3) Dwell time: 4–10 hours
      4) Dialysate drains by gravity: 20–40 minutes
      5) Four to five exchanges daily, 3–7 days a week
   c. Complications
      1) Peritonitis (rebound tenderness, fever, cloudy outflow)
      2) Bladder perforation (yellow outflow)
      3) Hypotension
      4) Bowel perforation (brown outflow)
   d. Advantages
      1) More independence
      2) Free dietary intake; better nutrition
      3) Easy to use
      4) Satisfactory control of uremia
      5) Least expensive dialysis
      6) Decreased likelihood of transplant rejection
      7) Closely approximates normal renal function

H. Urinary Tract Surgery
1. Kidney Transplantation
   a. Indicated for individual with irreversible end-

stage renal disease

   b. Requires well-matched donor
     1) Living donors: best donors are twin or family member
     2) Cadaver donors
   c. Preoperative management
     1) Regain normal metabolic state
     2) Tissue typing
     3) Immunosuppressive therapy
     4) Hemodialysis within 24 hours
     5) Teaching and emotional support
   d. **NURSING INTERVENTIONS** (postoperative management)
     1) Maintain homeostasis until kidney is functioning
     2) Administer immunosuppressive medications: azathioprine (*Imuran*), cyclosporin (*Sandimmune*), steroids
     3) Monitor for rejection: oliguria, edema, fever, tenderness over graft site, fluid and electrolyte imbalance, hypertension, elevated BUN, creatinine
     4) Monitor for infection;
     5) Maintain reverse isolation
     6) Provide emotional support

2. Urinary Diversion: remove bladder and transplant ureters into a pouch under the abdominal skin; can be either continent or incontinent; care is of a stoma plus general interventions

   a. **NURSING INTERVENTIONS**
     1) Monitor vital signs (hemorrhage and shock are frequent complications)
     2) Provide pain control
     3) Be alert for manifestations of paralytic ileus (very common)
     4) Provide adequate fluid replacement
     5) Weigh client daily
     6) Maintain function and patency of drainage tubes
       a) Indwelling catheter (dependent position, tape tubing to thigh)
       b) Nephrostomy tube
         (1) Never clamp
         (2) Irrigate only with order of 10 mL normal saline
         (3) Assess for leakage of urine
       c) Ureteral catheters
         (1) Each one drains ½ of the urinary system so expect only ½ of the urinary output from each one
         (2) Bloody drainage expected after surgery but should clear
         (3) Never irrigate
         (4) Surgical implant; make sure secure
         (5) Aseptic technique required

I. Benign Prostatic Hyperplasia (BPH)
1. Definition: enlargement of the prostate
2. Etiology: unknown, usually accompanies aging process in the male
3. Manifestations
   a. Difficulty starting stream/dribbling
   b. Urinary tract infection
   c. Nocturia; hematuria
   d. Decrease in size and force of urinary stream
   e. Differentiate from adenocarcinoma of the prostate with PSA test
4. Treatments
   a. Cystoscopy for diagnosis
   b. Urinary antiseptics
   c. Medications to promote urinary flow: terazosin hydrochloride (*Hytrin*), tamsulosin hydrochloride (*Flomax*), finasteride (*Proscar*)
   d. Prostatectomy
5. **NURSING INTERVENTIONS**
   a. Preoperative
     1) Maintain adequate bladder drainage (catheter) until the area heals
     2) Antibiotics as ordered
   b. Postoperative
     1) Observe for shock and hemorrhage
     2) Teach client to avoid heavy lifting for 6 weeks and avoid constipation; will cause a rebleed
     3) Monitor continuous bladder irrigation (CBI); expect bloody drainage; monitor intake and output carefully to ensure proper functioning
     4) Encourage fluid intake (at least 3000 mL/day)
     5) Assess for TUR syndrome (altered mental status, bradycardia, tachycardia and confusion) due to absorption of bladder irrigant through tissue planes of the wound
     6) Medicate for pain control: may need medication to decrease bladder spasms as well as narcotics
     7) Maintain catheter taped tightly to leg (for hemostasis at surgical site by catheter balloon); do not loosen, even though it may look painful; may cause bleeding
     8) Address sexual concerns
       a) Avoid sex for six weeks
       b) May have loss of sexual function or urinary control
       c) Psychological support needed
       d) Consider use of sildenafil citrate (*Viagra*) for treatment of erectile dysfunction

J. **Prostatitis**
1. Definition: inflammation of the prostate gland
2. Etiology
   a. Bacterial infection from urethra, kidneys, or bladder
   b. BPH
   c. Sexual activity
3. Manifestations
   a. Pain in perineum, rectum, lower back, abdomen, and penile head
   b. Chills/fever
   c. Urgency/dysuria/nocturia
4. **NURSING INTERVENTIONS**
   a. Acute
      1) Administer IV antimicrobials
      2) Educate client to avoid prolonged auto rides and sexual intercourse during acute inflammation
   b. Chronic
      1) Administer antimicrobials
      2) Maintain bed rest
      3) Administer antispasmodics
      4) Administer analgesics
      5) Provide sitz bath ➔ *soothing comfort*
      6) Administer stool softeners
      7) Promote adequate fluid intake

K. **Incontinence**
1. Types
   a. Urge: cannot hold urine when gets the stimulus to void
   b. Functional: cannot physically get to the bath-

room; doesn't know to go to the bathroom
   c. Stress: pressure such as coughing, straining, bearing down, laughing causes urine to escape; very common in middle-age women
2. **NURSING INTERVENTIONS** (general)
   a. Use adult incontinency devices
   b. Decrease fluids only after 6 p.m.
   c. Maintain toilet regimen: toilet routinely; use schedule
   d. Credé bladder as needed
   e. Monitor for signs of UTI
   f. Teach client Kegel exercises for stress incontinence
   g. Assure physical environment enhances ability to get to bathroom
3. Urine Retention
   a. Cause: actual obstruction of the urethra from acute or chronic causes; for example: edema, tumor, inflammation or inability of bladder to work; post-anesthesia, stroke
   b. **NURSING INTERVENTIONS**
      1) Stimulate bladder
         a) Stroke inner thigh
         b) Run warm water on abdomen
         c) Run water in sink
      2) Administer medications: bethanechol chloride (*Urecholine*) ➔ *gout* ➔ *muscle relaxant*
      3) Position client; near normal, upright
      4) Ensure adequate fluid intake

TABLE I-18.
SURGICAL APPROACHES FOR PROSTATECTOMY

APPROACH	ADVANTAGE	DISADVANTAGE	NURSING INTERVENTION
Transurethral (removal of prostatic tissue by instrument introduced through urethra)	Safer for client at risk; shorter period of hospitalization and convalescence	Not indicated for greatly enlarged prostate	Observe for hemorrhage, stricture, and incontinence
Open Surgical Removal			
- Suprapubic	- Technically simple	- Requires surgical approach through the bladder	- Strict aseptic care
- Perineal	- Offer direct anatomic approach	- Impotency and urinary incontinency; use drainage pads to absorb	- Avoid rectal tubes, thermometers, and enemas after perineal surgery
- Retropubic	- Most versatile procedure; affords direct visualization	- Cannot treat associated pathology in bladder	- Watch for evidence of hemorrhage

REVIEW OF NEUROLOGICAL SYSTEM DISORDERS

Neurological Assessment

A. History

B. Mental Status
1. Level of consciousness (alert, lethargic, obtunded, stupor, coma)
2. Orientation (person, place, time)
3. Affect
4. Mood
5. Speech (language, vocabulary, word-finding ability)
6. Cognition (judgment and abstraction ability)

C. Cranial Nerves (I thru XII)

D. Motor System
1. Muscles
   a. Size
   b. Symmetry
   c. Tone
   d. Strength
2. Coordination
3. Movement
   a. Voluntary control
   b. Tremors
   c. Twitches
   d. Balance and gait

E. Reflexes
1. Babinski
2. Corneal *- put your finger fo the eye*
3. Gag
4. Deep tendon (muscle-stretch)

F. Sensory System
1. Touch
2. Temperature
3. Superficial and deep pain

"Neuro-checks"

A. Level of Consciousness and Sensory Function

B. Client's Response

C. Pupil Check
1. Pupils are compared to one another for size, movement and response to light

2. Pupillary reaction is tested with a flashlight; expected reaction is a brisk constriction when the light is shone directly into the eye
3. Normal finding: Pupils equal and reactive to light (PERL)

D. Motor Type

E. Motor Strength

F. Reflexes

G. Vital Signs

H. Glasgow Coma Scale (normal 8–15; 7 or less indicates coma)
1. Best eye-opening response
   a. Spontaneously   =4
   b. To speech   =3
   c. To pain   =2
   d. No response   =1
2. Best motor response
   a. Obeys verbal command   =6
   b. Localizes pain   =5
   c. Flexion: withdrawal to pain   =4
   d. Flexion: abnormal (decorticate)   =3
   e. Extension: abnormal (decerebrate)   =2
   f. No response to pain on any limb   =1
3. Best verbal response
   a. Oriented x 3   =5
   b. Conversation   =4
   c. Speech: inappropriate   =3
   d. Sounds: incomprehensible   =2
   e. No response   =1

Diagnostic Procedures

A. Brain Scan
1. Obtain consent
2. Method: IV radioisotope accumulates in area of pathology
3. Explain procedure to client
4. Purpose: detects neoplasms, brain abscess, subdural hematoma

B. Lumbar Puncture (LP)
1. Obtain consent
2. Empty bladder and bowel
3. Position client in fetal position during LP
4. Needle inserted between two lower lumbar vertebrae, into the subarachnoid space
5. Withdraw cerebrospinal fluid *- flow*
6. After LP   *fast ↑ ICP*
   a. Position client horizontal
   b. Encourage fluid intake
   c. Check puncture site for redness, swelling,

clear drainage

   d. Assess movement of extremities

7. Normal cerebrospinal fluid (CSF) pressure

C. Computed Tomography (CT scan)

1. **NURSING INTERVENTIONS** (pre-procedure)
   a. Obtain consent
   b. Check for allergies
   c. Explain procedure (noninvasive, must remain still), can eliminate need for angiography
   d. If dye used, client must be NPO 4 hours before
   e. Assess for claustrophobia

D. Cerebral Arteriogram

1. Obtain consent
2. Method: dye injected into artery, and vascular system of brain visualized
3. Clear liquids before procedure
4. May have sedative
5. Void before procedure
6. Mark distal peripheral pulses
7. Warn client that they may feel warmth in face during the procedure
8. **NURSING INTERVENTIONS** (post procedure)
   a. Monitor for altered level of consciousness, sensory or motor deficits
   b. Check for hematoma
   c. Ice cap to decrease swelling
   d. Check peripheral pulses, color and temperature of extremities
   e. Maintain bed rest overnight
   f. Maintain involved extremity in extension

E. Myelogram

1. Method: contrast medium or air injected into spinal subarachnoid space by spinal puncture
2. **NURSING INTERVENTIONS**
   a. Obtain consent
   b. Maintain NPO 4 hours before procedure
   c. Keep client horizontal for 12 to 24 hours after procedure if oil based dye is used; head of bed raised 15 to 30 degrees if water based dye
   d. Monitor vital signs
   e. Monitor output
   f. Encourage fluid intake
   g. Monitor for fever, stiff neck and back pain

F. Electroencephalogram (EEG)

1. **NURSING INTERVENTIONS** (pre-procedure)
   a. Obtain consent
   b. Verify with primary health care provider which medications should be administered to client before EEG
   c. Withhold caffeine or sedatives before EEG
   d. Instruct client not to put any styling products (sprays, gels) in hair before EEG
   e. Verify if test is to be done awake, asleep, or

sleep-deprived

2. **NURSING INTERVENTION** (post procedure): assist client in cleansing hair

G. Electromyography (EMG)

1. Purpose: measure electrical activity of skeletal muscles
2. **NURSING INTERVENTIONS** (pre-procedure)
   a. Obtain consent
   b. Explain there will be some discomfort due to insertion of needle into skeletal muscles

H. Magnetic Resonance Imaging (MRI)

1. Magnet and computer produce three dimensional images of body parts
2. **NURSING INTERVENTIONS** (pre-procedure)
   a. Obtain consent
   b. Remove all metal objects, credit cards, body piercings

Increased Intracranial Pressure

A. Definition: increase in the amount of CNS tissue, size of cerebral blood vessels, or amount of cerebrospinal fluid; intracranial pressure greater than 15 mm Hg

B. Causes

1. Head injury
2. CVA
3. Brain tumor
4. Hydrocephalus
5. Bleeding post-surgery
6. Cerebral edema

C. Manifestations: may vary depending on cause and location; will affect the level of consciousness (LOC)

1. Lethargic, drowsy, stupor; motor and sensory changes
2. Headache; irritability
3. Nausea and vomiting, often projectile
4. Pupil changes: dilating, unequal, nonreactive
5. Changes in vital signs
   a. Widening pulse pressure; bradycardia with increased systolic BP is Cushing's Triad
   b. Irregular or decreasing respirations (Cheyne-Stokes respirations)

D. NURSING INTERVENTIONS

1. Monitor vital signs and "neuro-checks"
2. Keep head of bed elevated 30–45 degrees
3. Keep head in neutral position to enhance drainage
4. Avoid coughing, sneezing, suctioning
5. Maintain good respiratory exchange (hyperventilation causes CO_2 to decrease leading to vasoconstriction. This causes a decrease in the ICP; this

may be used as an intervention); administer oxygen to increase supply to brain

6. Monitor fluid intake and output; restrict fluids to prevent increased cerebral edema
7. Administer medications as ordered
   a. Avoid opiates and sedative (contraindicated)
   b. Barbiturates: for example: pentobarbital (*Nembutal*) may be ordered for uncontrolled increased intracranial pressure; client will require ventilatory support and close monitoring of cardiac status; may actually place the client in a barbiturate coma
   c. Acetaminophen (*Tylenol*) may be ordered for pain
   d. Administer osmotic diuretics: for example, mannitol (*Osmitrol*) and steroids: dexamethasone (*Decadron*) to decrease cerebral swelling
   e. May order antihypertensive medications or anticonvulsant medications
8. Use hypothermia as ordered to decrease metabolism
9. Monitor intracranial pressure; requires ICU care

Hyperthermia

A. Definition: body temperature above 105°F; can be caused by infection, cerebral edema, or heat; will increase intracranial pressure

B. Hypothermia Blanket
1. Protect skin
2. Manual temperature every two hours

C. NURSING INTERVENTIONS

1. Monitor vital signs
2. Monitor intake and output
3. Observe skin changes
4. Prevent shivering

Seizure Disorders

A. Definition: abnormal, sudden, excessive discharge of electrical activity within the brain

B. Classifications
1. Generalized (four types)
   a. Tonic-clonic (formerly grand-mal)
   b. Absence (formerly petit-mal seizures)
   c. Myoclonic
   d. Atonic ("drop-attacks")
2. Partial seizures (two types)
   a. Complex (loss of consciousness)
   b. Simple (no loss of consciousness)

C. NURSING INTERVENTIONS
1. During seizure

a. Maintain patent airway (turn to side after tonic phase)
   b. Protect from injury
   c. Do not restrain
   d. Do not put anything in client's mouth
   e. Turn client's head to side, prevent aspiration
2. Document: length of seizure, preceding aura, loss of consciousness, precipitating factors, incontinence, respiratory difficulty
3. Teach client: take medications, get adequate rest and exercise, diet, avoid alcohol
4. Administer anticonvulsants
   a. Phenytoin (*Dilantin*) side effects: gum hypertrophy, ataxia, diplopia, hirsutism; must visit the dentist routinely
   b. Carbamazepine (*Tegretol*) side effects: nystagmus, ataxia, blood dyscrasia
   c. Valproic acid (*Depakene*) and divalproex sodium (*Depakote*) side effects: nausea, bleeding problems, liver damage; monitor pulmonary and cardiac status
   d. Phenobarbital (*Luminal*) side effects: drowsiness
5. Monitor anticonvulsant levels; all anticonvulsants have variable absorption and excretion rates from one client to another; doses are tapered to maintain a therapeutic level
6. Seizure precautions for clients prone to multiple seizures and/or in poor control: bed rest with padded side rails; suction machine, oxygen at bedside; head of bed elevated; diazepam (*Valium*) available

D. Status Epilepticus:
1. Definition: An emergency condition in which the client has continuous seizures for 30 minutes or more; usually caused by sudden withdrawal of anticonvulsant medications (can lead to brain damage or death)
2. **NURSING INTERVENTIONS**
   a. Initiate standard seizure precautions
   b. Administer medications as ordered
      1) Lorazepam (*Ativan*) is the drug of choice; Dose: 4 mg IV q 2 minutes up to maximum dose of 8 mg
      2) Diazepam (*Valium*) may also be used in status epilepticus; Dose: 5–10 mg IVP q 10 minutes up to maximum dose of 30 mg
      3) Phenytoin (*Dilantin*) 500–1000 mg IV slowly
         a) No more than 50 mg/minute
         b) Do not mix with glucose; administer in saline only
         c) Monitor for bradycardia and heart block

Cerebrovascular Accident (CVA)

A. Definition: sudden loss of brain function resulting from a disruption of blood supply to the involved part of the brain causes; temporary or permanent dysfunction

B. Risk Factors
1. Hypertension
2. Smoking
3. Obesity
4. Hypercholesterolemia
5. Diabetes mellitus
6. Peripheral vascular disease
7. A-V malformation
8. Aneurysm
9. Hemorrhage (cerebral)

C. Manifestations: unlimited variety of neurological deficits depending on site and size of brain involvement
1. Middle cerebral artery
   a. Hemiparesis, hemiplegia
   b. Hemianopsia
   c. Aphasia (expressive, receptive, global)
2. Internal carotid
   a. Hemiplegia
   b. Aphasia
3. Right hemispheric lesion (tend to be foolhardy)
   a. Sensory: perception
   b. Visual: spatial
   c. Awareness of body space
   d. Great loss of functional skills
4. Left hemispheric lesion (tend to be overly cautious)
   a. Language
   b. Speech

D. NURSING INTERVENTIONS (initially same as management of unconscious client)
1. Maintain adequate airway
2. Monitor "neuro-checks" and vital signs routinely
3. Maintain fluid and electrolyte balance
4. Monitor for aspiration due to risk of dysphagia; feed slowly, from the front; place food on unaffected side
5. Provide psychological support due to emotional lability; understand and help family to cope
6. Establish means of communication due to aphasia (expressive, receptive, global): encourage client to talk; don't assume needs; don't speak in a loud voice; speak to client clearly and slowly
7. Participate in acute and rehabilitation phases
   a. Range of motion: prone to flexion contractures; keep extremities in position of extension or neutrality
   b. Hemiparesis, hemiplegia: will cause safety issues in the client; consult OT and PT

c. Hemianopsia: place articles where can see; encourages client to turn their head to actually be able to see items
d. Help client to achieve bowel and bladder control using regimen
e. Consult OT and PT to assist client with self-care deficits

Transient Ischemic Attacks (TIA)

A. Definition: temporary episode of neurological dysfunction lasting only a few minutes or seconds due to decreased blood flow to the brain; warning sign of stroke, especially in first 4 weeks after TIA; must heed warning sign and take care so that it does not lead to a stroke

B. Causes
1. Atherosclerosis
2. Microemboli from atherosclerotic plaque
3. Spasm

C. Manifestations
1. Sudden change in visual function
2. Sudden loss of sensory function
3. Sudden loss of motor function

D. Management: surgical carotid endarterectomy
1. Postoperative focus: assessing for neurologic deficits and respiratory distress
   a. Unable to swallow (vagus)
   b. Unable to move tongue (hypoglossal)
   c. Unable to raise arm, shoulder (spinal accessory)
   d. Unable to smile (facial)
   e. Respiratory distress
2. Anticoagulant therapy: dipyridamole (*Persantine*), aspirin (prevents platelet aggregation)

Spinal Cord Injury

A. Definition: partial or complete disruption of nerve tracts and neurons resulting in paralysis, sensory loss, altered activity, and autonomic nervous system dysfunction

B. Causes
1. Trauma (most common)
2. Infection
3. Tumors

C. Level of Injury (determines manifestations)
1. Cervical: causes quadriplegia
   a. Respiratory problems
   b. Paralysis of all four extremities
   c. Loss of bladder and bowel control
2. Thoracic injury: causes paraplegia

a. Loss of bladder and bowel control
b. Paralysis of lower extremities and major control of body trunk
3. Lumbar
a. Paralysis of lower extremities (remain flaccid)
b. Loss of bladder and bowel control

D. NURSING INTERVENTIONS

1. Immobilize client as ordered
   a. Spinal board
   b. Halo traction
   c. Gardner-Wells traction tongs or Crutchfield tongs
2. Provide care resulting from spinal shock (flaccid paralysis below level of injury followed by spastic reflexes)
3. Maintain respiratory function
4. Monitor for autonomic hyperreflexia or dysreflexia
   a. Life-threatening syndrome
   b. Sudden, severe hypertension secondary to noxious stimuli below cord damage
      1) Bowel or bladder distension
      2) Pressure ulcers or points
      3) Pain or spasms (labor pain)
   c. Remove stimuli to correct
   d. Symptoms
      1) Hypertension (250–300/100)
      2) Headache; flushing; nausea
      3) Blurred vision and restlessness
      4) Bradycardia
5. Initiate bladder management program
6. Initiate bowel regimen
7. Administer dexamethasone (*Decadron*) to reduce edema [→ steroid]
8. Consult with OT and PT regarding rehabilitation issues; self care deficits

Head Injury

A. Epidural Hematoma

1. Bleeding into space between skull and dura
2. Middle meningeal artery
3. Loss of consciousness, lucid interval, deterioration
4. Management: burr holes
5. Assess for signs of increased ICP

B. Subdural Hematoma

1. Bleeding below dura
2. Usually venous
3. Acute, subacute, or chronic
4. Management: craniotomy
5. Assess for signs of increased ICP

C. Basilar Skull Fracture

1. Bleeding from nose, ears [→ nose fracture]
2. Otorrhea, rhinorrhea or leaking CSF; differentiate between CSF and mucus by assessing sugar content of drainage
   [→ ear fracture]

3. Assess for signs increased ICP
4. Raccoon eyes (periorbital edema and ecchymosis)
5. Battle's sign (postauricular ecchymosis)
   [→ signs all the way to the back of the jaw]

Laminectomy

A. Definition: excision of a vertebral posterior arch (major symptom is back pain)

B. NURSING INTERVENTIONS

1. Observe for circulatory impairment
2. Observe for loss of sensation in lower extremities
3. Observe dressing for spinal fluid leakage and bleeding
4. Log roll client
5. Address sexual concerns
6. Institute measures to decrease infections at the site

Multiple Sclerosis

A. Definition: chronic, progressive disease of the CNS, characterized by small patches of demyelination in the brain and spinal cord (exact cause unknown)

B. Manifestations

1. Occurs in young adults 20–40 years of age
2. Nystagmus, blurred vision, diplopia [double vision]
3. Slurred hesitant speech
4. Spastic weakness of extremities/paresthesia
5. Emotionally labile/depression
6. Fatigue
7. Difficulty with balance
8. Intention tremors [→ overstressed]
9. Spastic bladder [→ for all the time]
10. MRI shows sclerotic patches through the brain and spinal cord

C. Management

1. No cure or specific treatment; long periods of remissions and exacerbation
2. During exacerbation: give corticosteroids (*ACTH*)
3. Stress management
4. Immunosuppressants - for example: azathioprine (*Imuran*) or beta-interferon (*Betaseron*)
5. Baclofen (*Lioresal*): for spasticity and tremors

NURSING INTERVENTIONS

1. Encourage active and normal life as long as possible
2. Teach client self-catheterization techniques
3. Promote daily exercise
4. Prevent injury
5. Educate client to avoid stressors that exacerbate condition, for example: infections
6. Teach client self-injection technique - for beta interferon (*Betaseron*)

Parkinson's Disease

A. **Definition:** progressive neurologic disorder affecting the brain centers responsible for control and regulation of movement: extrapyramidal tract; loss of pigmented cells of substantia nigra and depletion of dopamine

B. **Manifestations**
   1. Bradykinesia
   2. Rigidity
   3. Resting tremor
   4. Expressionless, fixed gaze; "mask-like"
   5. Drooling
   6. Constipation
   7. Depression
   8. Retropulsion, propulsion
   9. Slurred speech

C. **Stages**
   1. Unilateral flexion of upper extremity
   2. Shuffling gait
   3. Progressive difficulty ambulating
   4. Progressive weakness
   5. Disability

D. **Management**
   1. Drug Therapy
      a. Antiparkinsonian agent: levodopa (*Dopar*); side effects: hypotension, GI upset; administer on an empty stomach 1/2 to 1 hour before meals
      b. Antiparkinsonian agent: carbidopa (*Lodosyn*); side effects: hypokinesia, hyperkinesia, psychiatric manifestations
      c. Dopamine agonist: bromocriptine mesylate (*Parlodel*)
      d. Anticholinergic: benztropine (*Cogentin*); trihexyphenidyl (*Artane*); side effects: dry mouth, mydriasis, constipation, confusion
      e. Antiviral, antiparkinsonian: amantadine HCl (*Symmetrel*); side effects: tremor, rigidity, bradykinesia
   2. Stereotaxic thalamotomy to decrease tremors

E. **NURSING INTERVENTIONS**
   1. Initiate exercise program
   2. Initiate speech therapy
   3. Maintain nutrition
   4. Prevent constipation (add bran and psyllium to diet)
   5. Provide skin and oral care
   6. Maintain safety precautions (rubber-soled shoes, low heels, grab bars)
   7. Encourage self-care: energy conservation exercises; Velcro clothes; cane/walker
   8. Educate client about diet, medications, how to pre-

vent avoid falls
   9. Provide adequate lighting
   10. Use rocking chair to help to get up

Myasthenia Gravis

A. **Definition:** disorder affecting the neuromuscular transmission of the voluntary muscle of the body; loss of acetylcholine receptors on the postsynaptic membrane of the neuromuscular junction (cause unknown)

B. **Manifestations**
   1. Extreme muscular weakness: increased with fatigue and relieved by rest
   2. Early manifestations: diplopia, ptosis, dysphagia

C. **Management**
   1. Medication management
      a. Anticholinesterase drugs that increase the amount of acetylcholine in the neuromuscular function
         1) Pyridostigmine (*Mestinon*); Neostigmine (*Prostigmin*)
         2) Atropine is antidote
      b. Steroids: for example, prednisone (*Deltasone*)
   2. Thymectomy (excision of the thymus)
   3. Crisis
      a. Cholinergic; usually from overmedication; causes severe tremors
      b. Myasthenic; from infection or spontaneous; drooling and severe ptosis; can actually cause respiratory arrest
      c. Differentiate between the two with the Tensilon test: edrophonium (*Tensilon*) injected with a response expected in 30 seconds; if no response, it is cholinergic crisis

D. **NURSING INTERVENTIONS**
   1. Maintain patent airway
   2. Plan activities early in day to avoid fatigue
   3. Teach client: action of drugs, manifestations of crisis
   4. Give medications on time
   5. Be careful with drug interactions

Ménière's Disease

A. **Definition:** dilation of the endolymphatic system causing degeneration of the vestibular and cochlear hair cells   EAR

B. **Manifestations**
   1. Vertigo
   2. Tinnitus
   3. Sensorineural loss
   4. Pressure in the ear

C. **Management**
1. Bed rest in position of comfort
2. Salt-free diet
3. Vasodilators
4. Neuroleptics
5. Diuretics
6. Antihistamines *→ dry up*
7. Sedatives
8. Surgical division of vestibular portion of nerve or destruction of labyrinth

D. **NURSING INTERVENTIONS**
1. Assist in slowing down movement to avoid attacks
2. Prevent injury during attack
3. Keep room dark when photophobia present
4. Encourage client to stop smoking

Guillain-Barré Syndrome

A. **Definition:** an acquired acute inflammatory disease of peripheral nerves resulting in demyelination characterized by ascending, reversible paralysis

B. **Manifestations**
1. Disease usually proceeded by an infection (commonly Epstein Barr Virus): respiratory or GI
2. Initial manifestations: tingling of the legs that may progress to upper extremities, trunk and facial muscles; "ascending paralysis" is classic disease presentation
3. Progresses to paralysis, possible respiratory failure
4. Recovery after several months to one year; descending recovery: last lost, first recovered

C. **Management** *→ dialysis of blood*
1. Plasmapheresis
2. Steroids

D. **NURSING INTERVENTIONS**
1. Provide symptomatic care
2. Monitor respiratory, cardiovascular status
3. Provide physical and occupational therapy
4. Protect client from hazards of immobility

Detached Retina

A. **Definition:** occurs when the sensory retina separates from the pigment epithelium of the retina; vitreous humor fluid flows between the layers when a tear occurs in the retina; can be related to age and trauma

B. **Manifestations**
1. Gaps in vision preceded by sudden flashes of light
2. Feels like a curtain over field of vision

C. **Management**

1. Immediate bed rest
2. Avoid coughing, sneezing, straining
3. Surgical intervention: scleral buckling, photocoagulation, cryosurgery - *→ like a belt* *→ freezing*

D. **NURSING INTERVENTIONS:** (postoperative)
1. Maintain bed rest with both eyes bandaged for 24 hours
2. Avoid jarring or bumping head
3. Teach client self administration of eye drops on schedule

Cataract

A. **Definition:** lens of the eye becomes opaque

B. **Manifestations** *→ not clear, pearl color*
1. Visual loss is gradual
2. Distorted, blurred or hazy vision/photophobia
3. Cloudy lens

C. **Management:** surgical removal of the lens under local anesthesia, with intraocular lens implant

D. **NURSING INTERVENTIONS**
1. Preoperative (dilate the eye)
   a. Mydriatics
   b. Cycloplegics
2. Postoperative
   a. Operative eye kept covered
   b. Head of bed elevated 30–45°, do not turn client onto operative side *pressure*
   c. Teach client: avoid bending at waist, lifting, sneezing, coughing; keep fingers away from eyes
   d. Prevent vomiting/straining
   e. Report severe pain immediately; may indicate a major complication postop: glaucoma

Glaucoma

A. **Definition:** increased intraocular pressure; if uncorrected, may lead to atrophy of the optic nerve and eventual blindness

B. **Manifestations**
1. Acute (closed angle)
   a. Results from an obstruction to the outflow of aqueous humor
   b. Severe pain in and around eye
   c. Lights have a rainbow of colors around them
   d. Cloudy and blurred vision
   e. Pupils dilate
   f. Nausea and vomiting
   g. Within hours may develop GI, sinus, neuro, and dental manifestations
2. Chronic (open angle)

a. Insidious onset
b. Tired feeling in eye
c. Slowly decreasing peripheral vision
d. Halos around lights
e. Progressive loss of visual field

[handwritten: → sneaks up (hidden)]

C. Management
1. Administer medications
   a. Drug action
      1) Pupil contracts, iris is drawn away from cornea
      2) Aqueous humor may drain through lymph spaces (meshwork) into canal of Schlemm
   b. Types (avoid all anticholinergic medications)
      1) Pilocarpine hydrochloride (*Pilocar*); lasts 6–8 hours; drug of choice in glaucoma
      2) Acetazolamide (*Diamox*); decreases production of aqueous humor; side effect: gastric distress
      3) Mannitol (*Osmitrol*), intravenous (systemic); reduces intraocular pressure by increasing blood osmolality; indications: useful in treatment of acute attacks of pressure and preoperatively
      4) Isosorbide (*Isordil*), oral; cautions: safer than intravenous medication for cardiac clients; may cause diuresis, which is troublesome in men with prostatitis
2. Surgical care
   a. Procedures
      1) Iridencleisis
      2) Thermosclerectomy
      3) Trabeculectomy
   b. Local anesthetic usually used
3. **NURSING INTERVENTIONS**
   a. Promote safety when ambulating
   b. Administer stool softeners
   c. Teach client:
      1) Glaucoma is controllable, not curable
      2) Avoid emotional upsets, constrictive clothing, extreme exertion and lifting, colds
      3) Encourage moderate exercise, regular bowel habits, daily use of medicines, medical checkups and Medic Alert bracelet; monitor fluid intake

SECTION XI

REVIEW OF ONCOLOGY NURSING

Neoplastic Diseases

A. Characteristics
1. Etiology *[handwritten: → where does it come from / cause]*

a. Healthy cells transformed into malignant cells upon exposure to certain etiological agents: viruses, chemical and physical agents
b. Failure of immune response
2. Pathophysiology
   a. Rapid cell division
   b. Malignant cells metastasize
      1) Extending directly into adjacent tissue
      2) Permeating along lymphatic vessels
      3) Traveling through lymph system to nodes
      4) Entering body circulation
      5) Diffusing into body cavity
3. Classification of tumors
   a. Classified according to type of tissue from which they evolve
      1) Carcinomas begin in epithelial tissue (for example: skin, GI tract lining, lung, breast, uterus)
      2) Sarcomas begin in nonepithelial tissue (for example: bone, muscle, fat, lymph system)
   b. Type of cell in which they arise; cell type affects appearance, rate of growth, and degree of malignancy (for example: epithelial basal cells are basal cell carcinoma; bone cells are osteogenic carcinoma; gland epithelium are adenocarcinoma)
4. Staging
   a. Describes extent of tumor
   b. Describes extent to which malignancy has increased in size
   c. Indicates involvement of regional nodes
   d. Indicates metastatic development

B. Manifestations Suggesting Malignant Disease
(ACS 7 Warning Signs) – Client-Teaching mnemonic: "CAUTION"
1. Change in bowel or bladder habits
2. A sore that does not heal
3. Unusual bleeding or discharge
4. Thickening or lumps in breast or elsewhere
5. Indigestion or difficulty swallowing
6. Obvious change in wart or mole
7. Nagging cough or hoarseness

C. Cancer Therapy
1. Objective: to cure the client and to ensure that minimal functional and structural impairment results from the disease; if cure is not possible:
   a. Prevent further metastasis
   b. Relieve manifestations
   c. Maintain high quality of life as long as possible
2. Surgery
   a. Radical
   b. Prophylactic *[handwritten: → prevention]*
   c. Palliative *[handwritten: → comfort]*

3. Chemotherapy
   a. Drugs interfere with cell division; combination of drugs usually given
   b. Classification of drugs
      1) Alkylating agents: uracil mustard (*Nitrogen mustard*), cyclophosphamide (*Cytoxan*)
      2) Antimetabolite: fluorouracil (*5-FU*), methotrexate (*MTX*) (*Folex*)
      3) Antibiotics: doxorubicin hydrochloride (*Adriamycin*), bleomycin (*Blenoxane*), dactinomycin (*Actinomycin D*)
      4) Plant alkaloids: vincristine (*Oncovin*), vinblastine (*Velban*)
      5) Hormones: estrogen, progesterone, tamoxifen citrate (*Tamofen*)
      6) Miscellaneous: procarbazine (*Matulane*)
   c. Common side effects and interventions to counteract and cope with them
      1) Bone marrow depression: some is expected or drug is not working
         a) Leukopenia (decreased WBCs): measures to prevent infection; may need protective isolation; nadir: lowest WBC count; monitor WBC routinely; administer filgrastim (granulocyte colony-stimulating factor; GCSF) (*Neupogen*) to stimulate proliferation of white blood cells
         b) Anemia (decreased RBCs): care with activities; oxygen as needed; iron-rich foods; transfuse as needed; administer epoetin alfa, erythropoietin (*Epogen*) to enhance the rate of RBC production
         c) Thrombocytopenia (decreased platelets): prevent injury; watch for covert bleeding, transfuse as needed
      2) Alopecia: prevent if possible; help with body image changes; hair will return after therapy but may be a different color or texture
      3) GI tract problems: antiemetic medication prior to treatment; diet as tolerated; high-calorie supplements; small, frequent feedings; causes stomatitis so mouth washes are important as well as nonirritating foods and dental care; antidiarrheal medication or stool softeners may also be needed
      4) Elevated uric acid, crystal and urate stone formation: allopurinol (Zyloprim) therapy; increase fluid intake
      5) Specific drugs have specific toxic effects; most important are:
         a) Doxorubicin hydrochloride (*Adriamycin*): irreversible cardiomyopathy
         b) Cisplatin, cis-platinum (*Platinol*): renal toxicity
         c) Vincristine sulfate (*Oncovin*): peripheral neuropathy
   d. Emotional concerns: support client and family; support groups; help to live with this chronic disease
4. Radiation
   a. Purposes
      1) Curative (Hodgkin's disease)
      2) Palliative
   b. Types
      1) External: gamma rays
         a) **NURSING INTERVENTIONS**
            (1) Teach client about the procedure
            (2) Give antiemetic before treatment if nausea a problem; prochlorperazine edisylate (*Compazine*); ondansetron (*Zofran*)
            (3) Give pain medication before treatment if needed
            (4) Provide psychological support
            (5) Provide skin care: dermatitis 3–6 weeks after start of treatment; teach client to wash with water; avoid lotions, powders, sunlight
            (6) Treat "wet" reaction: cleanse with warm water; keep open; may use antibiotic cream
      2) Internal: cesium needles
         a) **NURSING INTERVENTIONS**
            (1) Observe time, distance and shielding because the client is radioactive
            (2) Follow institutional guidelines to protect yourself
            (3) Limit visitors; private room; face area of body to be irradiated toward the outside of the building
            (4) Very prone to inflammation in the site of radiation, for example: intrauterine may lead to proctitis and cystitis; oral insertion may lead to stomatitis
               (a) Observe for signs of complications
               (b) Treat specifically by resting the area; Foley
               (c) Alter diet as needed; increase fluids, low residue, soft, etc.
               (d) Administer medications to decrease inflammation as necessary; steroids, urinary antiseptics and

TABLE I-19.
NURSING INTERVENTIONS FOR CLIENT ON CHEMOTHERAPY

DRUGS	USES	SIDE EFFECTS	NURSING INTERVENTIONS
fluorouracil (5-FU)	Cancers of GI tract, breast, lung, uterus, ovary	Anorexia, nausea, bone marrow depression	Monitor CBC and platelets
mercaptopurine (6-MP)	Acute leukemia	Bone marrow depression	Monitor CBC and platelets
methotrexate (Folex) (Amethopterin, MTX)	Acute leukemia	Bone marrow depression	Methotrexate is excreted through the kidneys, so if renal function is impaired, the drug should not be given; folinic acid (Leucovorin) used to "rescue" non-cancerous cells after MTX treatment
chlorambucil (Leukeran)	Chronic lymphocytic leukemia	Bone marrow depression	Monitor CBC and platelets
cyclophosphamide (Cytoxan)	Acute lymphocytic leukemia	Bone marrow depression	Monitor CBC and platelets
mitomycin (Mutamycin)	Pancreas, stomach, breast cancer	Nausea, vomiting, bone marrow depression, severe skin reaction	Vitamin B_6 may reverse skin reaction
melphalan (Alkeran)	Cancers of the breast, ovary, testicles; multiple melanoma	Unpredictable bone marrow depression, nausea, vomiting, stomatitis	Monitor CBC and platelets; mouth care
vincristine sulfate (Oncovin)	Cancers of the breast and lung; acute leukemia	Alopecia, bone marrow depression	Monitor CBC and platelets; liquid diet for nausea

aesthetics

(5) If radiation source falls out, do NOT touch it with bare hands.
  (a) Use long forceps and put in lead container
  (b) Follow institution guidelines for radiation containment

REVIEW OF IMMUNOLOGIC DISORDERS

Acquired Immune Deficiency Syndrome (AIDS)

A. **Definition:** infectious disease characterized by severe deficits in cellular immune function; manifested clinically by opportunistic infection and/or unusual neoplasms
  1. Etiology: human immunodeficiency virus (HIV)
  2. Risk factors
    a. Unprotected intercourse with an infected or high-risk partner
    b. Intravenous drug abusers sharing needles
    c. Blood transfusions (hemophiliacs, surgical clients; blood supply testing for HIV began in 1985)
    d. Infants of infected mothers

The disease has a long incubation period, sometimes up to ten years or more; therefore, manifestations may not appear until late in the infection

3. Manifestations
   a. Malaise, weight loss
   b. Lymphadenopathy of at least 3 months
   c. Leukopenia (especially T_4 helper cells)
   d. Diarrhea
   e. Fatigue
   f. Night sweats
   g. Presence of opportunistic infections
      1) Pneumocystis carinii (major source of mortality)
         a) Cough
         b) Progressive SOB
         c) Low-grade fever
      2) Kaposi's sarcoma
         a) Purple-red raised lesions of internal organs and skin
         b) Poor prognosis
      3) Candidiasis
         a) Fungal infection
         b) Lesions usually in mouth
      4) Herpes viruses
         a) Genital and perirectal
         b) Cytomegalovirus (CMV)
      5) Cryptococcosis
      6) TB
      7) Diagnostic tests
         a) ELISA (enzyme-linked immunosorbent assay)
         b) Western blot
      8) **NURSING INTERVENTIONS**
         a) Provide respiratory support
            (1) Pulmonary toilet
            (2) Oxygen therapy
         b) Maintain fluid and electrolyte balance
         c) Prevent spread of infection through use of universal precautions
         d) Provide emotional support
         e) Provide skin care
         f) Provide high-nutrition, low-residue meals
         g) Teach clients about abstinence, safer sex practices, monogamy, hand washing, use of condoms
      9) Drug therapy: follow most current research findings, which are always being updated
         a) Azidothymidine (*AZT*)/zidovudine (*Retrovir*)
            (1) Side effects: bone marrow depression, anemia;
            (2) Drug of choice
            (3) Preventative effect for fetus if

given to pregnant mothers
   b) Interferon (Roferon)
   c) Pneumocystis pneumonia prophylaxis: Pentamidine (*Pentam 300*)
   d) Antifungals: metronidazole (*Flagyl*) and amphotericin B (*Fungizone*)
   e) Antituberculosis drugs as needed
   f) Acyclovir (*Zovirax*) herpes treatment
   g) Protease inhibitors: saquinavir (*Fortovase*), ritonavir (*Norvir*)
   h) Antivirals: zalcitabine, ddC, dideoxycytidine (*Hivid*), lamivudine (*Epivir*)

SECTION XIII

REVIEW OF BURNS

Assessment

A. **Extent of Body Surface**

		Adults	Children
1.	Rule of nines		
	a. Head and neck	9%	19%
	b. Anterior trunk	18%	36%
	c. Posterior trunk	18%	36%
	d. Arms (9%)	18%	18%
	e. Legs (18%)	36%	26%
	f. Perineum	1%	1%

B. **Depth of Burn**
   1. Partial thickness (formerly called first and second degree)
   2. Full thickness (formerly called third degree)

C. **Type of Burn**
   1. Thermal
   2. Chemical
   3. Electrical
   4. Radiation

D. **Preexisting Physical and Psychological Status of Client**
   1. Age
   2. Preburn weight
   3. Medical History

E. **Concomitant Injuries** — other injuries

Treatment

A. **Prehospital Care**
   1. Stop thermal process
      a. Stop drop and roll
      b. Cool water for 10 minutes
   2. Establish airway

3. Cover large areas with clean cloth to decrease pain *(→ large amts)*
4. Chemical burns: irrigate copiously *(not less than 15 minutes)*
5. Electrical burns: interrupt power source
6. Transport to emergency facility

B. Emergency Room
1. Establish and maintain client airway
2. Assessment
   a. Time of injury
   b. How injury occurred
   c. Cause of burn
3. Administer 100% oxygen if burn occurred in enclosed area
4. Maintain fluid balance
5. Insert Foley catheter *(→ I → O)*
6. Insert NG tube *(→ peristalsis)*
7. Administer tetanus toxoid *(→ skin (defense))*
8. Assist with escharotomy or fasciotomy if needed
   (→ dead skin & underlying tissue)

C. Hospital Care
1. Maintain patent airway
2. Maintain aseptic area
3. Provide fluid replacement therapy
   a. Goal is to maintain vital organ perfusion
   b. Shock phase: 24–48 hours
      1) Fluid shifts from plasma to interstitial space
      2) Hematocrit rises *(→ required part of my blood)*
      3) Metabolic acidosis
      4) Serum K$^+$ rises
      5) Fluid loss is plasma
      6) Protein loss
      7) Monitor vital signs
      8) Monitor urine output (need 50–100 mL/hr); oliguria occurs
      9) Fluid resuscitation:
         a) Parkland Formula (most common) 4 mL/kg/% burn (4 mL per kg times % burn)
         b) Give half of total fluids in first 8 hours
         c) Give second half over remaining 16 hours
   c. Post-shock phase (diuretic phase)
      1) Capillary permeability stabilizes and fluid shifts from interstitial spaces to plasma
      2) Observe for pulmonary edema
      3) Check vital signs, central venous pressure
      4) Monitor output
      5) Check lab values (electrolyte shifts such as low K+; high Na+)

(his during the phase)

D. NURSING INTERVENTIONS
1. Control client pain
   a. Medication (morphine sulfate/PCA pump/NSAIDS)
   b. IV administration due to poor absorption of tissues

2. Meet nutritional needs
   a. NPO until bowel sounds heard (usually has NG tube) *(paralytic ileus →)*
   b. Caloric needs high: 6,000–8,000 calories (consider TPN)
   c. High-protein diet *(↓ cooling)*
   d. Prevent stress ulcers: Maalox q 2 hours-omeprazole (Prilosec) or famotidine (Pepcid); Curling's ulcer, 2 weeks after burn
3. Prevent complications
   a. Infection
      1) Asepsis: reverse isolation
      2) Wound care (debridement, hydrotherapy)
      3) Antimicrobial therapy
   b. Contractures and deformities
      1) Range of motion initiated first post-burn day
      2) Positioning: position of good alignment (pressure garments and splints)
   c. Respiratory difficulty
      1) Airway
      2) C, T, DB (cough, turn, deep breathe)
      3) Assess for inhalation injury
      4) Give oxygen
   d. Emotional support
      1) Essential for long term adjustment
      2) Alteration in body image

Methods of Treating Burns

A. Open Air or Exposure Method
1. Allows for drainage of burn exudate
2. Eschar forms protective covering (may constrict circulation requiring escharotomy)
3. Use of topical therapy
4. Skin easily inspected
5. Range of motion easier
6. Asepsis essential
7. Disadvantages
   a. Painful
   b. Heat loss
   c. Difficult to manage burns of hands and feet

B. Occlusive (Pressure) Dressing
1. Less pain in first 48 hours, later more painful
2. Higher incidence of wound sepsis
3. Contractures may occur

C. Topical Antimicrobial
1. Silver sulfadiazine (*Silvadene*)
   a. Broad spectrum coverage including yeast
   b. Can be washed with water
2. Mafenide acetate (*Sulfamylon*)
   a. Broad spectrum coverage
   b. Penetrates tissue wall
   c. Never use a dressing

     d.   Breakdown of drug provides heavy acid load, may cause metabolic acidosis

     e.   Painful

3.   Silver nitrate (*Keratolytic*) (for small burns)

     a.   0.5 % solution on dressing B.I.D.

     b.   Dressings must be moist at all times

     c.   Hypokalemia, hyponatremia, hypochloremia

     d.   Discolors everything it touches

     e.   Poor penetration

     f.   Time consuming

4.   Gentamicin sulfate (*Garamycin*): 0.1 %

     a.   Cream penetrates wall

     b.   Nephrotoxic: monitor creatinine levels and BUN

D.   Biologic Dressings

1.   Allograft: same species, usually cadaver

2.   Xenograft, heterograft: animal (pig or dog)

3.   Amnion

4.   Autograft (self); pain control is necessary

     a.   Care of donor site

     b.   Care of graft site

E.   Pressure Garments

1.   Decreases scarring

2.   Wear 12–18 months

3.   Remove only to bathe

PSYCHIATRIC NURSING

UNIT CONTENT

SECTION I.   Overview 79
SECTION II.   Anxiety 85
SECTION III.   Schizophrenia 89
SECTION IV.   Mood Disorders and Associated Behaviors 91
SECTION V.   Personality Disorders 95
SECTION VI.   Chemical Dependence/Abuse 100
SECTION VII.   Organic Mental Disorders 103
SECTION VIII.   Eating Disorders 105
SECTION IX.   Developmental Disabilities 105
SECTION X.   Family Violence 107
SECTION XI.   Rape 108
SECTION XII.   Legal Aspects of Psychiatric Nursing 109

SYMBOLS

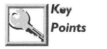 Key Points

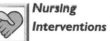 Nursing Interventions

 Points to Remember

OVERVIEW

A. Psychiatric Nursing: core, heart, basis, art of nursing
1. Interpersonal process
   a. Communication
   b. Caring
2. Goal
   a. Dealing with emotional responses to stress and crisis
   b. Satisfying basic needs
   c. Learning more effective ways of behaving
   d. Developing a healthy lifestyle
   e. Achieving a realistic and positive self-concept
3. Responsibilities
   a. Therapeutic relationship
   b. Therapeutic environment
4. Uses nursing process
   a. Assessment
   b. Diagnosis
   c. Planning
   d. Implementation
   e. Evaluation
5. Roles
   a. Counselor
   b. Teacher
   c. Advocate
   d. Leader, coordinator, manager

B. Theoretical Models of Treatment
1. Medical-biologic model
   a. Oriented to diagnosing mental disturbances as medical diseases with specific classifiable manifestations
      1) Causes
         a) Biochemical
         b) Psychological conditions
         c) Psychophysiological conditions
         d) Structural problems
      2) Diagnosis
         a) History
         b) Physical
         c) DSM classification of disorders
      3) Focus
         a) Accurate diagnosis
         b) Selection of treatment modalities
         c) Nurse's role is supportive, not therapeutic
   b. Treatment
      1) Physical or somatic
      2) Interpersonal
2. Psychoanalytical model (Sigmund Freud)
   a. Oriented to uncovering childhood trauma and repressed feelings that cause conflicts in later life

KEY INFORMATION
1) Psychopathology
   a) Alterations in psychosocial behavior
   b) Stress related behaviors
2) Structure of the mind
   a) Id: contains instinctual primitive drives
   b) Ego: mediates demands of primitive id and self-critical superego
   c) Superego: values and mores that guide behavior
   d) Conscious: ability to recall or remember events without difficulty
   e) Unconscious: memories and thoughts that do not enter awareness
3) Freud's psychosexual stages
   a) Oral 0–1 years
   b) Anal 1–3 years
   c) Phallic (oedipal) 3–6 years
   d) Latency 6–12 years
   e) Genital 12–young adult
b. Treatment modalities: clarify meaning of unconscious and conscious events, feelings and behavior to gain insight
   1) Transference (unconscious projection of feelings onto others)
   2) Countertransference
   3) Free Association
   4) Dream Analysis
   5) Catharsis (talking it out)
c. **NURSING INTERVENTIONS**
   1) Guidelines for understanding human behavior
   2) Determine adaptive/maladaptive personality traits
   3) Individualize teaching based on psychosexual development
3. Psychosocial developmental model: (Eric Erikson) psychosocial tasks that are accomplished throughout the life cycle; an individual who experiences failure in any stage is likely to have greater difficulty achieving success in future stages of development
   a. Uses an interdisciplinary approach to treatment; wellness is on a continuum
   b. Developmental stages (see table II-1.)
   c. **NURSING INTERVENTIONS**
   1) Identify client's present stage of psychosocial development
   2) Assist client to complete that stage (see table II-2)
   3) Set goals toward advancing through next stage(s)

TABLE II-1.
ERIKSON'S STAGES OF DEVELOPMENT

STAGE	TASK	BEHAVIOR
Infancy (0–18 mos)	Trust vs Mistrust	Hopefulness, trusting vs Withdrawn, alienated
Early childhood (18 mos–3 yrs)	Autonomy vs Shame, doubt	Self-control vs Compliance and compulsiveness, uncertainty
Late childhood (3–5 yrs)	Initiative vs Guilt	Realistic goals: explores, tests reality vs Strict limits on self-worry
School age (5–12 yrs)	Industry vs Inferiority	Explores, persistent, competes vs Incompetent, low self-esteem
Adolescence (12–20 yrs)	Identity vs Role diffusion	Sense of self vs Confusion, indecision
Young adulthood (20–25 yrs)	Intimacy vs Isolation	Commitment in love/work/play vs Superficial, impersonal
Adulthood (25–65 yrs)	Generativity vs Stagnation	Productivity, caring about others vs Self-centered and indulgent
Old age (65 yrs–death)	Integrity vs Despair	Sense of accomplishment vs Hopelessness, depression

TABLE II-2.
ERIKSON'S STAGES DEFINED

STAGE	DEFINITION
INFANCY (0 – 18 MOS) Trust vs. Mistrust	Babies learn to trust one consistent caregiver (not necessarily the mother)
EARLY CHILDHOOD (18 MOS – 3 YEARS) Autonomy vs. Shame & Doubt	Learning independence and self control; how to affect the environment with direct manipulation
LATE CHILDHOOD (3 – 5 YEARS) Initiative vs. Guilt	Personal exploration and setting goals that influence the environment; evaluating own behavior
SCHOOL AGE (5 – 12 YEARS) Industry vs. Inferiority	Developing sense of self & competency; learning to create and manipulate
ADOLESCENCE (12 – 20 YEARS) Identity vs. role diffusion	Integrating life experiences for a sense of self (trying new roles to see "what fits"; peer pressure creates tumultuous rebellions; examines own sexual identity
YOUNG ADULTHOOD (20 – 25 YEARS) Intimacy vs. isolation	Develop intimate or committed relationships; commit to work/ profession; seek balance in life
ADULTHOOD (25 – 65 YEARS) Generativity vs. Stagnation	Establishing and guiding next generation "giving back" to society with creativity; productivity and concern
OLD AGE (65 YEARS – DEATH) Integrity vs. despair	Life review (necessary); accepting one's life as fulfilling; worthwhile, successful; providing a legacy

4. Basic human needs model (Maslow): a hierarchy of needs; a belief that needs are fulfilled in a progressive order
   a. Levels
      1) Physical
         a) Air
         b) Food
         c) Sleep
         d) Sexual expression
      2) Safety
         a) Avoiding harm
         b) Feeling secure
      3) Love and belonging
         a) Group identity
         b) Being cared about
         c) Caring for others
         d) Play
      4) Self-esteem
         a) Self-confidence
         b) Self-acceptance
      5) Self-actualization
         a) Self-knowledge
         b) Satisfying, interpersonal relationships
         c) Environmental mastery
         d) Stress management

TABLE II-3.
MASLOW'S PYRAMID

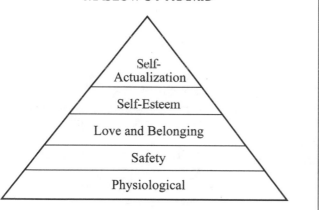

b. Treatment
   1) Interdisciplinary: shared roles
   2) Developmental: interpersonal view of the self
   3) Goal: fill needs in progressive manner
c. **NURSING INTERVENTIONS**
   1) Use needs and psychosocial development for assessment
   2) Prioritize care based on needs according to hierarchy
   3) Help client fulfill needs to relieve stress
   4) Help client advance through stages to become more able to fulfill own needs
   5) Help client develop new behaviors to reduce stress and prevent recurrences of mental illness and dysfunction

5. Behaviorist model (behavior modification): "maladaptive behavior is learned"
   a. Changes behavior by using learning theory: replaces nonadaptive behavior with more adaptive behavior
   b. Treatment
      1) Reconditioning: unlearning learned or maladaptive behavior
      2) Reinforcement: increases the probability of positive behavior recurring
         a) Positive reinforcement: per contract, use rewards to increase or reinforce desired behavior (for example: adding something such as food, attention, phone privileges)
         b) Negative reinforcement: per contract, extinguish undesirable behavior by removing aversive consequences (for example: removal of imposed restrictions)
      3) Positive punishment: decrease behavior by adding aversive consequences (for example: quiet time)
      4) Negative punishment: decrease behavior by withdrawing a reward (for example: privilege, such as an outing or calls)
   c. Main uses
      1) Children
      2) Severely regressed individuals
      3) Personality disorders
      4) Anxiety disorders such as phobias
      5) Eating disorders
      6) Mentally disabled clients
   d. **NURSING INTERVENTIONS**
      1) Assess behavior
      2) Implement specific behavioral interventions either negative or positive reinforcement (contracts, role-play, progressive relaxation)
      3) Emphasis is on positive reinforcement as a primary nursing intervention
      4) Evaluate progress; change behavioral interventions specific to client need

6. Community mental health model (psychosocial rehabilitation): individual interacting with environment
   a. Uses interdisciplinary team approach; nurse works as case manager and supervises the team
   b. Emphasis is on providing treatment services in the least restrictive setting
   c. Treatment Modalities
      1) Primary prevention: maintenance and promotion of health by teaching (for example: risk factors, medication management, health promotion and wellness)

2) Secondary prevention: early diagnosis and treatment (for example: crisis intervention, partial hospitalization, acute care hospitalization)

3) Tertiary prevention: rehabilitation, follow-up to avoid permanent disability (for example: psychiatric "Day Care")

d. **NURSING INTERVENTIONS**
1) Holistic care
2) Therapeutic use of self in the nurse/client relationship
3) Uses primary, secondary, tertiary prevention
4) Identify client needs, strengths, and community resources

C. Treatment Modes

1. Crisis intervention
   a. Definitions
   1) Crisis: a sudden, disequilibrating event in one's life when previous methods of problem solving are ineffective
   2) Crisis intervention: brief treatment used to help clients cope with or adapt to stressors
   b. Type of crisis
   1) Situational (unanticipated; for example: death, divorce, being fired)
   2) Transitional (maturational, anticipated; for example: birth, marriage)
   3) Cultural/social (for example: war)
   c. Responses to crisis
   1) Physiological (nervous system)
   2) Psychological (panic, fear, helplessness)
   3) Behavioral (extremes; talkative to withdrawn)
   d. Principles of crisis management
   1) Requires prompt intervention in calm, controlled atmosphere
   2) Focus on client strengthens positive coping skills
   3) Time limited (6–8 weeks)
   e. **NURSING INTERVENTIONS**
   1) Provide therapeutic interventions to keep client focused on immediate problem
   2) Set specific goals for resolution
   3) Help client develop more adaptive coping behaviors; sense of mastery
   4) Reinforce client's own responsibility to act (collaborate)

2. Group therapy
   a. Definition: collection of 7–10 individuals interacting together with a shared purpose
   b. Dynamics and concepts
   1) Content: work is done to problem solve and fulfill the group functions and goals
   2) Process: what is happening in the group;

interactions, seating, participation
3) Cohesiveness: feeling of belonging, helpfulness, problem solving, sharing
4) Norms: standards of behavior adhered to by group

c. **NURSING INTERVENTIONS**
1) Assume leadership role
2) Promote problem solving
3) Direct group towards common goals and tasks.
4) Set limits and prevents scapegoating within group
5) Clarify issues and promote consistency
6) Support members

d. Types of groups
1) Supportive, therapeutic
2) Psychotherapy
3) Task groups
4) Teaching groups
5) Psychotherapy
6) Peer support
7) Self-help groups
   a) 12 Step (Alcoholics Anonymous (AA), Al-anon, Alateen, Overeaters Anonymous)
   b) Recovery, Inc.
   c) Ostomy Clubs

3. Family therapy
   a. Definition: psychotherapy in which the focus is on the family as the unit of treatment, not just one individual
   b. Concepts
   1) Systems approach: member with the manifestations, illness
   2) Scapegoating: the object of blame or displaced aggression, usually one member of the family
   3) Family involvement is necessary for treatment
   c. **NURSING INTERVENTIONS**
   1) Help family reestablish communication between members
   2) Help family redefine roles and rules
   3) Clarify ambiguous communication patterns between family members
   4) Support individual family members
   5) Teach family problem solving techniques
   6) Help the family accept differences among the members

4. Milieu therapy
   a. Definition: management of the client's environment to promote a positive living experience and facilitate recovery (holistic approach)
   b. Concepts
   1) Client government: groups and meetings between client and staff to promote shared responsibility and cooperation

2) The environment in the facility is as close to the "real world" as possible and has potential for therapeutic value

c. **NURSING INTERVENTIONS**
   1) Guidance in developing new ways of relating and learning to cope more effectively
   2) Help client maintain strengths
   3) Management of day-to-day activities
   4) Provide a positive, therapeutic environment through environmental manipulation
   5) Assist in developing effective relationship and coping skills

5. Adjunctive therapies
   a. Definition: therapies used to aid assessment, increase social skills, encourage expression of feelings and provide opportunities to raise self-esteem, relieve tension and be creative
   b. Types:
      1) Dance: movement
      2) Recreational: picnic, volleyball
      3) Occupational: painting, hand work
      4) Art: clay, painting, drawing
      5) Alternative therapies: pet therapy, reminiscence therapy, music therapy

6. Interdisciplinary Team Approach
   a. Definition: A team with members of different disciplines involved in a formal arrangement to provide client services while maximizing educational interchange
   b. Members of the team:
      1) Nurse
      2) Primary Care Provider
      3) Social Work
      4) Psychologist
      5) Case Manager
      6) Occupational Therapist
      7) Recreational Therapist
      8) Job Coaches
      9) Mental Health Technicians

   c. **NURSING INTERVENTIONS:** The nurse works collaboratively with the interdisciplinary team to promote and maintain health

D. **Mental Health/Mental Illness Continuum** (see table II-4.)
   1. Mental health
      a. Positive attitude toward self
      b. Growth, development, self-actualization, autonomy
      c. Ability to cope with stress
      d. Reality perception and environmental mastery
   2. Mental Illness
      a. Inability to cope/manage stress
      b. Development of maladaptive behavior
      c. Disruption in ability to relate successfully with others
      d. Inability to meet basic needs in a socially acceptable way
   3. Defense mechanisms
      a. Definition: unconscious operations used to defend against anxiety or stress and relieve emotional conflict
      b. In contrast, coping mechanisms are conscious efforts to deal with daily frustrations and conflicts

KEY INFORMATION

   c. Unconscious defense mechanisms
      1) Denial: avoidance of disagreeable reality by ignoring or refusing to recognize it
      2) Rationalization: offering a socially acceptable or logical explanation for otherwise unacceptable impulses, feelings, and behaviors (for example: "I failed the NCLEX-RN because it is a poor test.")
      3) Displacement: transferring painful feelings

TABLE II-4.
MENTAL HEALTH/ILLNESS CONTINUUM

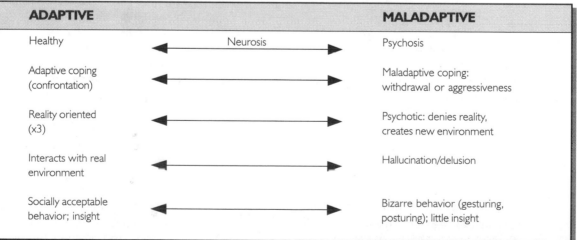

ADAPTIVE		MALADAPTIVE
Healthy	←— Neurosis —→	Psychosis
Adaptive coping (confrontation)	←——→	Maladaptive coping: withdrawal or aggressiveness
Reality oriented (x3)	←——→	Psychotic: denies reality, creates new environment
Interacts with real environment	←——→	Hallucination/delusion
Socially acceptable behavior; insight	←——→	Bizarre behavior (gesturing, posturing); little insight

to a neutral object (for example: you're angry at your brother so you kick the dog)

4) Projection: attributing own thoughts or impulses to another person (for example: "You made me take a wrong turn.")

5) Compensation: putting forth extra effort to achieve in areas of real or imagined deficiency (for example: an unpopular student excels as a scholar)

6) Reaction formation: involves displaying overt behavior or attitudes in precisely the opposite direction of unacceptable conscious or unconscious impulses (for example: feeling compassion for a person you dislike)

7) Identification: the unconscious adoption of characteristics of another, generally someone who possesses attributes that are admired or envied *wana be somebody else*

8) Sublimation: directing energy from unacceptable drives into socially acceptable behavior (for example: aggressive person becomes a star football player)

9) Regression: going back to an early level of emotional development (for example: becoming dependent on someone else for all decisions)

10) Undoing: a compulsive response that negates or reverses a previous unacceptable act (for example: washing hands [of guilt] after touching germs)

11) Introjection: incorporating the traits of others (for example: a depressed client causes the nurse to become depressed)

12) Isolation: splitting-off response in which person blocks feeling associated with unpleasant experience (for example: planning out funeral details of a loved one)

13) Splitting: viewing people as all good or all bad; failure to integrate positive and negative qualities

14) Repression: unconscious, involuntary forgetting of unacceptable or painful thoughts, impulses, feelings, or actions (for example: forgetting what was on a difficult exam)

d. Conscious defense mechanism: Suppression: deliberate forgetting of unacceptable or painful thoughts, impulses, acts

E. Nurse/Client Relationship: an interpersonal, collaborative helping process and organized sequence of events leading toward a mutually identified goal

1. Characteristics
   a. Professional vs. social
   b. Purposeful

c. Nonjudgmental
d. Designated setting and time
e. Organized sequence of events
f. Goal directed to facilitate client's growth vs. reciprocal
   1) Collaborative: contract that outlines and clarifies role expectations
   2) Confidential

2. Phases of the nurse/client relationship
   a. Preinteraction phase
      1) Gather data from secondary source
      2) No prejudgment
      3) Assess nurse's feelings
      4) Assess client's feelings
   b. Orientation phase: assessment
      1) Introduction: purpose, roles, responsibilities
      2) Establish trust
         a) Honest
         b) Nonjudgmental
         c) Empathetic
         d) Offer self
      3) Assess client
         a) Orientation
         b) Activities of daily living (degree of ability to perform)
         c) Physical status
         d) Memory (recent and remote)
         e) Emotional state
         f) Intellectual capacity
         g) Family history
         h) Spiritual history
         i) Alcohol and drug history (OTC and prescription)
         j) Identify problem
      4) Formulate contract
         a) Time of meeting
         b) Confidentiality
         c) Focus: goals that are behaviorally stated
   c. Working phase: planning and intervention
      1) Establish specific collaborative goals
      2) Explore thoughts, feelings, actions
      3) Establish nursing diagnosis
      4) Problem solve

KEY INFORMATION

      5) Communication tools
         a) Listening: nonverbal, use eye contact
         b) Offering self: "I'll stay with you."
         c) Focusing: on "here and now" and on the client
         d) Broad openings: "How are things going today?"
         e) Clarifying: "What does that mean to you?"
         f) Reflecting: directing back ideas,

feelings, and content, "You feel tense when you fight."

g) Empathy: stating a feeling implied by the client

h) Summarizing: "Today we have discussed…"

i) Silence: sitting, conveying nonverbal interest

j) Sharing perceptions: "You seem angry"

k) Restating: repeating the main thought "You are sad"

l) Validating: "Are you saying…"

m) Giving information (for example: answering a direct question, teaching)

6) Communication blocks

a) False reassurance: "Don't worry."

b) Agreeing and disagreeing: "I think you did the right thing."

c) Advice: "You should . . ."

d) Judging: "That was good."

e) Belittling: "Everyone feels like that."

f) Defending: "All the doctors here are great."

g) Approval: good or bad

h) Focus on nurse: "I feel that way, too."

i) Changing the subject

j) Ignoring a client

k) Changing client's words or assuming feelings

7) **NURSING INTERVENTIONS:**

a) Avoid communication blocks

b) Use open-ended questions and responses vs. closed

c) Avoid "why" questions that the client is unable to answer

d) Limit questions to one idea at a time

e) Communicate client's nonverbal communication: "I notice you are shaking your legs."

f) Avoid invading the client's space

g) Use touch carefully - can be interpreted as caring or as a threat

d. Termination phase: termination begins on admission or first contact. The nurse prepares the client for this eventuality during the first meeting

1) Evaluation of behavioral goals

2) Transfer to other support systems

3) Assess for separation reactions such as regression, acting out, anger, withdrawal

4) Help express and work through feelings

5) Be alert to nurse's response to separation

6) Do not promise to continue the relationship or schedule future appointments

what you did to get me, is what you should do to keep me...

SECTION II

ANXIETY

A. **Definition:** anxiety and apprehension are tension in response to a perceived physical or psychological threat (internal or external) resulting in feelings of helplessness and uncertainty

P perceiving you to peppu feels not good

B. **Responses**

1. Psychological

a. Fear

b. Impending doom

c. Helplessness

d. Insecurity

e. Low self-confidence

f. Anger

g. Guilt

2. Defense mechanisms

a. Displacement

b. Regression

c. Repression

d. Sublimation

3. Physiological: nervous system

a. Dry mouth

b. Elevated vital signs

c. Diarrhea

d. Increased urination

e. Palpitations

f. Diaphoresis

g. Hyperventilation

h. Fatigue

i. Insomnia

j. Sexual dysfunction

k. Irritability

l. Fidgeting, pacing

4. Behaviors

a. Fight or flight response

b. Talkative, giggly, angry, withdrawn

C. **Levels of Anxiety** (see table II-5.)
KEY INFORMATION

The initial nursing priority is to reduce the anxiety to a tolerable level since learning cannot occur until the client's anxiety is manageable.

D. **Maladaptive Responses to Anxiety**

1. Anxiety disorders: characterized by fear that is out of proportion to external events; attacks lasting minutes to hours

a. Panic disorders

1) Definition: sudden onset of intense apprehension, fear or terror (panic attacks)

2) Physical manifestations

a) Dyspnea

b) Palpitations
c) Chest pain
d) Faintness, dizziness
e) Fear of dying or going crazy (out of control)
f) Choking
g) Depersonalization or derealization
h) Hyperventilation

3) **NURSING INTERVENTIONS**
   a) Stay with client and remain calm
   b) Reassurance and support
   c) Remove anxiety-producing stimuli
   d) Have client take deep breaths
   e) Distract client from anxiety producing stimuli
   f) Provide a paper bag for hyperventilation

b. Phobic disorders
   1) Definition: persistent or irrational fear of a specific object, activity, or situation that leads to avoidance (for example: fear of flying)
   2) Types

a) Agoraphobia: fear of being away from a safe place or person in which there is no escape
b) Simple: irrational fear of object or situation
c) Social (Social anxiety disorder): irrational fear that social situations expose one to possible ridicule or embarrassment

3) Defense Mechanisms
   a) Repression
   b) Displacement
   c) Avoidance

4) **NURSING INTERVENTIONS**
   a) Teach client relaxation techniques
   b) Avoid major decision making
   c) Utilize behavior modification techniques
   d) No competitive situations
   e) Provide gradual desensitization experiences
   f) Assist client in verbalizing thoughts and feelings of anxiety

TABLE II-5.
LEVELS OF ANXIETY

LEVEL	PHYSIOLOGIC RESPONSE	COGNITIVE STATE	BEHAVIORAL CHANGES	NURSING INTERVENTIONS
Mild (+)	Slight discomfort, restlessness; tension relief; fidgeting, tapping	Perceptual field can be heightened; learning can occur	* - Restlessness (inability to work toward goal) * - Examine alternatives	* - Listen * - Promote insight, problem solving
Moderate (++)	Increased pulse, respirations, shakiness, voice tremors, difficulty concentrating, pacing	Perceptual field narrows; selective in attention	* - Focus on immediate events * - Benefits from guidance of others	* - Calm, rational discussion * - Relaxation exercises
Severe (+++)	Elevated BP, tachycardia, somatic complaints, hyperventilation, confusion	Perceptual field greatly reduced; attention scattered; cannot attend to events even when pointed out	- Feelings of increasing threat; purposeless activity * - Feeling of impending doom	* - Listen * - Encourage expression of feelings * - Concrete activity Reduce stimuli (channel energy into simple tasks)
Panic (++++)	- Immobility or severe hyperactivity; cool, clammy skin; pallor; dilated pupils; severe shakiness * - Prolonged anxiety can lead to exhaustion	- Perceptual field closed * - Hallucinations or delusions may occur * - Effective decision making is impossible	- Mute or psychomotor agitation * - May strike out physically or withdraw - Loss of control	* - Isolate from stimuli * - Stay with client * - Remain very calm * - Decrease demands * - Protect client safety * - Do not touch client
* Important				

c. Obsessive-compulsive disorders
  1) Definition: recurring obsessions or compulsions
    a) Obsessions: recurring thoughts of violence, contamination, doubt, and worry that cannot be voluntarily removed from consciousness.
    b) Compulsions: recurring, irresistible impulse to perform acts (for example: touching, rearranging, checking, opening and closing, washing)
    c) Obsessions and compulsions may occur together or separately
    d) Client's attempt to reduce anxiety
  2) Characteristics
    a) Irrational coping to handle guilt
    b) Feelings of inferiority and low self esteem
    c) Compulsion to repeat act
    d) Repeating act prevents severe anxiety
    e) Defense Mechanisms
      (1) Displacement
      (2) Undoing
      (3) Isolation
      (4) Reaction formation
  3) **NURSING INTERVENTIONS:** nursing interventions are aimed at reducing client anxiety
    a) Distract: substitute
    b) Do not interrupt compulsive act
    c) Schedule time to complete ritual; gradually decrease the time and number of times ritual performed
    d) Provide safety
    e) Maintain structure, schedules, activities
    f) Demonstrate acceptance of individual
    g) Encourage expression of feelings
    h) Antianxiety medications may be used to relieve manifestations
2. Somatoform disorders: physical manifestations and complaints without organic impairment (no real pathology, for example: soldiers paralyzed during war with no real injury)
  a. Conversion disorders (hysteria)
    1) Definition: alteration in physical function that is an expression of an unconscious psychological need
    2) Characteristics of manifestations
      a) Sensory: blindness, deafness, loss of sensation in extremities
      b) Motor: mutism, paralysis of extremities, ataxia, dizziness
      c) Visceral: headaches, difficulty breathing
      d) Convulsive disorder with atypical seizure response
      e) Little concern about manifestations: la belle indifference
      f) Defense mechanism: repression of conflict and conversion of anxiety into manifestations
      g) Primary gain: suppressing conflict
      h) Secondary gain: sympathy or avoidance of unpleasant activity gained
    3) **NURSING INTERVENTIONS**
      a) Redirect client away from manifestations
      b) Encourage client to express feelings
      c) Utilize stress reduction techniques
      d) Teach client relaxation techniques
      e) Understand the symptoms are real to the client
      f) Engage client in schedule of daily activities to decrease time spent focusing on symptoms and counter secondary gain
  b. Hypochondriasis
    1) Definition: exaggerated preoccupation with physical health, not based on real organic disorders, not pathology
    2) Characteristics
      a) Multiple manifestations
      b) Worried/anxious about manifestations
      c) Seeks medical care frequently from multiple healthcare providers
    3) **NURSING INTERVENTIONS**
      a) Help client express feelings
      b) Set limits on rumination
      c) Do not feed into the manifestations
3. Psychophysiological/psychosomatic disorders
  a. Definition: stress-related medical disorders with true pathology; psychosocial factors predispose client to episodes of illness and influence the progression of manifestations; can be fatal if not treated adequately. These disorders are characterized by increasing anxiety in addition to the physical manifestations. Clients are often first treated in medical facilities.
  b. Defense mechanisms
    1) Repression
    2) Introjection
  c. Types
    1) Migraine
    2) Ulcerative colitis
    3) Peptic ulcer
    4) Eczema
    5) Cancer
    6) Rheumatoid arthritis
  d. **NURSING INTERVENTIONS**
    1) Care for physical signs
    2) Educate client about body/mind

TABLE II-6.
ANTIANXIETY AGENTS AND ADVERSE REACTIONS

CHEMICAL CLASS	GENERIC NAME	TRADE NAME	MEDICATION ALERTS
Benzodiazepine compounds	- chlordiazepoxide	- Librium	- Benzodiazepines: Warn clients about sedating effects. Avoid activities requiring mental alertness. Monitor for signs of drug dependence. Withdrawal up to two weeks; risk for seizure.
	- diazepam - oxazepam - clorazepate - lorazepam - alprazolam - clonazepam - clomipramine HCL	- Valium - Serax - Tranxene - Ativan - Xanax - Klonopin - Anafranil	- Anafranil, commonly used for OCD, should be cautiously used in clients with cardiovascular disease and is potentially fatal in overdose
Mephenesin-like compounds	meprobamate	Miltown, Equanil	
Sedating antihistamines	hydroxyzine	Vistaril, Atarax	Antihistamines tend to cause drying and sedation
Beta-blockers	propranolol	Inderal	
(SSRI) Selective Serotonin Reuptake Inhibitors	paroxetine	Paxil	Shown to be effective with Social Anxiety Disorder. Allow 2-3 weeks to note effects
Anxiolytics	buspirone	BuSpar	BuSpar-non-sedating, allow 2-3 weeks to note effects. Do not use concurrently with alcohol or history of hepatic disease

ADVERSE REACTIONS	NURSING INTERVENTIONS
Dry mouth	Provide candies, fluids
Blurred vision	Will disappear within a week
Urinary retention	Monitor intake and output; for distention, run water
Drowsiness or sedation	Instruct client not to operate machines; do not give with other CNS depressants
Ataxia	Use side rails if needed; stay with client if out of bed
Tremors	Observe severity
Hypotension	Take frequent BP
Tolerance	Observe for proper usage and effect; withdraw gradually

DRUG INTERACTIONS

- CNS depressants: action potentiated; avoid alcohol, avoid concurrent use of MAOIs
- Tolerance does develop; discontinue slowly to minimize symptoms and rebound symptoms of insomnia or anxiety
- Elderly more vulnerable to adverse reactions; safety risk
- Possible paradoxical reactions in children and elderly
- Stopping suddenly could cause seizures or death

relationship

    3) Teach client relaxation techniques (for example: biofeedback imagery, progressive relaxation)

    4) Assist client to express thoughts and feelings

    5) Encourage self health promotion and regulation activities (for example: relaxation, exercise)

    6) Promote positive lifestyle changes

4. Dissociative disorders (hysterical neuroses)

    a. Definition: splitting off an idea or emotion from one's consciousness; "psychological flight" from anxiety (common with abused children)

    b. Types

      1) Multiple personality

      2) Psychogenic fugue

      3) Psychogenic amnesia

      4) Depersonalization

    c. **NURSING INTERVENTIONS**

      1) Assess client to rule out organic pathology

      2) Help client recognize when dissociation occurs

      3) Help client express feelings

      4) Initiate individual, group, and family psychotherapy

5. Somatic treatment for maladaptive responses to anxiety, insomnia, and stress-related conditions

6. Antianxiety agents: anxiolytic, minor tranquilizers (see table II-6.)

7. Expressive therapy for maladaptive responses to anxiety

    a. Client with poor concentration: group work, simple tasks

    b. Client with hyperactivity: decrease external stimuli, one-to-one interaction, walks, uncompetitive activities

KEY INFORMATION

Antianxiety medications are not a cure for anxiety, but a temporary means to reduce anxiety. Antianxiety medications can be highly lethal in overdose. Monitor suicidal clients closely. Elderly clients are easily sedated and at risk for fall with benzodiazepines.

SECTION III

SCHIZOPHRENIA

A. Definition: group of psychotic disorders characterized by regression, thought disturbances (including delusions and hallucinations), bizarre dress and behavior, poverty of speech, abnormal motor behavior, and withdrawal

B. Overview

1. Bleuler's four A's

    a. Autism: preoccupation with self and inner experience

    b. Affect: feeling tone is flat, blunted or inappropriate

    c. Ambivalence: conflicting strong feelings that may confuse, frighten or immobilize

    d. Loose association: disrupted or disorganized thinking

2. Appearance: disheveled

3. Other major manifestations

    a. Delusions: fixed false beliefs; can be paranoid, grandiose, or somatic delusions

    b. Hallucinations: sensory perceptions without any environmental stimuli (for example: hearing voices, seeing spiders, smelling foul)

    c. Illusions: misidentification of actual environmental stimuli; client may see an electrical cord as a snake

    d. Ideas of reference: personalizing environmental stimuli (for example: client believes static on telephone is wiretapping)

    e. Neologisms: made up words

    f. Circumstantiality: can't come to point, includes nonessential details

    g. Blocking: interrupt flow of speech due to distracting thoughts, words, ideas, subjects

    h. Regressive behavior: behavior appropriate at earlier stage of development

    i. Echolalia: repetition of words or phrases heard from another person

    j. Clanging: repeating words or phrases that sound the same but not related

    k. Pressured speech: words rush out quickly

    l. Poor interpersonal relationships

    m. Declining ability to work, socialize, care for self

4. Characteristics and defense mechanisms

    a. Depersonalization: feel alienated from self, no ego boundaries

    b. Projection

    c. Regression

    d. Denial

    e. Fantasy world

C. Schizophrenic Disorders

1. Types

    a. Disorganized: incoherent, severe thought disturbance, shallow, inappropriate, often silly behavior and mannerisms

    b. Catatonic (psychomotor)

      1) Stupor: lessening of response

      2) Excitement: increase in activity

      3) Waxy flexibility: bizarre posturing

      4) Negativism: doing the opposite of what is

being asked

    5) Mutism: continuous refusal to speak

    6) Severe withdrawal

  c. Paranoid (can be dangerous)

    1) Hallucination: grandiose or persecutory

    2) Delusions: persecution and grandeur

    3) Emotions: angry, suspicious, argumentative, mistrust, excessive religiosity of a punitive nature

  d. Undifferentiated

    1) Mixed characteristics

    2) Meets criteria of more than one type

2. **NURSING INTERVENTIONS**

  a. Provide physical care

  b. Promote client safety

  c. Increase client trust with a 1:1 nurse/client relationship

  d. Orient to reality

  e. Provide structure to the day

  f. Involve family

  g. Interactions should be simple and concrete; often nonverbal and short

  h. Help work through regressive behavior

  i. Decrease bizarre behavior, anxiety, agitation, aggression

  j. Deal with hallucinations

    1) Distract client

    2) Do not confront; do not deny

    3) Point out that you do not share the same perception, but acknowledge that the hallucination is real to client

    4) Seek to establish feelings

    5) Avoid leaving client alone (client will hallucinate more)

    6) Engage client in activities (for example: current events discussion groups)

  k. Provide least restrictive environment, avoid restraining

  l. Provide care in a firm matter-of-fact manner that allows participation

  m. Provide consistency, positive reinforcement, and unconditional acceptance of client

D. Paranoid Personality Disorder

  1. Definition: insidious development of a permanent and unshakable delusional system accompanied by preservation of clear and orderly thinking

  2. Characteristics

    a. Projection: unacceptable feelings are attributed to others

    b. Delusions of grandeur and/or persecution

    c. Ideas of reference (for example: personalizing environmental stimuli)

    d. Resistance to treatment

    e. Loneliness and distrust (failed Erikson's Stages)

    f. Refusal to eat

  g. Suspiciousness and fear

  h. Emotional expressions are appropriate to content of delusional system

  i. Argumentative and hostile

3. **NURSING INTERVENTIONS**

  a. Persecutory delusions

    1) Do not argue or confront

    2) Interject reality when appropriate

    3) Get to feeling level

    4) Discuss topics other than delusions

  b. Aggression and hostility

    1) Help client express self verbally

    2) Set limits and offer alternatives

    3) Keep at a safe distance

    4) Don't respond with aggression; use calm, controlled tone

    5) Use direct, simple statements

    6) Keep other clients away

    7) Decrease stimulation with time out

    8) Have back up and use speed when restraining

    9) Seclude as last resort

    10) Provide outlet for aggression

    11) Monitor

  c. Fear of being poisoned

    1) Serve food in containers

    2) Medications should be wrapped or in containers

    3) Do not covertly put meds in juice

    4) Open meds in presence of client

  d. Attempt to de-escalate client's aggression, allow opportunity to gain control

  e. Avoid verbal and nonverbal communication that could be interpreted as a threat

  f. Respect the client's personal space and avoid touching as they may strike out in response to fear and anxiety

  g. Attitude of superiority

    1) Small groups, ratio of one nurse to one client

    2) Activities that ensure success

    3) Limits without judging

    4) Increase self-esteem

    5) Descale, talk about feelings

E. Pervasive Developmental Disorders (usually seen in children)

  1. Autistic disorders

    a. Characteristics

      1) Lack of interest in human contact

      2) Compulsive need for following routines; distressed by slight environmental changes

      3) Abnormal or no social play

      4) Autoerotic behavior (for example: rocking, excessive masturbation)

      5) Abnormal nonverbal communication

6) Self-mutilation (for example: head banging)
7) Impaired ability to form peer relationships
8) Abnormal production of speech and content
9) Obsessional attachments to inanimate objects
10) Impaired ability to form peer relationships

b. **NURSING INTERVENTIONS**
1) Assess social and physical aspects of client
2) Assess family understanding and coping
3) Facilitate communication (verbal and/or nonverbal)
4) Maintain optimum level of functioning and prevent regression

2. Attention-deficit and hyperactivity disorder
a. Characteristics
1) Fails to complete task
2) Easily distracted
3) Difficulty concentrating
4) Acts before thinking, impulsive
5) Has difficulty sitting still

b. **NURSING INTERVENTIONS**
1) Assist to communicate effectively
2) Set stage for improving ego function
3) Help learn more adaptive coping behaviors
4) Initiate supportive and educative methods for assisting parent and child
5) Promote client safety when head banging or other self-destructive behaviors are exhibited
6) Techniques to use:
a) Play therapy
b) Cognitive-behavioral
c) Family therapy
d) Psychopharmacology: methylphenidate (*Ritalin*)

F. **Medications:** antipsychotics (for schizophrenic and paranoid behavior patterns); compliance is a problem secondary to adverse reactions
1. Block dopamine receptors
a. Target positive manifestations
1) Negativism
2) Combativeness
3) Disorganization
4) Hallucinations, delusions
5) Hostility
6) Suspiciousness
7) Seclusiveness
8) Self-care deficits
b. Negative manifestations not affected
1) Apathy
2) Withdrawal
3) Insight

4) Lack of interest
5) Blunted affect
6) Judgment
2. Antipsychotic agents (major tranquilizers or neuroleptic agents) (see table II-7.)
3. Drugs to control extrapyramidal reaction (CNS)
a. Commonly used
1) Trihexyphenidyl (*Artane*)
2) Benztropine mesylate (*Cogentin*)
3) Diphenhydramine (*Benadryl*)
b. Adverse reactions: anticholinergic
1) Blurred vision
2) Dry mouth
3) Constipation
4) Urinary retention
5) Drowsiness
6) Nervousness
7) Photosensitivity
8) Hypotension
4. Drug abuse potential with benztropine mesylate (*Cogentin*) and antihistamines
5. Benztropine mesylate (*Cogentin*) should not be given to clients with narrow angle glaucoma

SECTION IV

MOOD DISORDERS AND ASSOCIATED BEHAVIORS

A. **Depression and Elation**
1. Definition
a. Depression: mood state of gloom, despondency, and dejection with accompanying physical, cognitive and behavioral responses
b. Mania: predominant mood is elevated; great amount of activity
2. Continuum of emotional responses (see table II-8.)
3. Range and severity of moods
a. Grief: takes 2 years for full recovery; a normal process
1) Precipitating factors
a) Death in family
b) Separation
c) Divorce
d) Physical illness
e) Work failure
f) Disappointment
2) Stages (Kubler-Ross)
a) Denial
b) Anger
c) Bargaining
d) Depression
e) Acceptance

3) **NURSING INTERVENTIONS**
a) Accept client's stage

TABLE II-7.
ANTIPSYCHOTIC AGENTS AND ADVERSE REACTIONS

CHEMICAL CLASS	GENERIC NAME	TRADE NAME	MEDICATION ALERT
Phenothiazine, aliphatic	chlorpromazine	Thorazine	
Phenothiazine, piperidine	- thioridazine - mesoridazine	- Mellaril - Serentil	
Phenothiazine, piperazine	- fluphenazine - perphenazine - trifluoperazine	- Prolixin - Trilafon - Stelazine	
Thioxanthene, piperazine	thiothixene	Navane	
Butyrophenone	haloperidol	Haldol	
Dibenzoxazepine	- loxapine - clozapine	- Loxitane - Clozaril	- Clozaril is an effective antipsychotic especially in clients not responding to other neuroleptics - Clozaril requires weekly CBCs
Thienobenzodiazepine	- olanzapine - quetiapine - sertindole	- Zyprexa - Seroquel - Serlect	Zyprexa is mirrored after Clozaril with fewer adverse reactions. Does not require weekly CBCs
Benzisoxazole	risperidone	Risperdal	- Risperdal has fewer EPS and targets negative and positive symptoms - Can be used safely in the elderly

ADVERSE REACTIONS	NURSING INTERVENTIONS	MEDICATION ALERT
Sedation	Most common in low-potency antipsychotics; ask primary care provider if entire dose can be given at bedtime	Sedation is common in Thorazine and Mellaril
Extrapyramidal effects (EPS): parkinsonian symptoms (for example: fine hand tremors, pill rolling, drooling, muscle stiffness)	Report to the primary care provider; specific medication may be changed; antiparkinsonian medication is given to control manifestations	EPS is usually associated with high potency (Stelazine, Navane, Haldol, and Loxitane); least likely to have EPS with Mellaril
Dystonia: muscle spasm of the face and neck; eyes rolling back in head	Report to primary care provider; usually an antiparkinsonian medication is given and the antipsychotic medication is changed	Dystonia is most common in males taking Haldol, Prolixin, Stelazine
Akathisia: restlessness, inability to sit still	Call primary care provider; if treated with antiparkinsonian medications, may need to change antipsychotic medication	
Tardive dyskinesia: lip smacking, sucking, tongue protrusion, jerking of the head and neck, extension and flexion of the fingers, back and forth movement of spine, movement of the arms	Careful observation in early steps of treatment; discontinue medication at first sign to prevent permanent disability; Abnormal Involuntary Movement Scale (AIMS) is used to assess clients for permanent adverse reactions	

TABLE II-7.
ANTIPSYCHOTIC AGENTS AND ADVERSE REACTIONS (CONTINUED)

ADVERSE REACTIONS	NURSING INTERVENTIONS	MEDICATION ALERT
Anticholinergic - Dry mouth - Constipation - Urinary retention - Blurred vision - Nasal congestion - Orthostatic hypotension	- Provide candies, fluids - Laxatives, diet - Monitor intake and output - Client teaching: will disappear within a week - Increase humidity (showers help) - Monitor BP frequently, sitting and standing; caution client to stand up slowly	Thorazine, Mellaril, Risperdal, and Zyprexa have potential to cause orthostatic hypotension specially in the elderly
Hypotension	Monitor BP frequently, sitting and standing; caution client to stand up slowly	
Photosensitivity	Sunscreen; cover up with clothing	Thorazine: exposure to sun causes dark purplish pigmentation of skin
Agranulocytosis	Observe for sign of infection, or nosebleeds and report immediately if present; discontinue medication; weekly CBCs	Most often seen with Clozaril
Retinopathy	Sunglasses	Thorazine and Mellaril may cause retinopathy
Neuroleptic malignant syndrome (NMS) (Can be fatal)	Discontinue medication and report immediately if manifestations occur (altered consciousness, unstable BP&P, fever, muscle rigidity, diaphoresis and tremors) (EPS with fever)	All neuroleptics can cause NMS, an extreme emergency situation
Endocrine - Breast enlargement	- Yearly breast exams	- Neuroendocrine effects are most often seen with Mellaril; these symptoms are related to decreased hypothalamic function
- Decreased libido; ejaculatory incompetence	- Decrease dose or change to high-potency drugs	
- Appetite increase, weight gain	- Exercise/diet regimen	- Most common adverse effect of Zyprexa is weight gain; Seroquel is an alternative medication to use if client experiences extreme weight gain
DRUG INTERACTIONS		
- MAO inhibitors - Anticonvulsants		

b) Encourage expression of feelings
c) Help through stages by providing anticipatory guidance

KEY INFORMATION

4) Unresolved grief produces psychotic and neurotic manifestations such as chronic depression, psychosomatic disorders, acting out behavior

b. Moderate mood disorders
1) Types
   a) Dysthymia: chronically depressed mood
   b) Cyclothymic: cycles of depression and hypomania (not as severe as mania)
2) Characteristics: depression (dysthymia)
   a) Pessimism
   b) Insomnia or hypersomnia
   c) Social withdrawal
   d) Feelings of worthlessness, not caring, little pressure, irritability
   e) Low energy

c. Severe mood disorders
1) Major depression
   a) Weight gain or loss of over 10 pounds
   b) Sleep disturbances
   c) Loss of pleasure or interest in usual activities, including sex
   d) Low energy, fatigue
   e) Feelings of helplessness and hopelessness
   f) Decreased concentration
   g) Psychomotor retardation or agitation
   h) Anger turned inward
   i) Cannot make decisions
   j) Suicidal ideation
   k) Delusional about guilt, unworthiness, sin
   l) Social withdrawal
   m) Persistent physical manifestation such as headaches, digestive disorders, chronic pain
   n) Lack of self care

2) Mania's characteristics: client may be or display
   a) Extroverted
   b) Flight of ideas
   c) Accelerated speech
   d) Accelerated motor activity
   e) Anger turned outward
   f) Impulsive
   g) Arrogant, demanding, controlling behavior with underlying feelings of vulnerability and inadequacy
   h) Delusions of grandeur
3) Bipolar: alternate periods of depression and mania with a short period of "normalcy" in between
   a) Manic periods decrease over time
   b) Depressive periods increase
   c) Suicide potential greatest during period of "normalcy"

d. **NURSING INTERVENTIONS**
1) Depression
   a) Structure environment and time; promote client's physical well being
   b) Initiate suicide precautions
   c) Communicate with client to decrease loneliness
   d) Build trust, short frequent visits
   e) Discourage decision making: increase social skills
   f) Schedule nonintellectual activities such as leatherwork, sanding
   g) Encourage goal setting to provide success
2) Mania
   a) Provide for physical welfare
   b) Provide frequent small feedings, finger foods
   c) Protect from impulsive activity to promote client safety
   d) Reduce external stimuli (client responds to environment)
   e) Communicate calmly

TABLE II-8.
CONTINUUM OF EMOTIONAL RESPONSES

ADAPTIVE RESPONSES		MALADAPTIVE RESPONSES
- Sadness - Grief	- Dysthymic - Cyclothymic - Reactive - Exogenous	- Major depression - Bipolar disorder - Endogenous
No treatment ⟶ Psychotherapy ⟷ Medications		
Duration of illness increases ⟶		

f) Initiate milieu activities such as walks, ball tossing, creative writing, and drawing; avoid competitive games

3) Interventions are specific to client behavior for example:
   a) Depression: lack of sleep; reestablish sleep patterns
   b) Mania: weight loss; reestablish eating patterns (finger foods, decrease stimuli)

4) Priority nursing care is given to suicidal client (frequent interactions and monitoring)

5) Clients are most at risk for suicide between their depressive and manic episodes

e. Suicide
1) Definition: self-imposed death stemming from depression, especially hopelessness and negative feelings about the future

2) High-risk groups: depressed, hallucinating, delusional, organic mental disorders, substance abusers, adolescents, chronic or painful illness, elderly, sexual identity conflicts

3) Danger signs
   a) Specific plan (ask client for specifics)
   b) Giving away personal items, completing wills, finalizing personal or business matters
   c) Making amends
   d) Change in behavior in a depressed client
   e) Gesture or history of attempt
   f) Client indicates that he/she "feels better" or "has everything figured out"

4) **NURSING INTERVENTIONS**
   a) Initiate crisis intervention
   b) Take all gestures seriously
   c) Initiate suicide precautions
      (1) Stay with client
      (2) Establish safety contract
      (3) Remove sharp and harmful objects
   d) Maintain personal contact providing care, concern, neutral tone, hope, and goals
   e) Provide diversional activities with increasing numbers of people
   f) Safety is always the first priority

B. **Treatments**
1. Antidepressant agents (see table II-9.)

2. Antidepressant agents: MAO Inhibitors (see table II-10.)

3. Antimanic agents and mood stabilizers (see table II-11.)

4. Electroconvulsive therapy (ECT)
   a. Characteristics
      1) Used mainly with severely depressed clients
      2) Used after other methods have been tried and failed
      3) Grand-mal seizure induced by passing an electric current through the temporal lobes and hypothalamus for 0.1–1 second
      4) Slight grimace and/or plantar flexion and toe movement may be observable
      5) Dose: 6-20 treatments 3 times a week
   b. Medications
      1) General anesthesia
      2) Muscle relaxant succinylcholine chloride (*Anectine*)
      3) Atropine sulfate: to dry secretions and block vagal reflexes
   c. **NURSING INTERVENTIONS**
      1) Obtain informed consent
      2) NPO after midnight
      3) Take baseline vital signs, every 15 minutes postoperatively
      4) Remove prosthesis and jewelry
      5) Bladder emptied
      6) Reassure that memory loss is temporary up to 2 months
      7) Educate client and family for ECT as a treatment modality
      8) Prepare client and family for the temporary memory loss post-treatment
      9) Monitor client for decrease respirations as a potential adverse effect of Anectine
   d. Recovery period
      1) Monitor vital signs
      2) Maintain a patent airway
      3) Position on side to prevent aspiration
      4) Provide reorientation to person, place, time
      5) Assist to ambulate
      6) Resume ADLs as soon as possible
      7) Provide symptomatic treatment of residual headache or nausea

SECTION V

PERSONALITY DISORDERS

A. **Definition:** individual personality traits reflecting chronic, inflexible, and maladaptive patterns of behavior that impair social and occupational functions

TABLE II-9.
ANTIDEPRESSANT AGENTS

CHEMICAL CLASS	GENERIC NAME	TRADE NAME	MEDICATION ALERTS
Tricyclic antidepressants (more adverse reactions)	- imipramine - desipramine - amitriptyline - nortriptyline - protriptyline - doxepin - amoxapine	- Tofranil - Norpramin - Elavil - Aventyl - Vivactil - Sinequan - Asendin	Tricyclic antidepressants (TCAs) inhibit serotonin uptake from synaptic gap
Tetracyclic antidepressant	- maprotiline - mirtazapine	- Ludiomil - Remeron	
Newer antidepressants (fewer adverse reactions) (SSRIs)	- trazodone - fluvoxamine - bupropion HCl - fluoxetine - sertraline - paroxetine - venlafaxine HCL - citalopram	- Desyrel - Luvox - Wellbutrin - Prozac - Zoloft - Paxil - Effexor - Celexa	- Selective serotonin reuptake inhibitors (SSRI) act to inhibit reuptake of serotonin into CNS neurons. SSRIs have fewer adverse reactions, and can be used in elderly clients safely - Antidepressant medications usually take 2 - 3 weeks to become therapeutic. Fluoxetine (*Prozac*) may take 4 weeks.

ADVERSE REACTIONS	NURSING INTERVENTIONS	MEDICATION ALERTS
Anticholinergic effects (can be treated – usually clear in one week) - Dry mouth - Constipation - Urinary retention - Blurred vision - Aggravated glaucoma	 - Increase fluids, good oral hygiene - Bulk, diet, exercise, stool softeners - Urecholine, monitor intake and outflow - Corrective lenses or pilocarpine drops, large print - Ophthalmologist consult	All tricyclic and tetracyclic medications can cause dry mouth, constipation, blurred vision, drowsiness, and hypotension
Cardiovascular effects - Postural hypotension - Direct effects on the heart tachycardia, arrhythmia, conduction defects - Fluid retention: can lead to CHF	 - Take BP regularly, sitting and standing to cardiovascular effects - Use smaller divided doses in clients with known heart disease; avoid in those with cardiac conduction defects or recent MI - Check vital signs regularly; weigh client daily; check for fluid retention	Tricyclic antidepressants are potentially lethal in cases of overdose due
Allergic reactions - Rashes	- Observe and report to primary care provider	- Prozac most commonly causes skin rash

TABLE II-9.
ANTIDEPRESSANT AGENTS (CONTINUED)

ADVERSE REACTIONS	NURSING INTERVENTIONS	MEDICATION ALERTS
- Photosensitivity	- Provide sunscreen, protect skin with clothing, observe carefully	
- Insomnia	- Single morning dose	- Insomnia is common with Prozac
- Tremors and seizures	- Observe carefully; advise client to avoid caffeine	- Wellbutrin or Celexa should not be taken if there is a history of seizure disorder. Do not double dose if a dose is missed. Luvox, used to treat OCD, can also induce seizures and induction of a manic episode.
- Excessive perspiration	- Observe, report, provide comfort measures	
- Erection/orgasm difficulty (may cause noncompliance)	- Lower dose or switch to less anticholinergic preparation	
- Anxiety, restlessness	- Observe, report, may have to discontinue	

DRUG INTERACTIONS	ADVERSE REACTIONS	MEDICATION ALERTS
MAO inhibitors	14-day waiting period before changing from MAOI to antidepressant or vice versa	Do not use tricyclic or SSRIs concurrently with MAOIs
Antihypertensives and heart medications	Causes hypotension or hypertension	
Antacids	Inhibits absorption	
Antipsychotics	Potentiates anticholinergic effects	
CNS depressants/alcohol	Effects are potentiated	

TABLE II-10.
ANTIDEPRESSANT AGENTS: MAOI'S

CHEMICAL CLASS	GENERIC NAME	TRADE NAME
MAOI	- isocarboxazid - phenelzine - tranylcypromine	- Marplan - Nardil - Parnate

ADVERSE REACTIONS	NURSING INTERVENTIONS	MEDICATION ALERTS
Hypertensive crisis: elevated BP, palpitations, diaphoresis, chest pain, and headache that can lead to intracranial hemorrhage and death	Teach clients to avoid foods with high tyramine content such as aged cheeses, fermented foods, chocolate, liver, bean pods, yeast, sausage and bologna, beer, Chianti and vermouth wines; limit amounts of ETOH, sour cream, yogurt, raisins, soy sauce; teach clients to avoid OTC and prescription medications such as antidepressants, sedatives, cough and cold preparations, which interact to produce hypertensive crisis	Monitor client's BP and assess for complaint of headache

TABLE II-10.
ANTIDEPRESSANT AGENTS: MAOI'S (CONTINUED)

ADVERSE REACTIONS	NURSING INTERVENTIONS	MEDICATION ALERTS
Anticholinergic disturbances: dry mouth, constipation	Increase fluids, bulk in diet, and exercise	
CNS effects: drowsiness, fatigue, headache, restlessness	Some can be expected to last for a short period; increase activity, short afternoon nap	
Orthostatic hypotension (drop in BP due to change in position)	Monitor BP frequently, lying, sitting, standing; teach to rise slowly	
Delay in ejaculation/orgasm	Take dose in morning if sexual activity is in evening	
Insomnia	Give single morning dose; relax several hours before bedtime	

DRUG INTERACTIONS	ADVERSE REACTIONS	MEDICATION ALERTS
Tricyclic antidepressants	Hypertensive crisis	Must wait 2 weeks before changing to a different antidepressant medication
CNS depressants	Decrease liver function	
Dibenzoxepins	Hypertensive crisis	
Amphetamines	Potentiate action	
Antihypertensives (diuretics)	Decrease action	

TABLE II-11.
ANTIMANIA AGENTS AND MOOD STABILIZERS

CHEMICAL CLASS	GENERIC NAME	TRADE NAME	MEDICATION ALERTS

Lithium
- Blood level
  - .5–1.5 meq/liter: therapeutic
  - Above 1.5 meq/liter: toxic
  - 2.0 mEq/liter: lethal
	- Lithium	- Eskalith
		- Lithonate
		- Lithotabs
		- Lithobid
			- A client who is to start lithium therapy should be ruled out for thyroid, cardiac, and renal problems before initial therapy. Lithium should be discontinued prior to surgery, ECT, and during pregnancy. It is essential to monitor lithium levels routinely to maintain a therapeutic range.
			
			- ½ life = 24 hours

Anticonvulsants	- valproic acid	- Depakote	- Depakote should not be used in clients with liver or hepatic disease; must monitor LFTs, CBCs

TABLE II-11.
ANTIMANIA AGENTS AND MOOD STABILIZERS (CONTINUED)

CHEMICAL CLASS	GENERIC NAME	TRADE NAME	MEDICATION ALERTS
Anticonvulsants (continued)	- gabapentin - carbamazepine	- Neurontin - Tegretol	- Do not stop anticonvulsant medications suddenly; may have seizures

ADVERSE REACTIONS	NURSING INTERVENTIONS	MEDICATION ALERTS

- Initial effects of Lithium	- Interventions for all adverse reactions:
	  - Instruct client of short duration
	  - Observe client carefully for changes in manifestations
	  - Lithium work-up: renal, thyroid, EKG
	  - Check blood levels
	  - Regular physicals
	  - Lower doses in geriatric clients
		Teach client that initial adverse reactions are common

- Fine tremor	- Eliminate caffeine; adjust dose	
- Transient nausea	- Use of side rails; assist when up	
- Drowsiness, lethargy	- Avoid using machinery	
- Loose stools, abdominal discomfort	- Take with meals; change to slower release form	
- Polyuria		
- Thirst		
- Weight gain, fatigue		
- Toxic levels of Lithium - Causes: Elevated doses of medication; low Na levels; prolonged vomiting or diarrhea	Careful observation for and of blood levels as sodium decreases and lithium levels increase; hold doses and obtain blood level; liver function/hematology levels need to be monitored with valproic acid	- If Lithium toxicity is suspected and blood levels exceed 2.0, discontinue medications and begin fluid and electrolyte therapy - Discontinue Lithium therapy 48–72 hours preoperatively; prolongs the action of Anectine

- Results:
  - Vomiting
  - Diarrhea
  - Lethargy
  - Muscle twitching
  - Ataxia
  - Slurred speech
  - Coma, seizure, cardiac arrest		

DRUG INTERACTIONS	ADVERSE REACTIONS	MEDICATION ALERTS
- Diuretics - Antipsychotics - Sodium bicarbonate - ECT /surgery - Pregnancy	- Increase risk of lithium toxicity do not use with Haldol - Neurotoxicity, especially in elderly - Promote excretion, lowering serum level - May cause neurotoxicity - Crosses placental barrier	Use cautiously with neuroleptics

B. Causes

1. Genetic abnormalities
2. Learned responses
3. Deficiencies in ego and superego development
4. Unresponsive, inappropriate parent-child relationship
5. Early separation

C. Manifestations

1. Antisocial: sociopathic/psychopathic (Usually men)
   a. Superficial charm, wit, intelligence; manipulative, often seductive behavior
   b. Inability or refusal to accept responsibility for self-serving, destructive behavior
   c. Failure at school and work; delinquency, rule violations, inability to keep a job
   d. Repeated substance abuse
   e. Thefts, vandalism, multiple arrests
   f. Inability to function as a responsible person; no give or take
   g. Fights, assaults, abuse of others
   h. Impulsiveness, recklessness, inability to plan ahead
   i. Inappropriate affect: not sorry for violating others, no guilt
   j. Does not seek treatment
   k. Does not change with punishment
2. Borderline (usually women)
   a. Impulsive and unpredictable behavior in self-damaging areas: spending, sex, gambling
   b. Unstable and intense interpersonal relationships, rapid attitude shifts, idealization, devaluation
   c. Inappropriate, intense anger
   d. Manipulative, splitting behaviors
   e. Identity disturbance with uncertain self-image and imitative behavior
   f. Intolerance of being alone, chronic feelings of emptiness or boredom
   g. Unstable affect with mood swings
   h. Self-destructive behavior: suicidal gestures, self-mutilation, frequent accidents and fights

D. NURSING INTERVENTIONS

1. Be aware of own feelings
2. Approach client directly; confront
3. Reinforce appropriate behavior
4. Set limits
5. Protect other clients from verbal and physical abuse
6. Set clear rules and regulations with consequences for rule violation
7. Establish contract for behavioral changes
8. Initiate group treatment, help identify manipulative behavior
9. Recognize manipulative behaviors and be clear about boundaries and rules
10. Hold frequent interdisciplinary meetings to address client behaviors and to provide consistency in treatment
11. Encourage verbal expression of feelings
12. Encourage responsibility and accountability
13. Teach social skills

SECTION VI

CHEMICAL DEPENDENCE/ABUSE

A. Substance-Related Disorders

1. Definition
   a. Abuse: drug use leading to legal, social, and medical problems
   b. Addiction: refers to physical dependence
   c. Dependence: need resulting from continued use; results in mental and physical discomfort upon withdrawal of the substance
2. Contributing factors
   a. Genetic predisposition
   b. Peer pressure and social approval
   c. Low self-esteem
   d. Low frustration tolerance
   e. Availability
3. Defense mechanisms
   a. Denial
   b. Rationalization
   c. Intellectualization
   d. Projection
   e. Blaming
4. Behavioral effects
   a. Reduces anxiety
   b. Sense of well-being
   c. Inhibits self-control
   d. Dependence: physical and psychological addiction
   e. Tolerance: need for increasing amounts to achieve the same effect
5. Alcohol dependence and abuse
   a. General characteristics
      1) Abuse vs dependence
      2) Central nervous system depressant with progression from relaxation to slurred speech and impaired motor activities to stupor and anesthesia
      3) Physical effects occur in all systems
         a) Nervous system: psychosis, dementia, seizure disorders; Wernicke-Korsakoff's syndrome secondary to dementia; memory loss, ataxia, confusion (thiamine and niacin deficiency)

TABLE II-12.
SUBSTANCE ABUSE

DRUG	MANIFESTATIONS OF INTOXICATION	WITHDRAWAL SYNDROME	METHOD OF DETOXIFICATION
Hallucinogens: psychedelics, LSD, mescaline peyote, marijuana "gateway drugs"	Flushing of skin, dilated pupils, transient increase in pulse rate and blood pressure, hallucinations, psychosis, marked anxiety, depression, suicidal thoughts, confusion, paranoia	None	None required; "bad trips" can be treated with diazepam (Valium) or, more simply, by "talking down" through verbal reassurance and emotional support; flashbacks may occur for several months
Phencyclidine (PCP, angel dust)	Vertical or horizontal nystagmus, increased BP and heart rate, ataxia, marked anxiety, emotional liability, dysarthria, euphoria, agitation, delusions, grandiosity, irrationality, violence, synthesis (seeing colors when loud sound is heard); sensation of slowed time; can lead to dangerous behavior	None	Minimize social stimulation and control environment; administer ascorbic acid (Vit. C tabs or cranberry juice); do not "talk down"; treat with Valium if excited; if psychotic, admit to psychiatric unit and treat with antipsychotic medication
Stimulants: amphetamines, amyl nitrate, cocaine (see separate category)	Restlessness, irritability, anxiety, tachycardia, cardiac arrhythmia, paranoia, psychosis with clear sensorium, elation, grandiosity, psychotic behavior, perspiration or chills, nausea and vomiting, weight loss with prolonged use	- Use of high doses associated with a rapidly developing syndrome on withdrawal: - persecutory delusions - ideas of reference - aggressiveness and hostility anxiety - psychomotor agitation - suicidal - Prolonged, heavy use yields withdrawal syndrome after 2–4 days of depression and fatigue	None usually required; psychiatric hospitalization for severe withdrawal symptoms or addiction
- Cocaine/Crack No longer a "rich man's drug" - Same dose consistently can cause an overdose	Same as amphetamines; overdose: syncope, chest pain, seizures, death may result from cardiac and respiratory failure: high dose use: visual and tactile hallucinations and "cocaine bugs;" a "rush" of increased self-confidence and well-being, confusion, anxiety, paranoia; headache, palpitations followed by "crashing"	- Sleepiness, depression, lack of energy or motivation, poor concentration, irritability, "cocaine craving," psychosis - Can cause a stroke in the fetus	Hospitalization for high-dose "crack" or freebase use or the polyaddicted; others treated in outpatient programs

TABLE II-12.
SUBSTANCE ABUSE (CONTINUED)

DRUG	MANIFESTATIONS OF INTOXICATION	WITHDRAWAL SYNDROME	METHOD OF DETOXIFICATION
Opiates: heroin, morphine, Dilaudid, Demerol, Percodan, codeine, Opium, methadone	Mitosis, euphoria, drowsiness, dysphoria, apathy, psychomotor retardation, slurred speech, impaired attention or memory, impaired social judgment; chronic use can lead to malnourishment, criminal behavior, sexually transmitted disease, HIV/AIDS with IV drug use	Withdrawal begins after 8–12 hours and lasts 3—5 days; severity varies with extent of abuse; lacrimation, rhinorrhea, sweating, piloerection, diarrhea, yawning, mild hypertension, tachycardia, fever, insomnia, dilated pupils, restlessness, abdominal cramps, anxiety	Can be accomplished "cold turkey" or medically managed with anti-anxiety agents, methadone or clonidine (*Catapres*)
Sedative-Hypnotics: barbiturates, Equanil, Miltown, benzodiazepines, Ativan, Librium, Valium, Klonopin, Xanax	Mental impairment, confusion, nystagmus, and lack of motor coordination, ataxia, depression, dysarthria; frequently used by alternating with alcohol: which can lead to overdose	Weakness, insomnia, nausea postural hypotension develop within first 48 hours and last 5–7 days; seizures may occur at any time, especially within first few days; delirium may develop between the 3rd-7th days and last 3–5 days	Can be medical emergency; hospitalization required and pentobarbital or phenobarbital used to prevent precipitous withdrawal
Sleep Agents: Dalmane, Restoril, Halcion, Ativan	Can have paradoxical response, hyperactivity in elderly, children		

b) Cardiac: arrhythmias, myopathy, hypertension

c) GI: gastritis, cirrhosis, pancreatitis, hypoglycemia, ulcers, esophageal varices

d) Respiratory: COPD, pneumonia, cancer

e) Genitourinary system: fetal alcohol syndrome (there is no safe amount of alcohol in the pregnant women documented), decreased libido

f) Skin and skeletal: ulcers, spider angiomas, fractures

4) Psychological and social effects
   a) Erratic, impulsive, abusive behavior
   b) Poor judgment, loss of memory
   c) Family problems
   d) Depression, low self-esteem
   e) Suicide
   f) Job loss

b. Withdrawal
   1) Definition: physical manifestations developing 6–8 hours after abstinence from alcohol
   2) Manifestations (autonomic nervous system)
      a) Shakiness
      b) Anxiety
      c) Mood swings
      d) Insomnia
      e) Impaired appetite
      f) Some confusion
      g) Elevated vital signs

c. Delirium tremens (DTs)
   1) Definition: acute medical condition occurring usually 2–4 days after abstinence, potentially fatal
   2) Manifestations
      a) Confusion
      b) Disorientation
      c) Visual and auditory hallucinations
      d) Convulsions
      e) All manifestations of withdrawal

d. Treatment
   1) The best treatment for alcohol withdrawal is prevention or early detection and treatment
   2) Inpatient detoxification: 3–7 days; purpose is to medically manage withdrawal and prevent DTs

a) Antianxiety medications
b) Fluids and vitamins
c) Antidiarrheal medications
d) Symptomatic relief: analgesics, fluids, sleeping medications
e) Seizure precautions: anti-seizure medications, magnesium sulfate and sedation
f) Diet: high-protein, high-carbohydrate, low-fat
g) Decreased stimuli
h) Avoid restraints

3) DTs
a) Quiet moderately lit area
b) Decreased stimuli
c) Reality orientation

e. **NURSING INTERVENTIONS**
1) Administer medications and treatments as ordered
2) Observe for physical complications
3) Provide rest and nutrition
4) Observe for manifestations of depression and suicide
5) Provide firm limits
6) Be nonjudgmental
7) Monitor visitors
8) Assist in identifying use of defense mechanisms (denial)
9) Encourage rehabilitation programs and aftercare - for example: Alcoholics Anonymous (AA); alcoholism is characterized by periods of relapse and sobriety; prognosis: recovery not cure
10) Educate and support family; discuss support groups such as Al-Anon and Alateen

f. Aftercare
1) AA: 12-step program of sobriety
2) Disulfiram (*Antabuse*): medication used to prevent use of alcohol; aversion therapy
a) Sensitizes the client to alcohol
b) If alcohol is used, client suffers headache, vomiting, nausea, flushing, hypotension, tachycardia, dyspnea, chest pain, palpitations, confusion, respiratory and circulatory collapse, convulsions, death
c) Avoid drinking for 2 weeks after last dose
d) Warn client that alcohol is present in cough medicines, rubbing compounds, vinegars, aftershave lotions, and some mouthwashes

Substance Abuse

A. **Definition:** Substance abuse is the term used to designate the use of psychoactive drugs, including alcohol, to the extent of significant interference with the user's physical, social, and or emotional well-being. It is characterized by preoccupation with the drug and loss of control over its use. If the quantity and duration of abuse is sufficient, physical dependence may develop with tolerance and risk of a withdrawal syndrome when drug use is terminated. (see table II-12.)

B. **General characteristics**
1. Abuse vs. dependence
2. Effect on CNS depends on the type of substance
3. Psychological and social effects
   a. Isolation and withdrawal
   b. Family and work problems
   c. Loss of property
   d. Incarceration
4. Physical effects
   a. Endocarditis/AIDS
   b. Hepatitis B, C
   c. Pulmonary emboli
   d. Gangrene
   e. Malnutrition
   f. Trauma
   g. Psychosis

C. **Common drugs abused** (see table II-12.)

D. **Rehabilitation:** 30 days to 2 years; change lifestyle

E. **NURSING INTERVENTIONS**

1. Carry out medical regime
2. Observe for manifestations of withdrawal
3. Provide quiet, safe environment
4. Monitor visitors
5. Be nonjudgmental, accepting, firm attitude
6. Set limits
7. Monitor nutrition
8. Promote sleep
9. Refer for detoxification, rehabilitation, and aftercare
10. Support family in seeking help (Al-Anon)

SECTION VII

ORGANIC MENTAL DISORDERS

A. **Normal Aging**
1. Life-cycle changes
   a. Physical health
   b. Emotional: integrity, despair
   c. Intellectual changes
   d. Social changes such as retirement, widowhood

B. **Organic Mental Disorders** (OMD): psychological and behavioral problems resulting from organic conditions; may be reversible or irreversible

1. Delirium: acute brain syndrome; decreased attention and level of awareness; usually temporary and reversible; rapid onset; identifiable stressor
   a. Disturbance
      1) Disturbances in sleep and wakefulness
      2) Attention: easily distracted, illusions
      3) Restless and disoriented
      4) Difficulty concentrating
      5) Disorganized speech
   b. Causes
      1) Medical
      2) Surgical
      3) Pharmacological
      4) Neurological

2. Dementias
   a. Definition: sustained and often progressive intellectual impairment
   b. General manifestations
      1) Lingering
      2) Gradual, progressive
      3) Language disorders (for example: confabulation, blocking)
      4) Motor impairment (ataxia)
      5) Disintegrating personality and behavior
      6) Memory impairment (short term)
      7) Judgment impairment
      8) Thinking impairment (abstract)
      9) Degeneration (1–15 years post-onset)
   c. Types
      1) Wernicke-Korsakoff's syndrome (dementia associated with alcoholism)
         a) Memory (long or short term); impairment is predominant
         b) Confabulation
         c) Polyneuritis
         d) Flat affect
         e) Ataxia
         f) Confusion
         g) Learning impairment
      2) Alzheimer's disease (primary degenerative dementia)
         a) Onset: 45 years or older
         b) Gradually progressive and chronic
            (a) Orientation disturbance
            (b) Concentration decreases
            (c) Forget words
            (d) Denial
      3) Dementia
         a) Disorientation
         b) Anxiety, denial
         c) Delusions, hallucinations, paranoia
            d) Agitation
            e) Physical deterioration
      3) Multi-infarct dementia: difference from Alzheimer's is mainly its step-wise progression, rather than gradual decline; trauma induced (stroke, neurosurgery)

 3. **NURSING INTERVENTIONS:** allow as much independence as possible
   a. Manage physical manifestations
      1) Medical care: physical problems
      2) Adequate nutrition: provide finger foods, tolerate poor manners
      3) Exercise and rest: range of motion exercises, walks, naps, keep awake during the day
      4) Elimination: monitor intake and output, diet, limit fluids at bedtime, use stool softeners, toilet at regular intervals
   b. Assist client with activities of daily living
      1) Break down tasks into short simple steps
      2) Provide clear expectations
      3) Allow ample time
      4) Remain with client
      5) Assist with grooming and hygiene
      6) Matter of fact manner (avoid embarrassing client)
   c. Promote client safety (Evaluate and implement as needed)
   d. Optimize cognitive abilities
      1) Eliminate multiple stimuli
      2) Short, simple conversation (slow, distinct, soft voice)
      3) Consistency: establish routine, familiar caregivers
      4) Orient x 3
      5) Use visual cues such as pictures, labels, calendar, clock
   e. Provide opportunities for socialization
      1) Provide human contact
      2) Children
      3) Alternatives therapies
         a) Pet therapy
         b) Music therapy
         c) Reminiscence therapy
   f. Families
      1) Explain disorder
      2) Explain regression and provide activities such as photo albums, music, games
      3) Resources: Alzheimer's Disease and Related Disorders, Inc.
      4) Discuss need for family to obtain support, relief
      5) Counseling is necessary at times

It is important to remember that the basic principle underlying all care for the cognitively impaired is to facilitate the highest level of functionality possible while allowing as much independence as possible.

SECTION VIII

EATING DISORDERS

A. Anorexia/Bulimia
1. Definitions
   a. Anorexia: refusal to eat and relentless self-induced pursuit of thinness; up to 21% die
   b. Bulimia: binge-purge cycle of eating
2. Causes
   a. Adolescent struggle for independence and control
   b. Feelings of control are related to body
   c. Family problems: denial, conflict avoidance, enmeshment
   d. Society promotes thinness, dieting
3. Comparison (anorexia and bulimia) (see table II-13.)
   a. Obedient, bright, ambitious
   b. Perfectionist, type A personalities
   c. Low self-esteem
   d. Preoccupied with food
   e. Depression
   f. Manipulation
4. Effects
   a. Anorexia: holding in
      1) Skeletal muscle atrophy; emaciated, loss of fatty tissue
      2) Hypotension
      3) Constipation
      4) Susceptible to infections
      5) Blotchy, sallow skin
      6) Dryness and loss of hair
      7) Amenorrhea
      8) Electrolyte imbalance
      9) Cause of death: cardiac dysrhythmia; arrest
   b. Bulimia: letting go
      1) Electrolyte imbalance
      2) Dental caries
      3) Gingival infections, erosion of tooth enamel
      4) Susceptible to infections
      5) Bingeing
      6) Vomiting
      7) Use and abuse of laxatives and diuretics
5. **NURSING INTERVENTIONS**
   a. Recognize need for hospitalization
   b. Provide nutrition
      1) Monitor intake and output
      2) Vigilance 30–60 minutes after eating
      3) Help with relaxation prior to eating
      4) Enforce a behavior modification plan
      5) Positive reinforcement for weight gain
      6) Administer parenteral feedings as needed
   c. Teach coping skills
      1) Encourage recognition and verbalization of feelings
      2) Reinforce realistic perception of weight and appearance
      3) Acceptance of self-responsibility
      4) Limit setting and consistency
   d. Family
      1) Therapy
      2) Education
   e. Refer to self-help groups
      1) American Anorexia/Bulimia Association, Inc.
      2) Anorexia Nervosa and Associated Disorders (ANAD)

KEY INFORMATION

Recognize that many clients with eating disorders are extremely resistant to change, and progress may be slow. Remember the seriousness and life-threatening consequences of an eating disorder.

SECTION IX

DEVELOPMENTAL DISABILITIES

A. Definition: adaptive ability compromised by an alteration in the pattern or rate in stages of development during childhood: functional limitations in self-care, learning, mobility, self-direction, self-sufficiency in independent living; diagnosis based on IQ and socially adaptive behavior

B. Causes
1. Genetic
   a. Chromosomal
      1) Down's syndrome (trisomy 21): congenital mental retardation with motor involvement
      2) Klinefelter syndrome (XXY): gonadal defect with subnormal intelligence and social adaptation
   b. Errors of metabolism
      1) Phenylketonuria (PKU): accumulation of phenylalanine, which is toxic to the brain; retardation may be avoided by strict dietary avoidance of phenylalanine
      2) Tay-Sachs: inherited disorder of lipid metabolism causing mental retardation, blindness and muscle weakness
2. Acquired
   a. Prenatal: viruses, toxins

TABLE 11-13.
ANOREXIA/BULIMIA CONTRASTED

ANOREXIA	BULIMIA
- Younger (13 - 22)	- Older (20 – 30)
- Underweight	- Normal or slightly overweight
- Unable to maintain body weight at 85% of expected body weight	- Weight fluctuates considerably
- Introvert	- Extrovert
- Amenorrhea	- Amenorrhea
- Starvation	- Binge eating
- Don't admit abnormal eating patterns	- See patterns and fears loss of control
- Intense fear of becoming obese	- Hide food, hoard
- Prefers health foods	- Prefers high-calorie food
- Preoccupation with buying, planning, and preparing foods	- Repeated crash dieting, use of laxatives, diuretics, amphetamines
- Rigorous exercise	- Abuse of alcohol and/or drugs, petty crime, obsessive/compulsive disorder
- Electrolyte imbalance	- Electrolyte imbalance
- Still views self as overweight	- Aware that behavior is abnormal
- Cardiac arrhythmias	- Excessive dental caries-secondary to vomiting

b. Perinatal: anoxia, injury, prematurity
c. Post-natal: infections, poisons, trauma, deprivation

C. **Levels of Mental Retardation:** based on IQ level (normal range is 80–110)
1. Mild
   a. Social and communication skills
   b. Vocational skills, minimal self-support
   c. May be self-sufficient and independent as adult
   d. IQ range: 50–70
   e. Mental age of approximately 8 to 10 years
2. Moderate
   a. Can care for self
   b. Poor awareness of social conventions
   c. May learn to count
   d. May contribute to own support under close supervision
   e. IQ range: 35–49
   f. Mental age of approximately 5 to 6 years
3. Severe
   a. Poor motor and speech
   b. May learn simple work tasks

c. IQ range: 20–34
d. Mental age of a toddler
4. Profound
   a. Very limited, or no self-care ability
   b. IQ range: below 20
   c. Mental age of an infant

D. **Emotions:** client with a developmental disability has a full range of emotions and may be subjected to the full range of emotional illnesses

E. **NURSING INTERVENTIONS**
1. Know growth and development
2. Assess physical status
3. Denver development test
   a. Gross motor
   b. Language
   c. Fine motor
   d. Personal, social
4. Help parents with grieving; suggest parent support groups
5. Encourage early intervention programs
6. Encourage parents to get help and rest through respite care; make sure parents know all available resources (for example: medical, social, educational,

legal, community)
7. Prevention
   a. Health teaching such as nutrition, obstetrical care
   b. Immunizations
   c. Prenatal counseling and family planning
   d. Psychological needs

SECTION X

FAMILY VIOLENCE

(See also Unit IV, Section VI)

A. Definition: abuse of a violent physical or verbal nature within a family, which crosses socioeconomic, religious, racial, and cultural lines

B. Types of abuse
1. Physical: non-accidental use of force that results in injury, pain or impairment
2. Psychological: inflicting of mental anguish by threats, humiliation or fear
3. Sexual: any kind of non-consensual sexual contact
4. Neglect: failure of the caregiver to provide essential food, clothing, shelter or medical care. It may also include abandonment
5. Social: isolation
6. Material or financial (especially in elderly): may include theft or embezzlement of life savings

C. Abused Persons
1. Spouses
2. Children
3. Elderly

D. Risk Factors
1. Physical or cognitive impairment of the victim
2. Isolation of the victim
3. Caregiver stress
4. History of violence in the home
5. Pathology or mental incapacity of the abuser

E. Characteristics of Abuser
1. Low self-esteem
2. Substance abuser
3. Projects anger
4. Anxious
5. Depressed
6. Has come from an abusive household (victimization), was abused as child
7. Socially isolated
8. Impulsive, immature
9. Guilt ridden

F. Characteristics of Abused Persons
1. Adult victims often also were victims of child abuse
2. Accepts responsibility for others (co-dependency issues)
3. Helpless
4. Suicidal at times
5. Submissive
6. Frightened (may be harmed or killed)
7. Emotionally or physically dependent on abuser

G. General Manifestations of Abused Persons
1. Psychological manifestations
   a. Sleep disorders such as nightmares
   b. Headaches
   c. Anxiety or fear
   d. Depression
   e. Suicidal ideation
   f. Substance abuse
   g. Disruptive behavior at home, school, work
   h. Runaway behavior
   i. Frequent emergency room visits
   j. Anger or agitation
   k. Personality changes
   l. Hesitation to talk openly
   m. Withdrawal or resignation
2. Physical manifestations
   a. Unexplained fractures (especially spiral), bruises or burns
   b. Hunger and dehydration
   c. Poor hygiene
   d. Inappropriate dress
   e. Difficulty walking or sitting
   f. Missing essential aid items such as glasses, dentures, hearing aids
   g. Venereal disease or genital infection
   h. Repetitive hospital admissions or missed medical appointments
3. Financial manifestations (especially among elderly)
   a. Lack of knowledge about personal finances
   b. Reluctance to discuss finances
   c. Disparity between income and lifestyle
   d. Financial deprivation for essentials (for example: food, medical treatment, drugs, housing or clothing)
   e. Sudden withdrawals or closing of bank accounts

H. NURSING INTERVENTIONS

1. Be aware of the signs of abuse in children, spouses, and the elderly.
2. Recognize that many adult victims of abuse deny that it is occurring. They may be in denial due to isolation, shame or fear of reprisal.
3. Be ready to listen
4. Ask in detail about manifestations

TABLE II-14.
SIGNS OF ABUSE IN CHILDREN

TYPE	PHYSICAL	BEHAVIORAL
Physical abuse	- Multiple injuries and/or in various stages of healing - Unexplained bruises, burns, fractures or lacerations - Incongruence between explanation and injury - X-rays show numerous injuries	- Wary of strangers - Labile behavior - Depressed, frightened, stiff, rigid, distant, does not seek out parents
Physical neglect	- Appearance: poor hygiene and dress - Medical and physical problems unattended	- Fatigue - Withdrawal - Substance abuse
Sexual abuse	- Venereal disease - Pregnancy - Pain or itching in perineal area; difficulty walking or sitting	- Unusual sexual behavior or knowledge - Poor peer relations - Reports of sexual assault
Emotional abuse		- Decreased self-esteem - Lack of emotional response (no tears) - Hypochondriasis (vague complaints) - Slowed growth and development - Sleep disorders or neglect - Behavioral extremes - Delinquent (runs away)

5. Build trust
6. Be nonjudgmental
7. Offer the victim support in seeking help (for example: phone number of shelter)
8. Report suspected cases of child and elder abuse to the proper authorities (legal responsibility)
9. Encourage adult victims to file for an Order of Protection when appropriate
10. Assist to identify support system; identify resources for housing, money, legal aid, vocational counseling, crisis center for therapy

SECTION XI

RAPE

A. Characteristics
1. Crime of violence: force, penetration, lack of consent
2. Motives: power, anger, intimidation
3. Myths
   a. Provoked by victim's actions or mode of dress
   b. Victim promiscuous
   c. Women can avoid rape; cannot be raped against their will
   d. Rape is an impulsive act
   e. Elderly are not raped
   f. Women frequently get revenge by accusing men of rape
   g. Only women can be raped

B. Post-Traumatic Stress Disorder
1. Disorganization
2. Reorganization
3. Physical, emotional, and behavioral stress

C. NURSING INTERVENTIONS
1. Crisis intervention: "Rape Trauma Syndrome"
   a. Use empathetic, understanding approach
   b. Provide safe and secure environment
   c. Encourage verbalization about feelings
   d. Clarify what happened
   e. Offer support and reassurance
   f. Provide referrals for ongoing counseling
2. Emergency action
   a. Allow choices (loss of control)
   b. Get consent; offer comfort and provide privacy
   c. Take history "What occurred?" and allow client to verbalize feelings
   d. Physical examination: do not undress client until they agree, preferably after law enforcement has arrived
   e. Collect medical evidence (X-rays, specimens, photos) with assist of law enforcement authorities (must follow legal "chain of evidence" for future potential court action)
   f. Provide emotional support
   g. Medical follow-up for STDs, AIDS, VDRL
3. Help with psychological trauma
   a. Disrupted relationships

b. Phobias
c. Nightmares
d. Flashbacks
e. Family and sexual relations
f. Talking and working through feelings

SECTION XII

LEGAL ASPECTS OF PSYCHIATRIC NURSING

A. Types of Admissions
1. Voluntary
   a. Client admits him/herself
   b. Client consents to all treatment
   c. Client can refuse treatment, including drugs, unless danger to self or others
   d. Client can demand and receive discharge
2. Involuntary or judicial process
   a Initiated when someone files a petition
   b. Certification of the likelihood of serious harm to self or others, or unable to care for self
   c. At end of statutory time must be released, put on voluntary status, or have a hearing
3. If client is under 18, parents can confine with confirmation by a neutral fact finder

B. Judicial Precedents
1. Rights: unless incompetent, client maintains all previous rights
2. Right to treatment: efforts by staff consistent with medical knowledge
   a. Humane psychological and physical environment
   b. Qualified personnel and adequate nursing
   c. Individual treatment plan
3. Competency hearing

4. Least restrictive environment

C. Informed Consent Required
1. ECT
2. Medications
3. Seclusion
4. Restraint

D. Clients' Rights
1. Right to treatment (or to refuse treatment)
2. Access to stationery and postage
3. Access to unopened mail
4. Visits by primary care provider, attorney, clergy
5. Visits by other people (daily)
6. Keep personal possessions
7. Keep and spend money
8. Storage space for personal items
9. Telephone access
10. Hold property, vote, marry
11. Make wills, contracts
12. Educational resources
13. Sue, be sued
14. Challenge hospitalization

E. NURSING INTERVENTIONS: promote and provide care to the psychiatric client in the least restrictive environment

F. Insanity As A Defense
1. Insanity: determined in court; legal terminology
2. McNaughten rule: at the time of the crime, did the individual know the nature and quality of the act, or didn't know right from wrong?
3. Present
   a. Does client know right from wrong?
   b. Was client mentally ill at the time of the crime?
   c. Is client able to conform to the requirements of the law?
   d. Is the client able to assist in his or her defense?

WOMEN'S HEALTH NURSING

UNIT CONTENT

SECTION I.   Review of Female Reproductive Nursing 113
SECTION II.   Review of Labor and Delivery 118
SECTION III. Review of Postpartal Adaptations and Nursing Assessment 124
SECTION IV. Review of Reproductive Risks and Complications 125
SECTION V.   Nursing Care of the Neonate 128
SECTION VI. Review of High-Risk Newborn 130
SECTION VII. Nursing Care of the Gynecologic Client 131

SYMBOLS

 Key Points

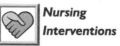 **Nursing Interventions**

Points to Remember

SECTION I

REVIEW OF FEMALE REPRODUCTIVE NURSING

Pregnancy

A. **Anatomy and Physiology of the Female Reproductive Tract**
1. External genitalia
   a. Mons pubis
   b. Labia majora
   c. Labia minora
   d. Clitoris
   e. Vestibule
      1) Urethral orifice
      2) Skene's glands
      3) Hymen and vaginal introitus
      4) Bartholin's glands
   f. Perineum
2. Internal genitalia
   a. Fallopian tubes
   b. Uterus
      1) Fundus
      2) Cervix
   c. Vagina
   d. Ovaries

B. **Fertilization and Fetal Development**
1. Conception (fertilization)
   a. Definition: union of sperm and ovum
   b. Conditions necessary for fertilization
      1) Maturity of egg and sperm
      2) Timing of deposit of sperm
         a) Lifetime of ovum is 24 hours
         b) Lifetime of sperm in the female genital tract is 72 hours
         c) Ideal time for fertilization is 48 hours before to 24 hours after ovulation
         d) Menstruation begins approximately 14 days after ovulation
      3) Climate of the female genital tract
         a) Vaginal and cervical secretions are less acidic during ovulation (sperm cannot survive in a highly acidic environment)
         b) Cervical secretions are thinner during ovulation (sperm can penetrate more easily)
   c. Process of fertilization (7–10 days)
      1) Ovulation occurs

2) Ovum travels to fallopian tube
3) Sperm travel to fallopian tube
4) One sperm penetrates the ovum
5) Zygote forms (fertilized egg)
6) Zygote migrates to uterus
7) Zygote implants in uterine wall
8) Progesterone and estrogen are secreted by the corpus luteum to maintain the lining of the uterus and prevent menstruation until placenta starts producing these hormones; (note: progesterone is a thermogenic hormone that raises body temperature, an objective sign that ovulation has occurred)
   d. Placental development
      1) Chorionic villi develop that secrete Human Chorionic Gonadotropin (HCG), which stimulates production of estrogen and progesterone from the corpus luteum (production of HCG begins on the day of implantation and can be detected by the sixth day)
      2) Chorionic villi burrow into endometrium, forming the placenta
      3) The placenta secretes HCG, human placental lactogen (HPL), and (by week three) estrogen and progesterone
   e. Fetal membranes develop and surround the embryo, fetus
      1) Amnion: inner membrane
      2) Chorion: outer membrane
      3) Umbilical cord
         a) Two arteries carrying deoxygenated blood to placenta
         b) One vein carrying oxygenated blood to fetus
         c) No pain receptors
         d) Encased in Wharton's jelly
         e) Covered by chorionic membrane
   f. Amniotic fluid
      1) Production origins
         a) Maternal serum during early pregnancy
         b) Fetal urine in greater proportion during latter part of pregnancy
         c) Replaced every 3 hours
         d) 800–1,200 mL at end of pregnancy
      2) Functions
         a) Protection from trauma and heat loss
         b) Facilitates musculoskeletal development by allowing for movement of the fetus

c) Facilitates symmetric growth and development
d) Source of oral fluid for fetus
g. Placental transfer of material to and from the fetus
1) Diffusion across membrane (for example: gases, water, electrolytes)
2) Active transport via enzyme activity (for example: glucose, amino acids, calcium, iron)
3) Pinocytosis: minute particles engulfed and carried across the cell (for example: fats)
4) Leakage: small defects in the chorionic villi cause slight mixing of material and fetal blood cells
5) Nutrients and wastes are exchanged in the placenta, but the blood does not intermingle

C. Fetal Development
1. Pre-embryonic: first two weeks
2. Embryonic: three to seven weeks
3. Fetal: eight to 40 weeks
   a. Full term: 38 to 42 weeks
   b. Preterm: less than 38 weeks
   c. Post-term: more than 42 weeks

D. Terminology
1. Gravida
   a. Definition: number of times pregnant, including present pregnancy
   b. Variations: primigravida, multigravida
2. Para
   a. Definition: number of pregnancies delivered after the age of viability, whether born alive or dead
   b. Variations: nullipara, primipara, multipara
3. Five-digit system
   a. G: gravida
   b. T: term infants
   c. P: preterm
   d. A: abortions
   e. L: living

Signs of Pregnancy

A. Presumptive (subjective)
1. Amenorrhea: missed periods
2. Nausea and vomiting: morning sickness, probably due to HCG; usually lasts about 3 months
3. Fatigue: first trimester
4. Urinary frequency: caused by enlarging uterus pressing on bladder
5. Breast changes: tenderness and tingling, nipples pronounced, full feeling, increased size, areola darker
6. Quickening: mother's perception of fetal movement around 16–18 weeks; fluttering sensation

B. Probable (objective)
1. Chadwick's sign: bluish coloration of the mucous membranes of the cervix, vagina, and vulva
2. Goodell's sign: softening of cervix; occurs beginning of the third month
3. Hegar's sign: softening of the isthmus of the uterus, between the body of the uterus and cervix; occurs about the sixth week
4. Enlargement of abdomen: uterus just above symphysis at 8–10 weeks; at umbilicus at 20–22 weeks
5. Braxton-Hicks contractions: painless contractions occurring at irregular periods throughout pregnancy; felt most commonly after 28 weeks
6. Uterine souffle: soft blowing sound; blood flow to placenta same rate as maternal pulse
7. Pregnancy test positive: HCG in serum and urine
8. Ballottement: can push fetus and feel it rebound
9. Pigmentation changes: increased pigmentation, chloasma, linea nigra, and striae gravidarum

C. Positive
1. Fetal heartbeat: by Doppler at 8–10 weeks
2. Fetal movements: felt by examiner
3. Fetal outline: on sonogram

Assessment of Date of Delivery

A. Nagele's rule: first day of last menstrual period (LMP) minus three months plus seven days; in most cases, add one year

B. Other parameters: fundal heights, quickening, sonograms

Physical Adaptations and Discomforts of Pregnancy

See Table III-1.

Teratogenic Effects on Fetal Development

A. Teratogen
1. Definition: nongenetic factor producing malformations of the fetus; greatest effect on those cells undergoing rapid growth, thus time is important
2. Types
   a. Chemical agents (for example: insecticides)

TABLE III-1.
ADAPTATIONS TO PREGNANCY

ADAPTATIONS TO PREGNANCY	TRIMESTER	INTERVENTIONS
G.I:		
- Nausea/vomiting	I	- Small frequent meals; eat crackers or dry toast before getting up in the morning; eat dry meals; drink liquids between meals
- Constipation, flatulence and heartburn	2, 3	- Exercise; increase fluid and fiber in diet; stool softeners if recommended by physician
- Bleeding gums	2, 3	- Use soft toothbrush for dental care
- Gallstones	2, 3	- Avoid fatty foods
- Heartburn	2, 3	- Small frequent meals; avoid spicy, fatty foods; no sodium bicarbonate as antacid; antacids as recommended by physician
Urinary Tract:		
- Frequency during first and third trimester due to pressure on bladder	I, 3	- Void when first urge felt; wear a pad if leaking
- Glomerular filtration rate (GFR) increases (glycosuria)		
- Increase in urinary infections	2, 3	- Increase fluid intake
Breasts:		
- Increase in size and nodularity, striae	I	
- Tenderness and tingling	I	- Wear good supportive bra
- Hypertrophy of Montgomery tubercles	2	
- Darkening of areola	2	
- Colostrum secreted	2, 3	
Vagina:		
- Epithelium undergoes hypertrophy and hyperplasia		
- Increased vascularity		
- Increased pH; good for growth of Candida (thrush)	I, 2, 3	- Report itching and burning to physician
- Increase in discharge; leukorrhea is common	I	- Promote cleanliness by bathing daily; avoid douching; avoid nylon undergarments
Respiratory System:		
- Increase in volume of up to 40–50% between 16–34th week		
- Diaphragm is pushed upward; ribcage flares out; breathing changes from abdominal to chest		
- Increase in oxygen consumption by 15%		

TABLE III-1.
ADAPTATIONS TO PREGNANCY (CONTINUED)

ADAPTATIONS TO PREGNANCY	TRIMESTER	INTERVENTIONS
Respiratory System (continued): - Stuffiness, epistaxis, and changes in voice occur as a result of increased estrogen levels	I	- Cool moist air may help; avoid over-the-counter decongestants and sprays
- Dyspnea	3	- Proper posture; sleep with head propped up
Skin: - Areola darkens - Abdominal striae, linea nigra - Diaphoresis - Chloasma: mask of pregnancy - Vascular spider nervi; chest, neck, arms, and legs	2, 3	Daily bathing; powder

Metabolism/Nutrition:
- Basal metabolic rate increased by 20%
 	
- Water retention: edema
 	
- Weight gain: 20–25 lbs. recommended
  - Adequate protein intake, especially for teens
  - Increase iron during last eight weeks
 	
- Pica: craving for nonnutritive substances
	2, 3
	
	2, 3
		- Elevate legs and feet when sitting; avoid prolonged standing; do not wear garters or clothing with restrictive bands around the legs; avoid crossing legs at knees
		
		- Eat well-balanced diet

Perineum: - Increased vascularity - Venous congestion of the perineum	2, 3	Kegel exercises
Cardiovascular: - Cardiac output increases by 30% - Blood volume progressively increases and peaks around 30–40 weeks at 47% above pre-pregnant state - Plasma volume increases greater than RBC and hemoglobin, resulting in "pseudo anemia" - Pulse rate increases by 10–15 beats/minute; BP drops slightly in second trimester due to peripheral dilatation effects of progesterone; returns to normal by third trimester		

TABLE III-1.
ADAPTATIONS TO PREGNANCY (CONTINUED)

ADAPTATIONS TO PREGNANCY	TRIMESTER	INTERVENTIONS
Cardiovascular (continued): - Varicose veins may develop	2, 3	Elevate legs; avoid standing for long periods of time; avoid constrictive clothing
Uterus: - Growth is influenced by estrogen - 500–1,000-fold increase in capacity - Cervical secretions form mucus plug		
Endocrine: - Increase in size and activity of thyroid - Increase in size and activity of anterior lobe of pituitary - Increase in size and activity of adrenal cortex - Increase in production of relaxin causes joint and back pain	2, 3	Pelvic rock; good body mechanics; supportive shoes

b. Radiation

c. Drugs: for example: alcohol, tetracycline (*Sumycin*), chemotherapeutic agents, phenytoin (*Dilantin*), narcotics, nicotine, megavitamins, warfarin (*Coumadin*), lead, lithium, carbamazepine (*Tegretol*), and mercury

d. Bacteria and viruses
1) Syphilis
   a) Spirochete does not cross placenta until after 18th week; treat as soon as possible; can treat later since penicillin does not cross placenta
   b) Can cause late abortions, stillbirths, and congenitally infected infants
2) Gonorrhea: causes injury to eyes at birth (ophthalmia neonatorum)
3) T.O.R.C.H.– severe effects on the fetus
   a) Toxoplasmosis: protozoan contracted by ingesting raw meat or feces of infected animal (for example: cats); pregnant women should not change cat litter boxes
   b) Rubella: first trimester most serious; causes congenital heart problems, cataracts, hearing loss; clients cannot receive the rubella vaccine during pregnancy as it is a live virus; if they receive the immunization in the postpartum period, they must understand that they should not become pregnant for at least three months
   c) Cytomegalovirus (CMV): member of the herpes family; causes congenital and acquired infection; principal organs affected: liver, brain, and blood
   d) Herpes simplex virus, Type 2 (HSV-2)
      (1) Transmitted to infant vaginally in intrauterine cavity or during delivery; do not deliver vaginally if active lesions are present
      (2) Affects blood, brain, liver, lungs, CNS, eyes, skin
      (3) Perinatal mortality: 96%; 50% of survivors have neurological or visual abnormalities
4) Chlamydia: causes conjunctivitis and pneumonia in the newborn
5) AIDS
   a) Transmitted via breast milk
   b) 30% chance of transmission in utero or during delivery
   c) Treatment of mother with zidovudine (*AZT*) while pregnant can reduce chance of transmission to fetus to approximately 8%

Emotional and Psychological Adaptations to Pregnancy

A. Stressors
1. Circumstances of pregnancy
2. Meaning of pregnancy to the couple
3. Responsibilities associated with parenthood
4. Resources available to family

B. Development Tasks of Pregnancy
1. First trimester: accept the biological fact of pregnancy; it is common to feel ambivalent early in pregnancy
2. Second trimester: accept growing fetus as a baby to be nurtured
3. Third trimester: prepare for the birth and parenting of the child

C. Emotional Responses
1. Self-concept related to body image
2. Mood swings related to biophysical and social changes
3. Ambivalence related to fear and anxiety
4. Sexual concerns related to biophysical changes

Prenatal Care

A. Assessment
1. Complete history
2. Lab work: complete blood count (CBC), blood type and Rh, Rubella, VDRL/FTA-ABS/RPR, hepatitis B surface antigen, HIV antibody (with client's consent), alpha fetal protein (AFP)
3. Vital signs, weight, urine test for protein and glucose
4. Physical exam: fundal height, fetal heart rate (FHR), fetal activity
5. Internal exam
   a. Adequate pelvic outlet, signs of pregnancy (First visit)
   b. Cervical changes, especially in last weeks (for example: "ripe cervix")
   c. Vaginal smear for Neisseria gonorrhea, chlamydia, group B strep, human papillovirus (HPV) cultures, and pap test
6. Psychosocial assessment

B. Health Teaching
1. Nutrition
2. Discomforts
3. Danger signs (The nurse must be able to differentiate potential complications from the normal discomforts or physical adaptations of pregnancy)
   a. Bleeding
   b. Rupture of membranes (ROM)
   c. Contractions (Braxton-Hicks contractions

usually go away when position is changed)
   d. Signs of pregnancy induced hypertension (PIH), toxemia
      1) Edema of hands and face, sudden weight gain
      2) Headache, blurred of vision, spots before eyes, dizziness
      3) Decrease in urinary output
   e. Burning on urination
   f. Fever
   g. Significant decrease in fetal activity
4. Childbirth education and alternative methods of birth
   a. Read method (Grantly Dick-Read)
      1) Natural childbirth
      2) Abdominal breathing
      3) Fear-tension-pain cycle
   b. Lamaze method
      1) Prepared childbirth
      2) Labor coach
      3) Chest breathing
   c. Leboyer
      1) Birth without violence
      2) Concerned with possible negative effect a traumatic birth can have upon an infant
   d. Birthing chairs
   e. Alternate positions
   f. Birthing rooms
   g. Birthing centers
   h. Delivery by midwife
   i. Home births
5. Rest and exercise

C. Ethical Issues
1. Rights of fetus
2. Fetal tissue or organs for transplants
3. In vitro fertilization
4. Fertility drugs (multiple pregnancy)
5. Intrauterine surgery

SECTION II

REVIEW OF LABOR AND DELIVERY

Components of Labor

A. Power (Uterine Contractions)
1. Frequency: from the beginning of one contraction to the beginning of the next contraction
2. Duration: from the beginning of one contraction to the end of that same contraction
3. Intensity: strength of contraction, measured with fingertips lightly on the fundus (mild, moderate, and strong); accurate measurement can only be made with an internal monitor

4. Regularity: establish a pattern that increases in frequency and duration
5. Effacement: thinning of cervix, 0–100%
6. Dilatation: opening of cervix, 0–10 cms

B. Passenger (Fetus)
1. Lie: relationship of the cephalocaudal axis of the infant to the cephalocaudal axis of the mother
   a. Transverse lie
   b. Longitudinal lie
2. Presentation: body part of the passenger that enters the pelvic passageway first is called the "presenting part"
   a. Cephalic
      1) Vertex: occiput (most common)
      2) Brow: sinciput
      3) Face: mentum
   b. Breech
      1) Complete: sacrum
      2) Frank
      3) Footling
   c. Shoulder
3. Position: relationship of the landmark on the presenting fetal part to the front, sides, and back of the maternal pelvis
   a. Pelvis is divided into six areas anterior, transverse, or posterior; left or right side
   b. Fetal landmarks are: occiput (O), mentum (M), sacrum (S), and scapula (Sc)
   c. Most common is left occiput anterior (LOA)
4. Attitude or habitus: to the relationship of the fetal parts to one another, usual is "fetal position"
5. Station: the relationship between the presenting part and the ischial spines; O-station is engagement
6. Cardinal movements of descent
   a. Descent
   b. Flexion
   c. Internal rotation
   d. Extension
   e. External rotation or restitution

C. Passageway (Maternal Pelvis)
1. False pelvis helps support pregnant uterus
2. True pelvis forms bony canal; inlet, pelvic cavity, outlet
3. Types
   a. Gynecoid: normal female (50%), best for delivery
   b. Android: normal male (20%), not favorable
   c. Platypelloid: flat female pelvis (5%), not favorable
   d. Anthropoid: apelike (25%), favorable
4. Cephalo-pelvic disproportion (CPD)

D. Psyche
1. Physical preparation for childbirth
2. Cultural heritage
3. Previous experience
4. Support systems
5. Self-esteem

Fetal Assessment

A. Sonogram
1. Purpose
   a. Locate placenta
   b. Diagnose multiple pregnancy
   c. Identify some congenital anomalies
   d. Determine gestational age
2. **NURSING INTERVENTIONS**
   a. Assure that client has a full bladder
   b. Provide client education

B. Fetal Monitoring
1. Purpose
   a. Determine fetal heart rate (FHR): normal is 110–160 BPM
   b. Recognize periodic changes in FHR
   c. Determine frequency and duration of contractions
2. Types
   a. Auscultation with fetoscope; palpation
   b. External electronic monitoring
   c. Internal electronic monitoring
      1) Provides actual intrauterine pressures
      2) Provides beat-to-beat variability of the FHR, which is an indication of the sympathetic and parasympathetic nervous system status
3. Periodic changes
   a. Early decelerations: head compression
   b. Variable decelerations: cord compression
   c. Late decelerations: uteroplacental insufficiency
   d. Accelerations: usually a sign of fetal well-being
4. Variability
   a. Long-term
   b. Short-term

C. Non-Stress Test (NST)
1. Purpose
   a. Assess fetal well-being
   b. Look for increase in FHR (accelerations) with fetal activity (reactive NST)
2. A non-reactive, non-stress test is NOT reassuring

D. Contraction Stress Test
1. Types
   a. Oxytocin challenge test (OCT)

b. Nipple stimulation test
2. Purpose
   a. Look for three contractions in 10 minutes
   b. No late decelerations determines fetal well-being
3. A negative CST IS reassuring

E. Biophysical Profile
1. Purpose
   a. Determine fetal well-being after questionable NST
   b. Determine amount of amniotic fluid
 2. **NURSING INTERVENTIONS**
   a. Provide client education
   b. Provide emotional support

F. Amniocentesis (performed after 16th week)
1. Purpose
   a. Determine fetal anomalies, sex, fetal maturity
   b. Determine lecithin-sphingomyelin (L/S) ratio, bilirubin levels, creatine levels
2. **NURSING INTERVENTIONS**
   a. Provide client education

b. Assess for premature labor, hemorrhaging
c. Provide RhoGAM for Rh negative client

G. Chorionic Villi Sampling
1. Purpose
   a. Determine fetal anomalies, genetic defects
   b. Early test: 8–10 weeks
2. **NURSING INTERVENTIONS**
   a. Provide client education
   b. Provide RhoGAM for Rh negative client

Signs of Impending Labor

A. Lightening → *babies dropped, relieved*

B. Braxton-Hicks Contractions → *up walking stops, getting ready for childbirth*

C. Weight Loss (one to three pounds)

D. Cervical Changes → *dilate + effaced*

E. Increase in Back Discomfort → *hands + knees and rock back + forth*

TABLE III-2.
STAGES OF LABOR

STAGES	CHARACTERISTICS	INTERVENTIONS
- First Stage: "stage of dilatation") begins true labor; ends with complete cervical dilatation; composed of of three phases	- Duration: *1st pregnancy* primigravida 3.3–19.7 hours; multigravida 0.1–14.3 hours	- Admission; assessment: medical and OB history, vital signs, FHRs, signs of labor, weight, vaginal exam (if no active vaginal bleeding)
- Latent phase	- 0–4 cm dilatation; mild to moderate contractions q 15–20 min, lasting 10–30 seconds; backache, cramping, bloody show; mother talkative, cheerful, anxious	- Diversional activities; time contractions; assess maternal-fetal status; pelvic rock; promote hydration; use breathing patterns; evaluate labor progress
- Active phase	- 5–7 cm dilatation; strong contractions q 3–5 minutes, lasting 30–60 seconds *Pt voiding, proper diurises if bladder is full*	- Assess maternal-fetal status; backrubs; comfort measures; mother may feel apprehensive; provide encouragement; provide analgesia or anesthesia if requested and is appropriate; promote hydration and elimination; keep perineum clean; promote rest between contractions; evaluate labor progress
- Transitional phase *(the gitters prob to have a baby)*	- 8–10 cm dilatation; strong contractions of 2–3 min, lasting 50–90 seconds; legs may cramp; nausea/vomiting, perspiration on forehead and upper lip; dark, profuse bloody show; mother may have amnesia between contractions, is irritable, anxious, and self-oriented	- Assess maternal-fetal status; provide much reassurance; provide comfort measures; pant/blow with pushing urges; be supportive and help mother maintain control with breathing; evaluate labor progress *3–20 hr*

completely dilated 10 and effaced

TABLE III-2.
STAGES OF LABOR (CONTINUED)

STAGES	CHARACTERISTICS	INTERVENTIONS
- **Second stage:** ("stage of delivery") begins with complete dilatation of the cervix and ends with delivery	- Duration: primigravida .3–1.9 hrs; multigravida .9–.69 hours; contractions 2–3 minutes, lasting 50–90 seconds; client has urge to push and is exhausted	- Assess maternal-fetal status; coach pushing; promote comfort; record time of delivery, episiotomy/lacerations, medications, or anesthetics; evaluate labor progress
- **Third stage:** ("placental stage") begins with delivery of infant; ends with delivery of placenta	- Mild contractions continue until placenta expelled, normally within 30 minutes; client may have to push to help expel placenta	- Assess maternal status, blood loss; note time of placenta delivery; administer an oxytocic after placenta separation, if ordered; promote bonding
- **Fourth stage:** ("stage of recovery") the first hour after delivery or until stable	- Cramping uterine discomfort; rubra vaginal discharge with small clots; discomfort if episiotomy done; client feels happy, relieved, excited	- Assess vital signs (BP, P and R) fundus, lochia, bladder and perineum q 15 min. for 1st hr., q 30 min. second hr.; temp. x1; encourage hydration and elimination; promote comfort; ice to perineum if painful; promote bonding

normal blood loss 500cc
for contractions uterus closed

F. Bloody Show → *mucous plug is coming out of the cervix*

G. Rupture of Membranes → *baby to deliver*
   1. Client should contact primary care provider
   2. **NURSING INTERVENTIONS**
      a. Monitor FHR
      b. Check for prolapsed cord
      c. Test vaginal secretions for alkalinity with Nitrazine paper → *blue*
      d. Watch for signs of infection/meconium → *baby poo!*

H. Sudden Burst of Energy

Stages of Labor

Analgesia in Labor

It is important to make nursing assessments of the mother, fetus, and labor status before administering analgesia in labor. Given too early, analgesia can slow down labor. Given too close to delivery, analgesia can result in respiratory depression of the newborn. Ideally, active labor (at least 4 cm) should be established before analgesics are administered.

TABLE III-3.
MEDICATIONS USED IN LABOR AND DELIVERY

NAME: GENERIC (TRADE)	USE
1. Oxytocin (Pitocin)	- Induces labor, stimulates labor, or contracts uterus after delivery
2. Methylergonovine maleate (Methergine)	- Contracts uterus after delivery *don't give for inducing labor*
3. Ritodrine hydrochloride (Yutopar)	- Treats premature labor *stops contractions*
4. Terbutaline sulfate (Brethine)	- Treats premature labor *relaxes smooth muscle*
5. Hydralazine hydrochloride (Apresoline)	- Treats high blood pressure
6. Magnesium sulfate (Epsom Salt)	- Controls convulsions when used with PIH; treats premature labor
7. Calcium gluconate (generic only)	- Antidote for magnesium sulfate toxicity
8. Rh(D)immune globulin (RhoGAM)	- Prevents sensitization of Rh⁻ mother carrying Rh⁺ fetus
9. Naloxone HCl (Narcan)	- Treats respiratory depression
10. Betamethasone (Celestone)	- Stimulates lung development in premature infant *steroid*
11. Prostaglandin E₂ gel (Prepidil)	- Softens and thins cervix

TABLE III-4.
ANALGESIA/ANESTHESIA FOR LABOR AND DELIVERY

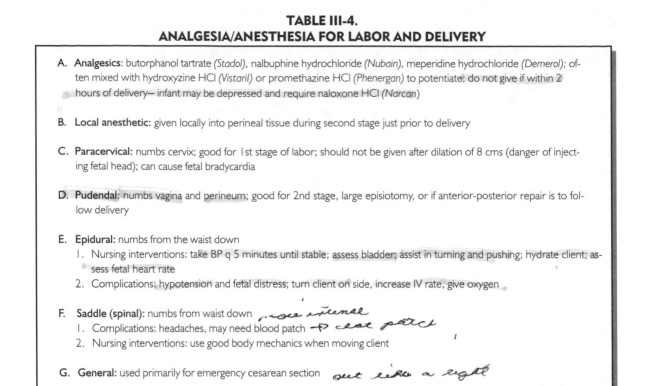

A. **Analgesics**: butorphanol tartrate *(Stadol)*, nalbuphine hydrochloride *(Nubain)*, meperidine hydrochloride *(Demerol)*; often mixed with hydroxyzine HCl *(Vistaril)* or promethazine HCl *(Phenergan)* to potentiate; do not give if within 2 hours of delivery— infant may be depressed and require naloxone HCl *(Narcan)*

B. **Local anesthetic**: given locally into perineal tissue during second stage just prior to delivery

C. **Paracervical**: numbs cervix; good for 1st stage of labor; should not be given after dilation of 8 cms (danger of injecting fetal head); can cause fetal bradycardia

D. **Pudendal**: numbs vagina and perineum; good for 2nd stage, large episiotomy, or if anterior-posterior repair is to follow delivery

E. **Epidural**: numbs from the waist down
   1. Nursing interventions: take BP q 5 minutes until stable; assess bladder; assist in turning and pushing; hydrate client; assess fetal heart rate
   2. Complications: hypotension and fetal distress; turn client on side, increase IV rate, give oxygen

F. **Saddle (spinal)**: numbs from waist down
   1. Complications: headaches, may need blood patch
   2. Nursing interventions: use good body mechanics when moving client

G. **General**: used primarily for emergency cesarean section

Complications During Labor and Delivery

A. Fetal Distress
1. Etiology
   a. Uteroplacental insufficiency
      1) Acute uteroplacental insufficiency
         a) Excessive uterine activity associated with oxytocin *(Pitocin)*
         b) Maternal hypotension: epidural, venacaval compression, supine position, internal hemorrhage
         c) Placental separation: abruptio, previa
      2) Chronic uteroplacental insufficiency
         a) PIH
         b) Diabetes
         c) Postmaturity
   b. **NURSING INTERVENTIONS**
      1) Position client on left side
      2) Start IV or increase rate
      3) Administer oxygen
      4) Notify primary care provider
      5) Monitor FHR continuously

B. PROM (Premature Rupture of Membrane)
1. Etiology
   a. Infection
   b. Trauma
2. **NURSING INTERVENTIONS**
   a. Assess FHR
   b. Assess for infection
   c. Assess for prolapsed cord

C. Umbilical Cord Compression
1. Etiology
   a. Prolapsed cord
      1) Causes: abnormal presentation, inadequate pelvis, presenting part at high station, multiple gestation, prematurity, PROM, polyhydramnios
      2) Complications: fetal asphyxia
      3) **NURSING INTERVENTIONS**
         a) Keep hand in vagina; push presenting part away from cord
         b) Continuously assess fetal welfare by pulsation of the cord
         c) Place client in Trendelenburg or knee-chest position
         d) Prepare for c-section; type and cross match blood; start IV; obtain consent
   b. Nuchal cord (cord around neck)

D. Premature Labor
1. Etiology
   a. Chronic pyelonephritis
   b. Incompetent cervix
   c. Multiple pregnancy
   d. History of premature births
   e. Sepsis
   f. Placental disorders
2. **NURSING INTERVENTIONS**

a. Place client on bed rest

b. Assess for signs of infection; monitor vital signs, FHR

c. Administer ritodrine HCl (*Yutopar*), terbutaline (*Brethine*) or magnesium sulfate as ordered to stop premature labor

d. Provide emotional support

e. Administer betamethasone (*Celestone*) to promote fetal lung development

f. Delivery if near term

e. trauma

E. Emergency Childbirth

1. Have mother pant, unless breech

2. Support perineum

3. If membranes not ruptured, do so

4. Feel for cord around infant's neck; gently slip over head

5. Clear out mucous; keep infant dry and warm

6. Do not cut cord

7. Deliver placenta: expect gush of blood and lengthening of cord; save placenta

8. Massage client's uterus to shrink it; place infant on client's breast

F. Amniotic Fluid Emboli

1. Definition: amniotic fluid in blood stream

2. Often happens at delivery

3. Emergency situation, often fatal

no long LABOR

G. Dystocia

1. Definition: prolonged, difficult labor

2. Etiology

a. Dysfunction of uterine contractions

b. Abnormal position

c. Cephalopelvic disproportion (CPD)

d. Maternal exhaustion

3. **NURSING INTERVENTIONS**

a. Depends upon cause

b. Can vary from rest to c-section

Operative Obstetrics

A. Episiotomy

1. Definition: incision made into the perineum during delivery

2. Purpose

a. To spare muscles from overstretching/lacerations; to avoid difficulty holding urine in later life

b. Limit pressure on infant's head

3. **NURSING INTERVENTIONS**

a. Assess for healing, infection, laceration of the anal sphincter (4th degree tear), hemorrhage

b. Teach Kegel exercises

B. Forceps

1. Definition: obstetric instrument used to aid in delivery

2. Indications

a. Poor progress

b. Fetal distress

c. Persistent occiput posterior position

d. Exhaustion (maternal)

3. **NURSING INTERVENTIONS**

a. Assess infant for intracranial hemorrhage, facial bruising, facial palsy

b. Assist with delivery as needed

c. Check FHR before traction is applied

4. Complications

a. Lacerations to cervix or vagina

b. Rupture of the uterus

c. Compression of cord

C. Vacuum Extraction

1. Definition: an OB procedure using a suction cup to aid in delivery

2. Indications

a. Poor progress

b. Fetal distress

c. Occiput posterior/occiput transverse position

d. Exhaustion (maternal)

3. **NURSING INTERVENTIONS**

a. Assess FHR every 5 minutes

b. Assess for cerebral trauma

c. Inform parents that caput will disappear in a few hours

D. Cesarean Section (c-section)

1. Definition: incision into abdominal wall and uterus to deliver fetus

2. Types

bikini Line

a. Low transverse: decrease chance of uterine rupture with future pregnancies; less bleeding after delivery

b. Classical: good for emergency delivery; provides more room

3. Indications

a. Fetal distress

b. Cephalo-pelvic disproportion (CPD)

c. Placenta previa, abruptio

d. Uterine dysfunction

e. Prolapsed cord

f. Diabetes   *babies big*

g. Toxemia   *mother's having PIH*

h. Malpresentation

4. **NURSING INTERVENTIONS**

a. Postoperative assessment

b. Postpartum assessment

5. Vaginal birth after c-section (VBAC): current accepted standard of care

E. Induction of Labor

1. Definition: process of initiating labor
2. Indications
   a. Maternal disease: cardiac, PIH
   b. Placental malfunctions (example: partial previa)
   c. Fetal conditions (for example: anomaly, death)
   d. Post maturity
3. Methods used to soften cervix
   a. Prostaglandin E_2 gel
   b. Laminaria (natural cervical dilation, made from seaweed; left in place 6-12 hours): be alert for contraindications such as asthma, nonreassuring FHR, pelvic infection, ROM, vaginal bleeding
4. Methods used to initiate induction
   a. Oxytocin (*Pitocin*)
   b. Rupture of membranes (ROM) (amniotomy)

5. **NURSING INTERVENTIONS**
   a. Assessment of FHR
   b. Assess for prolapsed cord, ruptured uterus
   c. Stop oxytocin (*Pitocin*) if contraction lasts longer than 90 seconds or at signs of fetal distress

SECTION III

REVIEW OF POSTPARTAL ADAPTATIONS AND NURSING ASSESSMENT

A. Physical Assessment

1. Fundus
2. Lochia
3. Breasts
4. Episiotomy
5. Bowels/hemorrhoids
6. Bladder
7. Signs of infection
8. Homan's Sign

B. Puerperium

1. Definition: period of time during which the body adjusts and returns to a near pre-pregnancy state; usually lasts six weeks, can last up to one year
2. Uterus (involution)
   a. Fundus is at umbilicus after delivery; 1 fingerbreadth above umbilicus 12 hours after delivery; decreases 1 fingerbreadth a day; by 10th day, is at symphysis pubis
   b. Fundus involutes faster if client breast feeds infant
3. Lochia
   a. Definition: vaginal discharge following delivery

   b. Color
      1) Rubra (1–3 days)
      2) Serosa (3–10 days)
      3) Alba (3–6 weeks)
   c. Odor: if foul smelling, may indicate infection
   d. Amount: moderate at first, will increase with activity
   e. Afterpains: due to involution of uterus; more severe with multiple births (example: twins), polyhydramnios; administration of oxytocin, breastfeeding
   f. Menstruation: resumes in about 6–8 weeks in non-nursing mothers; and can vary with nursing mothers
4. Breasts
   a. Engorgement
      1) Non breast feeding: don't stimulate
         a) Ice
         b) Supportive bra
         c) Pain meds
      2) Breast feeding
         a) Frequent hot showers
         b) Frequent feedings
         c) Massage
5. Perineum
   a. Episiotomy or laceration
      1) Edema
      2) Pain
   b. **NURSING INTERVENTIONS**
      1) Sitz baths
      2) Sprays or ointments
      3) Kegel exercises
6. Gastrointestinal
   a. Sluggish bowels
   b. Increased appetite
   c. Hemorrhoids
   d. **NURSING INTERVENTIONS**
      1) Administer stool softeners
      2) Instruct client to increase dietary fiber and fluids
      3) Suggest sitz baths, witch hazel pads for comfort
7. Urinary tract
   a. Lessened sensation of bladder fullness
   b. Urinary retention
   c. Difficulty urinating
8. Temperature
   a. First 24 hours, there can be an increase up to 100.4°F due to dehydration; exhaustion
   b. WBC normally elevated
9. Skin diaphoresis
   a. Diuresis
   b. Night sweats
   c. Increased output

10. Postpartal chill
    a. Neurologic or vasomotor response to impending delivery
    b. Normal immediately following delivery
11. Cardiac
    a. Puerperal brachycardia
    b. May occur in 1st 10 days of postpartum secondary to decreasing blood volume

Psychological Adaptation

A. **Self-Concept**
1. Body image
2. Fatigue
3. Discomfort

B. **Maternal Role:** Reva Rubin's stages
1. Taking-in phase: lasts about 2 days; mother focused on self; passive, dependent, fingertip touching
2. Taking-hold phase: increasing independence, ready to learn
3. Letting-go phase

C. **Postpartum Depression**
1. Mood swings, depression
2. Usually peaks on 5th day, if lasts longer than 10 days, notify primary care provider
3. Related to hormonal changes and fatigue; if continues, must seek professional help

Complications During the Postpartum Period

A. **Hemorrhage**
1. Definition: loss of more than 500 mL of blood, or blood loss of more than 1% of body weight after delivery
2. Etiology
    a. Early: atony
    b. Late: retained placenta
    c. Lacerations, hematomas
3. **NURSING INTERVENTIONS**
    a. Atony: massage fundus first, assess bladder, administer oxytocic medications; (prostaglandin F2a) (carboprost tromethamine) may be ordered if these measures don't stop the bleeding; do not give to clients with asthma; PID; cardiac, pulmonary, renal or hepatic conditions
    b. Retained placenta, lacerations and hematoma: surgery may be necessary

B. **Thromboembolic Disease**
1. Etiology

a. Normal changes in blood during pregnancy
b. Stasis
2. **NURSING INTERVENTIONS**
    a. Assess temperature, positive Homan's sign
    b. Ambulate to prevent stasis
    c. Elevate client's leg; provide heat, blood thinner, antibiotics
    d. Do not rub

C. **Infection** (temp above 101°F)
1. **NURSING INTERVENTIONS**
    a. Assess for signs of infection; check vital signs, pain, chills, lochia
    b. Administer antibiotic therapy
2. Complications
    a. Pulmonary embolism
    b. Peritonitis
    c. Pelvic cellulitis FLUID IN BETWEEN PELVIC TISSUES

SECTION IV

REVIEW OF REPRODUCTIVE RISKS AND COMPLICATIONS

Pregnancy

A. **High-Risk Pregnancy**
1. Younger than 16 and older than 35 years of age
2. Above gravida 4 FOUR PREGNANCIES
3. Over or underweight
4. Drug and alcohol abuse; smoking
5. Previous blood transfusions
6. Poverty income level
7. Less than high school education
8. Unmarried
9. Unwanted pregnancy
10. Little prenatal care
11. Difficulty conceiving
12. Medical problem or pregnancy induced disease
13. Multiple pregnancy (greater the number of fetuses, the greater the risk)

B. **Medical Problems**
1. Cardiac problems
    a. Pathophysiology
        1) Pregnancy expands plasma volume, which increases cardiac output and causes an increased work load on the heart
        2) Can result in congestive heart failure or death
    b. Prognosis
        1) Occurs in 1% of all pregnant women
        2) Danger of maternal death

a) When blood volume peaks at end of 2nd trimester (30–50% increase in volume)
b) During labor: increase of up to 20% from "milking" effect of contractions
c) During delivery: due to sudden increase in volume at birth when uterus contracts fully

c. Prenatal care
1) Prevent infection
2) High-protein diet, restrict weight gain, do not limit salt unless ordered *→ DIURETIC*
3) Monitor for anemia
4) Anticoagulant therapy: use heparin, NOT warfarin sodium (*Coumadin*) *→ PO*
5) Decrease activity, encourage rest, reduce stress

d. Labor and delivery
1) Avoid frequent changes of position
2) Avoid pain by use of medication, epidural
3) Avoid c-section; deliver vaginally with epidural and forceps
4) ECG, FHM and oxygen
5) Monitor IV carefully
6) Use oxytocin (*Pitocin*) with caution

e. Postpartum
1) Critical time: first 48 hours after delivery (congestive heart failure)
2) Watch for hemorrhage if oxytocin (*Pitocin*) not used
3) Monitor intake and output (cardiac failure)
4) No stockings
5) Assess for infection: prophylactic antibiotics may be given (prevent endocarditis)
6) Plan for discharge: client will need help; ability to breast feed

2. Diabetes mellitus
a. Pathophysiology affecting pregnancy
1) Maternal insulin: does not cross placenta; by 12 weeks fetus makes insulin, but this does not lower blood sugar level (maternal control)
2) First trimester: fetus draws large amounts of glucose for growth, so maternal need goes way down; may not need any insulin
3) Second trimester: HPL and other hormones secreted by the placenta after the 18th week of pregnancy have anti-insulin effect; need for insulin will increase

b. Prenatal care
1) Blood sugar control imperative for good outcome; assess maternal Hgb A_1C
2) High incidence of congenital anomalies and still births if client not in good glucose control

c. Labor and delivery
1) Assess infant for maturity and well-being by amniocentesis, stress and nonstress testing, estriol levels
2) C-section after 37 weeks may be necessary if placenta deteriorates

d. Postpartum
1) Insulin: need drops rapidly after delivery of placenta
2) Assess infant for hypoglycemia
3) Assess client for infection *→ crying) Trembling*

e. Complications
1) PIH
2) Polyhydramnios
3) Hypo/hyperglycemia
4) Fetal death *→ SYMPTOMS ABORTIONS*
5) Macrosomia (dystocia) *Problem ē uterus*
6) Spontaneous abortion

3. Gestational diabetes (2nd to 3rd trimester)
a. May be controlled by diet alone
b. 10–15% of clients need insulin
c. Normal after delivery; increased risk of being diabetic later in life

C. **Hyperemesis Gravidarum**
1. Definition: excessive vomiting
2. Etiology: may be hormonal or psychological
3. **NURSING INTERVENTIONS**
a. Monitor intake and output
b. Administer IV fluids
c. Introduce foods slowly
d. Decrease stress; psychiatric care if necessary
e. Assess for metabolic alkalosis (check for breath odor) *→ FRUITS*

D. **Polyhydramnios**
1. Definition: excessive amniotic fluid
2. Etiology
a. Maternal diseases (toxemia, diabetes)
b. Fetal malformation (esophagus not complete)
c. Erythroblastosis *moms blood killing babies blood*
d. Multiple pregnancies
3. Treatment
a. Relieve pressure by amniocentesis
b. Delivery

E. **Abortion**
1. Definition: expulsion of the fetus, usually before 20 weeks gestation (spontaneous or induced)
2. Etiology
a. Abnormal fetus
b. Infection
c. Anomaly of reproductive tract
d. Injury
e. Unwanted pregnancy

3. Terminology
   a. Spontaneous: miscarriage
   b. Therapeutic: termination of a pregnancy by medical intervention
   c. Criminal: abortion done outside medical facilities; against the law

4. **NURSING INTERVENTIONS**
   a. Save all pads and any tissues passed
   b. Assess for shock, infection, DIC, thrombophlebitis
   c. Administer RhoGAM if Rh negative
   d. Provide emotional support: do not give false encouragement (grieving necessary)

F. **Ectopic Pregnancy**
1. Definition: pregnancy that occurs outside the uterus; usually in the fallopian tube, but can be on the ovary, abdomen or interligaments
2. Etiology
   a. Malformation of tubes
   b. Pelvic inflammatory disease (PID)
   c. Tumors
   d. Adhesions secondary to surgery or endometriosis
3. Manifestations
   a. Sharp abdominal pain (rupture of tube)
   b. Shock
   c. Mild manifestations initially (little or no bleeding)
4. Diagnosis and treatment
   a. Culdocentesis (blood doesn't clot)
   b. Removal of tube; may need blood transfusion

5. **NURSING INTERVENTIONS**
   a. Watch for shock
   b. Provide usual postop care
   c. Provide emotional support; fear of happening again (only one tube remains)

G. **Hydatidiform Mole/Molar Pregnancy**
1. Definition: abnormal degeneration of the products of conception
2. Possible etiology (actual cause is unknown)
   a. Abnormal ova
   b. Protein deficiency
3. Manifestations
   a. Bleeding: spotting to profuse; pass tan-colored, grape-like clusters (anemia secondary to blood loss)
   b. Severe nausea and vomiting
   c. Increased levels of HCG (continues to increase)
   d. Signs of pregnancy induced hypertension (PIH) before 24th week
   e. Uterus enlarges at a rapid rate
4. Diagnosis and treatment
   a. Lab values for increased HCG
   b. Sonogram ←Dultrasound

c. Remove products by D&C (do not induce labor)
   d. Follow client closely for possible cancer; discourage client from becoming pregnant until cancer is ruled out (at least one year)
5. **NURSING INTERVENTIONS**
   a. Provide usual postop care: watch for hemorrhage
   b. Explain to client importance of close follow-up for cancer

H. **Incompetent Cervix**
1. Definition: defect in the cervix that prevents carrying a pregnancy to term
2. Manifestation: client has repeated 2nd trimester spontaneous abortions
3. Treatment: surgical procedures to close cervix (Shirodkar)
4. Prior to delivery: suture removed

I. **Pregnancy Induced Hypertension** (PIH)
1. Definition: hypertensive disorder of pregnancy occurring after the 20th week or early post partum
2. Pathophysiology: increased sensitivity to angiotensin II causes cyclic vasospasms leading to vasoconstriction; this is responsible for most or all symptoms of PIH
3. Terminology
   a. Pre-eclampsia: mild or severe depending upon degree of manifestations; IV hydralazine (*Apresoline*) is drug of choice for preeclampsia
   b. Eclampsia: convulsions occurs
4. Manifestations
   a. Edema: mild to severe swelling of hands, face; pitting of legs (or sacrum)
   b. Proteinuria: from 1 gm/24 hours to 5 gm or more/24 hours
   c. Hypertension: from 140/90 (or increase of 30/15 above base) to 160/110 or increase in systolic of 50 above base
   d. Decrease in urinary output (must have at least 30 mL/hour)
   e. Weight gain from edema
   f. Headaches, visual disturbances, vasospasm
   g. Hemoconcentration
   h. Epigastric pain
   i. Hyperreflexia
5. Occurrence
   a. Primigravida with age extremes (<16, >40)
   b. Any chronic medical condition that affects the vascular system (for example: diabetes mellitus, chronic hypertension, kidney disease, cardiac disease)
   c. Family history

d. Multiple pregnancies (for example: twins, triplets)

e. Dietary deficiencies, especially protein

 6. **NURSING INTERVENTIONS** (depends upon degree of illness; status can change very quickly)

a. Assess vital signs, weight, edema, protein in urine

b. Provide diet high in protein, adequate fluid intake, do not restrict salt unless ordered

c. Promote bed rest, controlled environment, lying on left side

d. Monitor intake and output

e. Institute seizure precautions (have suction and oxygen ready)

f. May have to stabilize client and deliver baby

   1) Check reflexes, then give magnesium sulfate ($MgSO_4$); have calcium gluconate at beside (must be given slowly)

   2) Assess for precipitous delivery and abruptio placenta

7. HELLP syndrome: hemolysis, elevated liver enzymes, and low platelet count

J. Abruptio Placenta

1. Definition: premature separation of the placenta from the uterus

2. Etiology

a. Trauma

b. PIH

c. Multiparity

d. Cocaine use

3. Manifestations

a. Bleeding: either internal or external

b. Board-like abdomen, severe pain, tenderness, lack of contractions

c. Bradycardia or no fetal heart rate (uteroplacental insufficiency)

4. Treatment

a. Usually immediate c-section

b. Treat for blood loss

 5. **NURSING INTERVENTIONS**

a. Observe for shock

b. Monitor vital signs, FHR

c. Assess for diffuse intravascular coagulation (DIC), infection, anemia

K. Placenta Previa *Painless*

1. Definition: placenta attaches low in the uterus, either near or covering the cervical os

2. Etiology

a. Older mothers

b. Multiparity

3. Types

a. Total: completely covers cervix

b. Partial: partial covering of cervical os

c. Low lying: near to cervical os

4. Manifestations: painless, bright red bleeding after the 7th month (bleeding may be intermittent)

 5. **NURSING INTERVENTIONS** (depends on type, severity, and gestational age)

a. Can vary from bed rest to immediate c-section, may need blood

b. Observe for hemorrhage; count pads; monitor vital signs and FHR; be prepared for emergency c-section; provide emotional support

c. Do not perform vaginal exams

SECTION V

NURSING CARE OF THE NEONATE

A. Initial Care of Newborn

1. Maintain patent airway by suction, position

2. Maintain temperature: dry, place baby on mother or under radiant heat source

3. APGAR score: performed at one and five minutes after birth

a. Five areas scored: heart rate, respiratory effort, muscle tone, reflex irritability, color

   1) 7–10: good

   2) 3–6: moderately depressed

   3) 0–2: severely depressed

4. Eye prophylaxis: silver nitrate ($AgNO_3$), erythromycin or tetracycline (protects against infections caused by chlamydia & gonorrhea)

5. Identification

6. Vitamin K (*AquaMEPHYTON*)

B. Vital Signs

1. Temperature range is 97–99°F; if too high: dehydration, sepsis, brain damage, overheated; if too low: infection, brain stem injury, cold

2. Heart rate range is 120–150 beats/minute, dependent upon state; murmur is common at first from transient patent ductus arteriosus

3. Respirations

a. 30–50/minute

b. Distress: nasal flaring, intercostal or xiphoid retractions, expiratory grunt, tachypnea

4. BP is 80/40 at birth, 100/50 by the 10th day

C. Head

1. Measure head circumference

2. Assess fontanels

a. Posterior: triangular shaped, closes at 8–12 weeks

b. Anterior: diamond shaped, closes at 18 months
c. Bulging: increased intracranial pressure; depressed: dehydration
3. Molding
4. Caput succedaneum (edema of soft scalp tissue)
5. Cephalohematoma (hematoma between periosteum and skull bone)

D. Eyes
1. Blue-gray color
2. Strabismus is common ("cross-eye")
3. Small hemorrhage (clears in a few weeks)
4. Cataracts

E. Ears
1. Low-set ears are associated with anomalies
2. Infants hear acutely as mucous is absorbed

F. Nose
1. Patency: infants are obligatory nose breathers; can smell
2. Symmetry

G. Mouth
1. Sucking reflex
2. Epstein pearls (small white epithelial cysts along midline of hard palate)
3. Thrush (white patches that adhere to tongue, palate, and Buccal mucosa)
4. Palate intact

H. Breast
1. Engorgement
2. Amount of breast tissue

I. Abdomen
1. Measure abdominal circumference
2. Palpate for masses
3. Umbilical cord
   a. Three vessels (one vein, two arteries) "AVA"
   b. Will fall off in 10 days; assess for infection

J. Skin
1. Normal variations
   a. Acrocyanosis: immature circulation (cyanosis of hands and feet)
   b. Milia (tiny white papules on face, distended sebaceous glands)
   c. Toxic erythema (pink papular rash on trunk)
   d. Vernix (white, cheese-like substance)
   e. Mongolian spots: birth marks (irregular areas of pigmentation)
   f. Lanugo (fine, downy hair on forehead, shoulders, back)
2. Color

K. Skeletal
1. Clavicles
2. Hips (Check for congenital hip dysplasia; feel for "Ortolani click")

L. Genitals
1. Female
   a. Swollen
   b. Pseudo menstruation
   c. Vaginal tag
2. Male
   a. Swollen
   b. Hypospadias (opening on underside of penis)
   c. Phimosis (stenosis that prevents foreskin from being retracted back; leads to problems with urination; treatment: circumcision)
   d. Testicles

M. Elimination
1. Void in first 24 hours: pink stains from urates
2. Patent rectum: meconium during first 24 hours

Assessment for Gestational Age

A. Physical Assessment (first 24 hours): for full-term infant
1. Resting posture
2. Vernix distribution (very little)
3. Skin
4. Nails
5. Lanugo (very sparse)
6. Sole creases (present at full term)
7. Skull firmness
8. Breast tissue
9. Ear formation and cartilage (firm; springs back)
10. Genitalia
11. Recoil

B. Neurological Exam (after 24 hours)
1. Ankle dorsiflexion
2. Square window sign
3. Popliteal angle
4. Heel-to-ear maneuver
5. Scarf sign (contraindicated if fractured clavicle is suspected)
6. Neck extensors
7. Neck flexors
8. Horizontal position
9. Major reflexes
   a. Sucking: response to nipple
   b. Rooting: touch cheek and neonate will turn head to that side
   c. Grasping: touch palm, fingers curl
   d. Moro: "startle" reflex

e. Tonic neck: turn head to one side in supine position: arm and leg on that side will extend, but flex on opposite side

C. Care of Newborn

1. Weigh daily: initial loss of 10% is normal; new-borns should regain birthweight by the two-week visit
2. Nutrition: record daily intake and number of wet and dry diapers
3. Regulate temperature
4. Circumcision: discuss options with parents
   a. Permit signed
   b. Assess for hemorrhage, infection
   c. Required or forbidden by some cultures, religions or ethnic groups
5. Tests
   a. Phenylketonuria (PKU): lack of enzyme to convert phenylalanine to tyrosine, Guthrie test: 24 hours after first milk feeding, again in 4–6 weeks
   b. Dextrostix: assess blood sugar level
   c. Cultures: if possible infection
6. Parent education: general care such as feeding, bathing, dressing, cord, and circumcision care
7. Promote attachment
8. Assess need for parental support after discharge

SECTION VI

REVIEW OF HIGH-RISK NEWBORN

Premature Newborn

A. Definition: gestational age of less than 37 weeks, regardless of weight

B. Physical Adaptation

1. Respiratory
   a. May lack surfactants
   b. At risk for respiratory distress syndrome (RDS)
      1) Retractions
      2) Nasal flaring
      3) Expiratory grunt
      4) Tachypnea
      5) Needs mechanical ventilation, oxygen, continuous positive airway pressure (CPAP)
2. Nutrition (fluid and electrolyte)
   a. May lack gag and sucking reflex if under 34 weeks
   b. Fed by gavage or hyperalimentation
3. Circulatory

a. Patent ductus arteriosus is common
b. Persistent fetal circulation

4. Complications
   a. Hypothermia
   b. Hypocalcemia
   c. Hypoglycemia
   d. Hyperbilirubinemia
   e. Birth trauma
   f. Sepsis
   g. Intracranial hemorrhage
   h. Necrotizing enterocolitis
   i. Apnea

 5. **NURSING INTERVENTIONS**
   a. Monitor vital signs
   b. Maintain temperature
   c. Assess hydration, nutrition
   d. Promote attachment and bonding between parents and newborn

Small for Gestational Age (SGA)

A. Definition: any newborn who falls below the tenth percentile on the growth chart at birth

B. Etiology

1. Placental insufficiency
2. PIH
3. Multiple pregnancy
4. Poor nutrition
5. Smoking, drugs, alcohol
6. Adolescent pregnancy

C. Complications

1. Perinatal asphyxia
2. Meconium aspiration syndrome
3. Hypoglycemia
4. Hypothermia
5. Infections

NURSING INTERVENTIONS

1. Support respirations
2. Provide neutral thermal environment
3. Provide adequate nutrition
4. Observe for complications
5. Protect from infection
6. Support parents; promote bonding

Large for Gestational Age (LGA)

A. Definition: newborn whose weight is at or above the 90th percentile (could still be premature)

B. Etiology

1. Diabetes
2. Genetic predisposition
3. Congenital defects

C. Complications

1. Birth trauma (for example: fractured clavicle)
2. Hypoglycemia
3. Polycythemia
4. If mother diabetic, same risk and care as premature infant

D. NURSING INTERVENTIONS

1. Assess for trauma
2. Assess for congenital abnormalities
3. Assess for hypoglycemia, especially if infant of diabetic mother (IDM)

Postmature Infant

A. Definition: gestational age of over 42 weeks

B. Physical Findings

1. Dry, parchment-like skin
2. Longer, harder nails
3. Profuse scalp hair
4. Absent vernix
5. Loose skin (2° fat wasting) with long thin body

C. Complications

1. Progressive aging of placenta
2. Difficult delivery
3. High perinatal mortality

Jaundice (Hyperbilirubinemia)

A. Causes

1. Physiological
   a. Never seen during first 24 hours; usually appears by third day
   b. Immature liver
2. Bruising
3. ABO incompatibility (Mother is O, baby is A, B, or AB)
4. Rh incompatibility (erythroblastosis fetalis)
   a. Rh⁻ mother and Rh⁺ baby
   b. Kernicterus (bilirubin encephalopathy) can lead to brain damage, anemia, hepatosplenomegaly
   c. Treatment
      1) Phototherapy, sunlight, exchange transfusion
      2) RhoGAM administered at 28 weeks gestation and within 72 hours of delivery
      3) Note: RhoGAM also given to all Rh negative mothers who abort after the 8th week of gestation
5. Breast feeding

Substance Abuse and the Newborn

A. Drug Dependent

1. Manifestations of withdrawal
   a. Early manifestation: irritability
   b. Sneezing, nasal stuffiness
   c. High-pitched, weak cry
   d. Tremors
   e. Perspiration
   f. Feeding problems (weak suck)
   g. Transient tachypnea
2. NURSING INTERVENTIONS
   a. Prevent overstimulation to prevent possible seizures
   b. Swaddle; hold infant firmly
   c. Administer medications as ordered
   d. Provide small, frequent feedings (may need to gavage)

B. Fetal Alcohol Syndrome

1. Etiology: consumption of alcoholic beverages during pregnancy
2. Manifestations
   a. Feeding problems (weak suck)
   b. Distinctive facial features (microcephaly, small eyes, thin upper lip)
   c. CNS dysfunction (including mental retardation and seizures)
   d. Physical defects (limb anomalies, hyperactivity, cardiocirculatory defects, deafness)
   e. Withdrawal manifestations
3. NURSING INTERVENTIONS
   a. Protect infant from injury
   b. Administer medications
   c. Monitor fluid therapy
   d. Decrease stimuli
   e. Provide support for parents to care for possibly difficult infant
   f. Provide social service referral

SECTION VII

NURSING CARE OF THE GYNECOLOGIC CLIENT

↳ female only!

Vaginal Infections

A. Candidiasis (Yeast)

1. Manifestations
   a. Cheese-like discharge
   b. Itching
2. Etiology and Risk factors
   a. HIV positive client
   b. Client on antibiotics

Diabetes!

 3. **NURSING INTERVENTIONS**
   a. Administer nystatin (*Mycostatin*)
   b. Discuss importance of cleanliness with client
   c. Ensure that both partners are treated

B. **Trichomoniasis** (sexually transmitted) *Parasite*
   1. Manifestations
      a. Frothy, yellow discharge *dead fish!*
      b. Itching
      c. Burning
 2. **NURSING INTERVENTIONS**
   a. Administer metronidazole (*Flagyl*); (not in first trimester) no alcohol consumption
   b. Ensure that both partners are treated

C. **Condyloma** (sexually transmitted)
   1. Caused by human papillovirus
   2. Manifestations: presence of soft grayish-pink lesions on perineum (genital warts)
   3. **NURSING INTERVENTIONS**
      a. Assist with application of podophyllum resin
      b. Assist with cryosurgery with liquid nitrogen or laser (carbon dioxide laser) surgery
      c. Educate client of increased risk for cervical cancer
      d. Instruct client of need for close follow-up with pap smears

Cancer

A. **Cervical**
   1. Manifestations
      a. Bleeding between periods or after intercourse, douching *white*
      b. Leukorrhea *flow*
      c. Pap smear
   2. Treatment
      a. Hysterectomy *removal of uterus*
      b. Radiation
      c. Laser surgery
      inside uterus

B. **Endometrium**
   1. Manifestations
      a. Post-menopausal bleeding
      b. Abnormal bleeding
   2. Treatment
      a. Radium
      b. X-ray therapy
      c. Hysterectomy **NURSING INTERVENTIONS**
         1) Assess for grieving
         2) Preop teaching
         3) Provide postop care
         4) Assess psychosexual needs

C. **Ovarian** *Ca-125*
   1. Manifestations (usually late in diagnosing)
      a. Back discomfort
      b. Ascites
   2. Treatment: oophorectomy

D. **Breast**
   1. Manifestations
      a. Nontender lump (often in upper outer quadrant of breast)
      b. Dimpling
      c. Asymmetry
      d. Nipple changes (bleeding or retraction)
   2. Treatment
      a. Mastectomy (lumpectomy, simple or radical)
      b. Radiation
      c. Chemotherapy
   3. **NURSING INTERVENTIONS**
      a. Instruct client of need for close follow up
      b. Educate client about breast self-examination (BSE): most accurate if performed 1 week after last menstrual period; mammography
      c. Provide emotional support/grieving

Uterine Disorders

A. **Myomas** *→ tumor*
   1. Definition: benign fibroid tumors of the uterine muscle
   2. Etiology: African-Americans over age 30 who have never been pregnant
   3. Manifestations
      a. Pain
      b. Hypermenorrhea
   4. Treatment: myomectomy

B. **Endometriosis**
   1. Definition: endometrial tissue located outside of uterus
   2. Manifestations
      a. Severe dysmenorrhea
      b. Lower abdominal pain, pain during intercourse, back and rectal pain
      c. Abnormal bleeding
   3. Treatment
      a. Oral contraceptives (hormone therapy)
      b. Surgery
      c. Pregnancy

Tubal Disorder

A. **Pelvic Inflammatory Disease** (PID)
   1. Etiology
      a. Infections
      b. Venereal disease

2. Manifestations
   a. Vaginal discharge: foul smelling, purulent
   b. Pain in abdomen, lower back
   c. Elevated temperature, nausea, vomiting

 3. **NURSING INTERVENTIONS**
   a. Administer antibiotic therapy
   b. Educate client

Menopause

A. **Definition:** complete cessation of menstruation for ~~one year~~

B. **Manifestations**
   1. Hot flashes
   2. Palpitations
   3. Diaphoresis
   4. Osteoporosis

C. **NURSING INTERVENTIONS**
   1. Assess psychosocial response
   2. Discuss merits of estrogen therapy, including prevention of osteoporosis, heart disease
   3. Alternative therapies (diet, exercise, calcium supplements)

Infertility

A. **Definition:** decreased capacity to conceive

B. **Etiology**
   1. Abnormal genitalia
   2. Absence of ovulation
   3. Blocked fallopian tubes
   4. Altered vaginal pH
   5. Sperm deficiency or decreased motility
   6. Infection

C. **Diagnosis**
   1. Assessment of male
   2. Assessment of female

D. **Management**
   1. Medication
      a. Clomiphene citrate (*Clomid*) or menotropins (*Pergonal*); associated with multiple births
      b. Hormone replacement
   2. Artificial insemination
   3. In vitro fertilization → *petri dish*
   4. Surrogate parenting

E. **NURSING INTERVENTIONS**
   1. Provide emotional support
   2. Provide client education

Contraception

A. **Nursing Assessment**
   1. Determine client's knowledge about and previous experience with family planning
   2. Determine client's need for genetic counseling
   3. Identify infertility problems
   4. Educate client that no method except condom protects against STDs + abstinence

B. **Types**
   1. Natural (rhythm) method
      a. Use of calendar, basal body temperature and cervical mucus
      b. **NURSING INTERVENTION:** teach method
   2. Oral contraceptives
      a. Side effects similar to pregnancy: initial discomforts, hypertension, clotting problems, fluid retention
      b. Contraindicated if client is:
         1) Over 35
         2) Hypertensive
         3) A smoker
         4) Has a history of clotting disorder
      c. **NURSING INTERVENTIONS**
         1) Teach method
         2) Assess for complications (increased BP)
   3. Injectable contraceptive: Medroxyprogesterone acetate (*Depo-Provera*)
      a. Long-acting contraceptive
      b. Administered every three months via IM injection
   4. Intrauterine device (IUD)
      a. High risk of PID, ectopic pregnancy, perforation of uterus; periods may be heavy (anemia)
      b. **NURSING INTERVENTIONS**
         1) Instruct client in the need for follow-up
         2) Client should get regular pap tests
         3) Teach client to feel for strings frequently
   5. Mechanical barriers
      a. Diaphragm
         1) **NURSING INTERVENTIONS**
            a) Teach client how to insert diaphragm
            b) Teach client how to use spermicidal jelly with diaphragm
            c) Teach client to leave in 6–8 hours after intercourse
            d) ~~Teach client to have diaphragm refitted if client gains or loses weight; after childbirth~~
      b. Condom
         1) **NURSING INTERVENTIONS:** female condom (vaginal sheath)
            a) Teach client to use with spermicide
            b) Protects against STDs, including HIV
         2) **NURSING INTERVENTIONS:** male condom

a) Teach client to leave space at end
b) Teach how to prevent slipping or tearing during removal
c) Protects against STDs, including HIV

c. Cervical cap: can be left in place up to 12 hours

6. Chemical barriers (spermicides)

a. **NURSING INTERVENTIONS**
   1) Teach client about possible allergic reactions
   2) Teach client how to clean equipment
   3) Warn client not to douche for 6–8 hours after intercourse

7. Sterilization
   a. Tubal ligation

removing the spermicide

1) **NURSING INTERVENTIONS**
   a) Discuss permanency
   b) Discuss methods of obstructing tubes

b. Vasectomy
   1) **NURSING INTERVENTIONS**
      a) Discuss permanency
      b) Warn client of need for negative sperm count three times before attempting unprotected intercourse

8. Unreliable methods
   a. Withdrawal/coitus interruptus
   b. Douching

NOTES

UNIT FOUR

PEDIATRIC NURSING

UNIT CONTENT

SECTION I.   Growth and Development 137
SECTION II.   The Hospitalized Child 145
SECTION III.   Nursing Care of the Child with Congenital Anomalies 147
SECTION IV.   Nursing Care of the Child with an Acute Illness 154
SECTION V.   Nursing Care of the Surgical Child 159
SECTION VI.   Nursing Care for Pediatric Accidents 160
SECTION VII.   Nursing Care of the Child with Chronic or Long-Term Problems .. 162
SECTION VIII.   Nursing Care of the Child with an Oncological Disorder 166
SECTION VII.   Nursing Care of the Child with an Infectious Disease 170

SYMBOLS

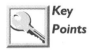
Key Points

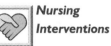
Nursing Interventions

Points to Remember

SECTION I

GROWTH AND DEVELOPMENT

Characteristics of Development

A. Lifelong Process

B. Critical Periods

C. Proximodistal (development of fine motor skills)

D. Cephalocaudal ("head to tail" development)

Lifespan and Development of the Infant

Birth–12 months
1. Physical characteristics
   a. Height: increases by 50% in first year
   b. Weight: birth weight doubles at 6 months; birth weight triples at 12 months
   c. Head: 70% of adult size at birth; 80% of adult size by end of first year
      1) Posterior fontanel: closes by 2 months of age
      2) Anterior fontanel: closes between 12 to 18 months of age
         a) Bulging: classic sign of increased intracranial pressure
         b) Sunken: classic sign of dehydration
   d. Dentition
      1) Drools at four months
      2) Primary teeth: By 12 months: six primary teeth (age of child in months minus 6 = number of teeth) (see table IV-1.)
      3) **NURSING INTERVENTIONS**
         a) Avoid medications that may stain teeth (example: tetracycline, iron)
         b) Avoid phenytoin (*Dilantin*): causes gingivitis and gingival hyperplasia
         c) Teach parents that increased drooling, finger sucking, biting on objects are all indicators of teething
         d) Inform parents that cool or cold items are soothing (teething ring)
         e) Use acetaminophen (*Tylenol*) for continued irritability
         f) Educate parents that once dentition occurs, avoid nighttime bottle with juice or formula - it increases the incidence of dental caries ("bottle mouth" caries)
   e. Reflexes
      1) Rooting (disappears by 3–4 months)
      2) Tonic neck (disappears by 3–4 months)
      3) Palmar grasp (disappears by 3–4 months)
      4) Moro (disappears by 3–4 months)
      5) Sucking (continues through infancy)
      6) Stepping (disappears by 3–4 months)
   f. Vital signs
      1) Pulse ranges from 100–140 beats/minute, may even be as high as 160 beats/minute depending upon activity
      2) Respirations range from 30–40 beats/minute
      3) Immature thermoregulatory mechanisms
      4) Crying will increase all vital signs
2. Nutrition
   a. Infant feeding
      1) Allow infant to set own schedule
      2) Breast or bottle feeding depends upon mother's preference
      3) Vitamin supplements as ordered usually begun around 3–4 months (vitamin D and iron); fluoride supplements for breast-fed infants
      4) Caloric requirements range from 110 to 120 calories/Kg/day
   b. Introduction of solid foods
      1) Physiologic readiness
         a) Tongue extrusion reflex (fades by about four months)
         b) Digestive enzymes

TABLE IV-1.
SCHEDULE OF PRIMARY TOOTH ERUPTION

ERUPTION	LOWER	UPPER
Central incisor	6 months	7–1/2 months
Lateral incisor	7 months	9 months
First molar	12 months	14 months
Cuspid	16 months	18 months
Second molar	20 months	24 months

c) Motor skills: sit with support; head and neck control

d) Interest in solid food

2) Nutritional guidelines

   a) Solids usually begun around 4–6 months

   b) Introduce foods one at a time, at every 4–7 days (observe for allergy)

   c) Sequence usually followed at one month intervals:

     (1) Rice cereal (good source of iron; avoid wheat) → *push for allergies*

     (2) Fruits and vegetables (yellow, then green)

     (3) Meats (begin with chicken, turkey)

     (4) Egg yolks (avoid egg whites)

   d) Begin table foods around 8–12 months

     (1) Avoid nuts, foods with seeds, raisins, popcorn, grapes (risk for aspiration)

     (2) Finger foods enhance thumb-finger apposition

   e) When switching from formula to cow's milk, avoid skim milk (not enough fat); infant needs whole milk

   f) As amount of solids increases, reduce quantity of milk (no more than 30 oz/day)

   g) Never mix food, medication with the formula

   h) Avoid sweeteners such as honey or corn syrup (risk of botulism)

c. Weaning

1) Usually begins around 4–6 months with sips from a cup; can use training cup with sipper tube and/or handles

2) Introduce cup gradually

3) Remove one bottle or breast feeding at a time; remove nighttime feeding last

4) By 12–14 months, should be able to drink from a cup

d. Nutritional concerns

1) Colic

   a) Seen in infants younger than 3 months

   b) Paroxysmal abdominal pain associated with crying and accumulation of gas

   c) Associated with overfeeding, air swallowing, maternal insecurity

   d) **NURSING INTERVENTIONS**

     (1) Feed slowly with frequent burping

     (2) Avoid excessive feedings

     (3) Increase TLC between mother and baby

     (4) Teach various feeding and holding techniques

2) Iron deficiency anemia

   a) Result of poor diet or low-iron stores in the newborn

   b) Seldom seen in first six months due to iron stores inherited from mother

   c) Most frequently seen in children between 6 months and 1 year who ingest large quantities of milk

   d) RBCs appear microcytic and hypochromic

   e) Prevention: use of an iron-fortified formula and/or cereal

   f) Ferrous sulfate (*Feosol*) is the drug of choice

   g) **NURSING INTERVENTIONS**: client education

     (1) Administer between meals

     (2) Administer with citrus juice for greater iron absorption

     (3) Teach parents that liquid preparations may stain teeth (use dropper or straw, then rinse mouth with water)

     (4) Inform parents that iron may cause tarry stools

3. Activity/rest

a. Normal infants sleep 14–16 hours a day

b. Nocturnal pattern of sleep develops by 3–4 months

4. Motor skills

a. 2 months

1) Smiles socially

2) Differentiated cry

3) Turns head from side to side

b. 3 months

1) Follows object 180° horizontal and vertical (20/100 visual acuity at birth)

2) Discovers hands

3) Reaches for object

4) Lifts head off bed; bears weight on forearms

c. 4 months

1) Recognizes familiar objects; moves extremities in response

2) Sits with support

3) Reaches for object

4) Laughs aloud

5) Begins to recognize parent

6) Rolls back to side

7) Almost no head lag

d. 5–6 months

1) Rolls over completely

2) Bangs with object held in hand

3) Vocalizes displeasure when object taken away
4) Rakes object
5) No head lag
   e. 6–8 months
   1) Holds own bottle (6 months)
   2) Transfers toy (7 months)
   3) Pincer grasp begins (8 months)
   4) Shows a fear of strangers: "stranger anxiety"
   5) Sits alone (8 months)
   6) Creeps and crawls (9 months)
   f. 10–12 months
   1) Pulls self to feet (9 months)
   2) Stands alone
   3) Walks with help
   5) Uses spoon, with spilling
   6) Cruises (9 months); crawls well (10 months)
   7) Claps hands on request
   8) Imitates behavior
   9) Smiles at image in mirror
5. Language development
   a. Vocalizes (distinct from crying) by 3–4 months
   b. Recognizes "no" by 9 months; own name by 10 months
   c. Two to three words in addition to "mama", "dada" by 12 months
6. Developmental stages
   a. Psychosocial development (Erikson)
      1) Trust vs. mistrust
      2) Quality of caregiver/child relationship
   b. Cognitive development (Piaget)
      1) Sensorimotor phase
         a) Reflexive
         b) Imitates and recognizes new experiences
      2) Object permanence
         a) Understands that self and object are separate (10 months)
         b) Will search for lost object (12 months)
         c) Separation anxiety (8–12 months)
7. Play
   a. Solitary *alone*
   b. Characteristics
      1) 0–3 months: verbal, visual, tactile stimuli
         a) Toys should be brightly colored, washable, of various sizes, shapes, and textures
         b) Enhance eye-hand coordination
            (1) Mobiles, cradle gyms
            (2) Busy box, toys with faces
         c) Stimulate auditory senses (examples: rattles, music box)
      2) 4–6 months: initiates, recognizes new experiences
         a) Mobility increasing

b) Hand coordination increasing
c) Memory begins
d) Types of toys
   (1) Mirrors to see image
   (2) Chewable, large toys
   (3) Brightly colored rattles, beads
   (4) Squeeze toys, teething rings
   (5) Remove cradle gym to avoid accidents
      3) 6–12 months
         a) Increasing self-awareness
         b) Repeats pleasurable activities
         c) Object permanence
         d) Imitates behavior at 10 months; "peek-a-boo"
         e) Increased desire to explore
         f) Types of toys
            (1) Large boxes, kitchen utensils
            (2) Water play with supervision
            (3) Texture play: sand, dirt
            (4) Pouring, filling, dumping
            (5) Playing with food (beginning of self-feeding)
   c. Safety measures
      1) Toys should be large; short strings
      2) Constructed of nontoxic materials
      3) Always supervise
      4) Inspect toys for problems
         a) Rough edges
         b) Parts that can be pulled off and swallowed or aspirated
8. Health maintenance
   a. Safety
      1) Avoid overstimulation, rough handling
      2) Limit-setting should involve redirecting behaviors to safer activities
   b. Immunizations (see table IV-10.)
      1) Hepatitis B: birth, two months, six months
      2) DTaP, IPV, HIB: two, four, and six months (timing of 3rd IPV optional)
      3) Acetaminophen (*Tylenol*) given prophylactically to lessen fever from DTaP
      4) Pertussis held if temperature > 105°F after previous DTaP or if child has history of neurologic disorder
   c. Infant restraints
      1) Semi-reclining seat that faces rear until 20 lbs/10kg
      2) Use car seat belt to anchor restraint
      3) Middle of car's back seat is the safest area
      4) Infant restraints should not be used in front seat, especially with passenger-side airbags
   d. Aspiration of foreign objects
      1) Common problems include food, buttons from clothing, baby powder, and older sibling's toys

2) Emergency measures for choking infant
   a) Five back blows, five chest thrusts (repeat until successful)
   b) No blind finger sweep
9. Health deviations
   a. Accidents (leading cause of death over one year of age)
      1) Falls (depth perception develops by 7–9 months)
      2) Suffocation/aspiration/drowning
      3) Burns
   b. Caregiver Education
      1) Childproof environment
      2) Constant supervision
      3) Anticipatory guidance
         a) Put gates at top and bottom of stairs
         b) Put pots on back burners of stove
         c) Place electrical cords out of reach
         d) Put safety plug covers in all electrical outlets
         e) When feeding, do not prop bottle
         f) Never lead alone on bed or table top
         g) Avoid infant walkers
         h) Avoid plastic bags
         i) Use infant restraints
         j) Supervise by any source of water
   c. SIDS (Sudden Infant Death Syndrome)
      1) Cause unknown; multiple theories
      2) Infant at risk
         a) Mostly males, ages 2-4 months
         b) Preterm infants with apnea problems
         c) Multiple births
      3) Occurs during sleep, usually in winter months
      4) Caregiver education
         a) Infant should sleep in supine or side lying position, not prone
         b) Firm mattress, no pillow; avoid overheating during sleep
         c) Lower incidence if breast fed

Lifespan and Development of the Toddler

12 months–36 months
1-3mos.

1. Physical characteristics
   a. Appearance is potbellied, long legged, clumsy
   b. Slowing rate of growth for height and weight (adult height = approximately double height at 2 years)
   c. Dentition
      1) By 2-1/2 years: all 20 primary teeth
      2) Adult should brush child's teeth by age 2
      3) 1st visit to dentist by age 2
   d. Vital signs
      1) Pulse: ranges from 80–110 beats/minute
      2) Respirations: range from 25–35/minute
      3) Blood pressure: average is 100/70
2. Nutrition
   a. Growth lag (100 kcal/kg)
   b. Expresses independence through food preferences; food fads are common
   c. Wants to feed self; very ritualistic, messy
   d. Space meals with frequent nutritious snacks (cheese, PB & J)
   e. Small portions (physiologic anorexia)
   f. Fluid requirements: 115 mL/kg/day (3 cups whole milk/day)
3. Activity/rest
   a. Sleeps 10–12 hours with naps
   b. Routines and rituals are reassuring
   c. Nightmares and night terrors are possible
4. Motor skills
   a. 13–16 months
      1) Uses spoon and cup, but will spill
      2) Walks without help (since about 13 months)
      3) Climbs up and down stairs with buttocks
      4) Mimics housework
      5) Stacks 2–3 blocks (15 months)
      6) Throws and drops things (15 months)
      7) Loves containers of all kinds
   b. 16–18 months
      1) Runs clumsily; falls often
      2) Throws ball overhand
      3) Pulls and pushes toys
      4) Uses spoon and cup without spilling
      5) Removes clothes (for example: shoes, socks)
      6) Jumps in place
      7) Kicks small ball
   c. 2 years
      1) Walks up and down stairs
      2) Runs well
      3) Turns knobs to open door; unscrews lids
      4) Dresses self in simple clothing
      5) Builds tower of 5 blocks
      6) Turns pages of a book
      7) Climbs
   d. 2-1/2 to 3 years
      1) Holds crayon with fingers
      2) May have daytime bowel and bladder control
      3) Strings beads
5. Language development
   a. Ten words by 18 months
   b. May say "no" when agreeing (means "yes")
   c. Uses two to three word phrases by 2 years; vocabulary of 300 words; verbalizes needs (toileting, food, drink); uses pronouns
   d. Gives first and last name by 2-1/2 years
6. Developmental stages
   a. Psychosocial development (Erikson)

1) Autonomy vs. shame and doubt (1–3 years)
   a) Egocentric *(ME)*
   b) Negativism and temper tantrums
   c) Uninhibited at showing independence
2) Gains control over bodily functions
  b. Cognitive development (Piaget)
   1) Sensorimotor (12–24 months)
      a) Objects are cause of action
      b) Separation anxiety
   2) Preoperational (24 months–4 years)
      a) Concrete thinking begins
      b) Egocentric
      c) Symbolic play
7. Play
  a. Parallel play
   1) No sharing
   2) Ownership determined by possession of object
   3) Short attention span
  b. Types of activities
   1) Gross motor
      a) Jungle gym
      b) Push pull toys
      c) Tricycle (2-1/2–3 years)
   2) Fine motor
      a) Crayons, paints, paper
      b) Building blocks
      c) Musical toys
   3) Enjoys being read to
8. Health maintenance
  a. Toilet training (18 months–2 years)
   1) Physiologic readiness (sphincter control at approximately 18 months)
   2) Imitation; potty chair
   3) May not be complete until 4 to 5 years of age (nocturnal control often delayed)
  b. Discipline
   1) Toddlers are negative and ritualistic
   2) Limits must be simple and consistent
  c. Safety
   1) Precautions
      a) Childproof the environment
      b) Supervise at all times
      c) Child restraints (may switch to forward facing car seat when child weighs approximately 20 lbs/10 kg)
   2) Immunizations (see table IV-10.)
      a) MMR: 15 months
      b) HIB: 15 months
      c) DTaP, IPV: 18 months
      d) Varicella zoster (chicken pox): after 12 months

9. Health deviations
  a. Accidents
   1) Motor vehicles: passengers, pedestrians
   2) Burns
   3) Drowning/suffocation/aspiration
   4) Falls
   5) Poisoning
      a) Have syrup of ipecac in the home
      b) Have phone number for poison control and emergency room posted by telephone
      c) Lock up all medications and potentially toxic substances
      d) Use child resistant caps appropriately
      e) Never refer to medication as candy
  b. Anticipatory guidance
   1) Supervise closely near any source of water
   2) Store flammables, lighters out of reach
   3) Use child restraints in vehicles
   4) Avoid easily aspirated foods

Lifespan and Development of the Preschooler

3–5 Years

1. Physical characteristics: Average four year old is 40 inches and 40 pounds
2. Nutrition
  a. Growth lag (90 kcal/kg)
  b. Encourage finger foods (for example: cheese, fruit)
  c. Food jags are common
3. Activity/rest
  a. May give up nap but needs quiet time
  b. Peak time for sleep disturbances
   1) Refusal to go to bed
      a) Child resists bedtime; comes out of room frequently
      b) **NURSING INTERVENTIONS**
         (1) Stress need for a consistent bedtime
         (2) Help parents' identify strategies to ignore attention seeking behaviors
         (3) Suggest that they avoid bringing child into parents' bed (consider client's culture)
         (4) Promote use of a transitional object (for example: blanket, toy)
   2) Nighttime fears
      a) Child resists bed because of fears (for example: dark, "monsters")

b) **NURSING INTERVENTIONS**
   (1) Tell parents to calmly reassure child
   (2) Suggest that the use of a night-light may be helpful
   (3) Suggest that parents monitor bedtime television viewing

4. Motor skills
   a. Three years
      1) Dresses with supervision; needs help with buttons
      2) Rides tricycle
      3) Climbs stairs with alternate feet
      4) Pours fluid from a pitcher
   b. Four years
      1) Hops and skips on one foot
      2) Walks upstairs without use of handrail; alternates feet walking downstairs
      3) Uses scissors
      4) Laces shoes but cannot tie
   c. 5 years
      1) Skips and hops on alternate feet
      2) Walks backwards
      3) Can master two-wheel bike/roller skates
      4) Uses simple tools, prints name
      5) May master tying shoes

5. Language development
   a. Three years
      1) Vocabulary of 900 words
      2) Talks constantly regardless of whether anyone is listening
      3) Complete sentences
   b. Four years
      1) Vocabulary of 1,500 words
      2) Questions constantly
      3) Exaggerates; tells "tall tales"
      4) May stutter
      5) May pick up profanity
   c. 5 years
      1) Vocabulary of 2,000 words
      2) Uses all parts of speech
      3) Speech 100% intelligible to others although some sounds may still be imperfect

6. Developmental stages
   a. Psychosocial development (Erikson)
      1) Initiative vs guilt (3-6 years)
         a) Vigorous behavior — aggressive
         b) Limit testing
      2) Child develops a conscience
   b. Cognitive development (Piaget)
      1) Preoperational (2-7 years)
         a) Egocentric in thought and behavior
         b) Concrete, tangible thinking
         c) Vivid imagination
            (1) Magical thinking (for example: thoughts can cause events)

      (2) Peak age for fears
   c. Socialization
      1) 3 years
         a) May have an imaginary friend
         b) Increased ability to separate from parents
      2) 4 years
         a) May be bossy and impatient
         b) Privacy and independence become important
      3) 5 years
         a) Less rebellious; more responsible
         b) Cares for self and hygiene needs with minimal supervision
   d. Sexuality
      1) Knows own sex and sex of others by three years
      2) Masturbation is normal, healthy expression, if not excessive
      3) Sexual exploration demonstrated in playing doctor
      4) Answer questions honestly and simply

7. Play
   a. Cooperative play beginning
      1) Enjoys loud, physical activities
      2) More socialization during play
      3) Self-criticism or boasting evident
   b. Purposes of play
      1) Increase coordination
      2) Decrease tension, anxiety
      3) Deal with fantasies
      4) Enhance self-esteem
      5) Sense of power, control
      6) Increase knowledge of self
   c. Materials
      1) Physical: bat, ball, sand box, sled, bike, puzzles
      2) Dramatic: dress-up clothes, dolls, costumes; imitate adult behavior
      3) Creative: pens, paper, crayons, paint, scissors, playdough, chalk

8. Health maintenance
   a. Safety
      1) Maintain safe environment
         a) Automobile safety: Use of car seat until approximately 4 years, 40 lbs; may depend on local laws; use of booster seat for smaller children.
         b) Immunizations (see table IV-10.)
            (1) Pre-kindergarten boosters given at five years (DTaP, IPV, MMR)
            (2) May catch up on "missed" immunizations required for school attendance
      2) Anticipatory Guidance
         a) Lock up flammables, medications,

and toxic substances
- b) Supervise at all times
- c) Teach water safety; swimming lessons
- d) Teach traffic (pedestrian) safety

b. Discipline
- 1) Consistent limit setting
- 2) "Time-out" for misbehavior
  - a) Effective if used consistently
  - b) Time out = one minute per year of child's age

Lifespan and Development of the School-Age Child

6–12 Years

1. Physical characteristics
   a. Grows 1–2 inches/year
   b. Gains 3–7 pounds/year
   c. Pubescent changes may begin to appear
      1) Girls: by approximately 10–12 years
      2) Boys: by approximately 12–14 years
   d. Vital signs approach adult normals
      1) Pulse: ranges from 60–80 beats/min
      2) Respirations: range from 18–20/min
      3) Blood pressure: averages 90–110/55–60
   e. Dentition
      1) Permanent teeth begin erupting about six years (see table IV-2.)
      2) 32 permanent teeth by 18 years of age

TABLE IV-2.
SCHEDULE OF PERMANENT TOOTH ERUPTION

ERUPTION	AGE
First molar	5 1/2–6 years
Medial incisor	6–7 years
Lateral incisor	7–8 years
Cuspid	10–12 years
Bicuspid	10–11 years
Bicuspid	11–12 years
Second molar	12–13 years

      3) May wear braces (orthodontia)
2. Nutrition
   a. Influenced by peers, mass media in food selections
   b. "Junk food" (empty calories), "fast food" preferred, encourage nutritious snacks
   c. Obesity possible if inadequate exercise
3. Activity/rest
   a. Sleeps 8–10 hours/day with vivid dreams
   b. Somnambulism (sleep walking) is common
4. Motor skills
   a. Gross-motor skills
      1) Roller skates/bicycles/skateboards/scooters
      2) Competitive sports
      3) Swimming
   b. Fine-motor skills
      1) Cursive writing
      2) Musical instruments
      3) Arts and crafts
      4) Learns keyboarding skills
5. Language development
   a. Masters all sounds by 7-1/2–8 years
   b. Uses telephone, computer to communicate with peers
   c. Reads and writes
6. Developmental stages
   a. Psychosocial development (Erikson)
      1) Industry vs inferiority (6–12 years)
         a) Primary tasks relate to learning skills, activities
         b) Afraid of failure; embarrassed by poor grades
      2) Child develops self-esteem
   b. Cognitive development (Piaget)
      1) Concrete operations (7–11 years)
         a) Classifies and sorts; enjoys collecting
         b) Concrete logic and problem solving
         c) Less egocentric
      2) Inductive thinking
   c. Socialization
      1) Prefers peers of same age and sex
      2) Responds positively to rewards
      3) Belonging is important: enjoys scouts, clubs, team sports; may join a gang
      4) Cliques may become evident (9–10 years)
      5) May be left alone for short periods (10–12 years); depends on maturity of child
   d. Sexuality
      1) Preadolescents need specific, age-appropriate information about puberty, physical changes (10–12 years)
      2) Answer questions openly and honestly
      3) Develops interest in opposite sex (10–12 years)
7. Play
   a. Cooperative
   b. Characteristics
      1) Clubs or gangs (8-12 years)
      2) Best friends (9–10 years)
      3) Secrets
   c. Suggested play activities
      1) Table games
      2) Collections
      3) Computer or video games
      4) Community sports/group activities
      5) Creative: dance, art, music
8. Health maintenance

a. Safety
   1) Prevention
      a) Focus on teaching child to be safe
      b) No longer under parental supervision at all times
   2) Immunizations
      a) MMR booster (if not given pre-kindergarten) at 11–12 years
      b) Varicella zoster (chicken pox) for susceptible children (can be given anytime after 1 year of age)
b. Common problems
   1) Swearing
   2) Lying
   3) Cheating
   4) Stealing
   5) Nail biting
   6) Sibling rivalry
      a) Often jealous of younger/older sibling
      b) Encourage parent not to become involved except in case of physical/emotional harm
c. Discipline
   1) Avoid punitive measures
   2) Consistency
   3) Withdrawal of privileges
   4) Time out
d. Stress and coping
   1) School-age children face enormous societal pressures
   2) Do not have cognitive skills to deal with these pressures
   3) Professionals need to be aware that sleep problems, enuresis, changes in appetite, or behavioral problems may be indicative of inadequate coping

9. Health deviations
   a. Accidents
      1) Motor vehicles (use seat belts)
      2) Fractures due to increased activity (use helmets and other protective gear)
      3) Firearms (increasing in frequency)
      4) Drowning
   b. School phobia
      1) Fear or dread of school
      2) Manifestations
         a) Nausea, vomiting and/or abdominal pain on school mornings
         b) Abrupt onset
         c) Manifestations subside when child is at home
      3) Etiology
         a) Teacher/child mismatch
         b) Fear of failure
         c) Bully
      4) Treatment
         a) Identify cause
         b) Support child in attending school daily
         c) Professional (psychiatric) help may be required in severe cases

Lifespan and Development of the Adolescent

12–18 years

1. Physical characteristics
   a. Very individualized
   b. By 17 years, 100% of adult stature
   c. Vital signs reach adult norms
   d. Dentition
      1) Third molars (wisdom teeth) by approximately 18 years
      2) Orthodontia in progress or completed
   e. Sexual maturation/puberty
      1) Female
         a) Breast enlargement (approximately 11 years)
         b) Pubic hair
         c) Growth spurt
         d) Menarche (onset of menstruation)
            (1) Approximately 11 years of age
            (2) Ovulation approximately 6 months–1 year after menarche
      2) Male
         a) Body hair growth
         b) Growth of external genitalia
         c) Growth spurt/increased muscle mass
         d) Voice changes
         e) Ejaculation/nocturnal emission
2. Nutrition
   a. Growth spurt
   b. Increased protein, iron, and calcium needs
3. Activity/rest
   a. Sleep needs increase due to growth demands
   b. Tire easily
4. Motor skills
   a. Risk takers
   b. Sense of indestructibility
   c. General increase in physical and psychomotor skills enhances self-esteem
5. Language development
   a. Sophisticated ability to communicate via verbal and written word
   b. Use of slang prominent
6. Developmental stages
   a. Psychosocial development (Erikson)
      1) Identify formation vs. identify diffusion (12–18 years)
         a) Identify future career goals
         b) Incorporate physical changes into identity
   b. Cognitive development (Piaget)

1) Formal operations (11+ years)
2) Abstract thinking (ability to hypothesize)
c. Socialization
1) Emancipation from family
2) Peer group major influence; has strong need to belong
3) Employment
4) Less adult supervision
d. Sexuality
1) Establishes sexual identity and orientation
2) Experiments with intimate relationships
3) Common issues
a) Sexually transmitted diseases
b) Human immunodeficiency virus (HIV)
c) Adolescent pregnancy
7. Recreation
a. Reflects psychosocial needs
b. Group activities with mixed sexes
c. May include dating, sports
d. Suggested recreational activities for hospitalized adolescent
1) Computer or video games
2) Cards
3) Portable CD player
8. Health maintenance
a. Safety
1) Accident prevention
a) Focus on educating adolescent to make safe choices
b) Be alert to signs of depression, substance abuse
2) Immunizations
a) Tetanus-diphtheria (Td) needed every 10 years
b) Hepatitis B series if not previously administered
c) 2001 CDC recommendation is for Meningococcal vaccine for college bound freshmen who will be living in dormitories
b. Discipline
1) Increased independence
2) Consistency
c. Stress and coping
1) Faced with enormous societal pressures
2) Feels pressure to belong, conform, achieve
3) Common reactions to stress
a) Early adolescent: mood swings and self-focused
b) Middle adolescent: increased rebellious behavior
c) Later adolescent: better coping skills
4) Common problems
a) Runaways
b) Eating disorders
c) Substance abuse

(1) Nonprescription, illicit, or street drugs
(2) Alcohol
(3) Tobacco
9. Health deviations
a. Accidents
1) Motor vehicles
a) Driver's education
b) Drunk driving
2) Firearms
3) Spinal cord injuries
4) Drowning
b. Homicide
c. Suicide

SECTION II

THE HOSPITALIZED CHILD

Stress of Hospitalization

A. **Potential Regression** → fall back!
1. Usually healthy adaptation to hospitalization
2. Respect child's use of this defense mechanism
3. Assist child to achieve past developmental levels

B. **Child's Reaction to Hospitalization** (Age/developmental specific)
1. Protest: strong, conscious need for parent; may be confused, frightened, crying
2. Despair: mourning period; may be withdrawn, apathetic
3. Denial: represses true feelings; feels parent has failed; interested in surroundings but not mom

C. **Developmental Influences on Stress of Hospitalization**
1. Infant: trust versus mistrust
   a. 0–6 months: loss of consistent care giver
   b. 6–12 months: strong need for mother; separation anxiety
2. Toddler: autonomy versus shame and doubt
   a. Separation anxiety, loss of significant other, inconsistency
   b. Loss of mobility due to restraints, crib
3. Preschooler: initiative versus guilt
   a. Separation anxiety
   b. Threats to body integrity may cause increased aggression
   c. Concept of illness
      1) Magical thinking (believes that feelings and thoughts can cause illness)
      2) May believe illness or hospitalization is punishment
4. School-age child: industry versus inferiority

a. Loss of control
b. Separation from: peers, school, after school activities
c. Concept of illness
   1) Perceives an external cause for illness
   2) May view illness as a result of "doing something wrong"
   3) Understands difference between acute and chronic illness
5. Adolescent: identity versus role diffusion
   a. Threats to body image
   b. Loss of control
   c. Separation from peers, school, activities
   d. Concept of illness
      1) Believes self to be invulnerable
      2) Understands internal cause of disease
      3) Best cooperates with treatment plan if understands immediate benefits

D. Stress of Hospitalization on Family
1. Shock and Denial
   a. Allow verbalization of feelings; recognize and accept defense mechanisms
   b. Enhance coping strategies
   c. Allow family to stay with child as much as possible; open visitation policy
   d. Explain that regressive behavior is normal and expected
   e. Explain that separation anxiety is normal and expected
2. Adjustment
   a. Encourage communication between family and medical personnel
   b. Encourage family participation in decision making and care giving

E. Reaction to Pain
1. Rule of thumb: assume that if a procedure would be painful for an adult, it is also painful for a child
2. **NURSING INTERVENTIONS** (strategies for pain management)
   a. Age-appropriate assessment
      1) Ask child with age-appropriate language
      2) Use pain rating tool (for example: Baker-Wong Faces)
      3) Developmental assessment of pain
         a) Infant
            (1) Generalized body response of rigidity, thrashing
            (2) Loud crying, facial expression
            (3) May sleep to avoid pain experience
         b) Toddler
            (1) Localized response: will withdraw from pain

(2) Physical resistance after painful stimulation
c) Preschooler
   (1) Verbalizes pain
   (2) Attempts to avoid painful stimulus
   (3) May view pain as punishment
d) School-aged child
   (1) Verbalizes pain
   (2) Stalling behavior; vocal protest
   (3) Recognizes physical cause of pain
e) Adolescent
   (1) Sophisticated verbal expression of pain
   (2) Less resistance offered: physical, vocal
   (3) Understands physical and psychological pain
b. Use of pharmacologic control methods
   1) Weight-appropriate (mg/kg) dosages
   2) Oral and IV routes preferred over IM; child will avoid "shot" and not be medicated
   3) Conscious sedation: midazolam (*Versed*), fentanyl citrate (*Sublimaze*) for painful procedures
   4) PCA (patient-controlled analgesia) appropriate for children who understand cause and effect (approximately seven years)
   5) Eutectic mixture of local anesthetics (*EMLA*) cream is a topical anesthetic that can be applied as a thick dollop and covered with a transparent dressing approximately one to two hours prior to a procedure (venipuncture, injection) to lessen the pain
c. Use of non-pharmacologic control methods
   1) Distraction
   2) Relaxation
   3) Kinesthetic (rocking) stimulation

F. Strategies for Stress Reduction
1. Prehospital preparation, preoperative teaching and tour
2. Specially trained pediatric staff
3. Use of outpatient facilities eliminates need for overnight hospitalization and separation
4. Therapeutic Play
   a. Purposes
      1) Mastery of situation
      2) Ego strengthening
      3) Deal with fears, anxiety and the unknown
   b. **NURSING INTERVENTIONS**
      1) Play with child appropriate to developmental level and illness

2) Allow child to set the pace of play
3) Provide a variety of play materials
4) Reflect back the child's feelings
5. Communication Strategies
   a. Appropriate for situation
   b. Clear and consistent
   c. Communicate in an age appropriate manner with the child
      1) Verbal
      2) Nonverbal

SECTION III

NURSING CARE OF THE CHILD WITH CONGENITAL ANOMALIES

Congenital Heart Defects

A. Hemodynamics of Fetal Circulation

1. Ductus venosus: carries oxygenated blood from placenta to inferior vena cava; partially bypasses liver; closes by approximately 8th week of life
2. Ductus arteriosus: bypasses flow of blood through lungs by shunting oxygenated and unoxygenated blood from pulmonary artery to aorta; closes 7–10 days after birth
3. Foramen ovale: connects right and left atria; allows blood to flow from right atrium to left atrium, thereby bypassing the right ventricle and pulmonary circuit; closes by 2–3 months
4. Transition to newborn circulation
   a. At first breath, lungs expand which increases blood flow to pulmonary system
   b. Pulmonary vascular resistance is decreased and systemic vascular resistance increases
   c. These changes lead to the closure of the ductus venosus, ductus arteriosus and foramen ovale

B. Characteristics

1. Unknown etiology (always consider genetic factors in addition to intrauterine infection, radiation, or drugs)
2. Incidence is 1 in 1,000 live births (accounts for 50% of all deaths in first year of life); may be associated with other birth defects, syndromes
3. May not be diagnosed while hospitalized in newborn nursery
4. Clinical signs include:
   a. Neonate and infant
      1) Cyanosis: especially circumoral and acrocyanosis; cyanosis on exertion (examples: feeding, crying)

2) Dyspnea: especially on exertion
3) Failure to thrive
4) Frequent upper respiratory infections
5) Feeding difficulty
6) Weak or muffled cry
   b. Older child
      1) Cyanosis and dyspnea (as above)
      2) Impaired growth
      3) Fatigue
      4) Digital clubbing
      5) Squatting
      6) Polycythemia: increased RBC count to compensate for impaired gas exchange; increases oxygen-carrying capacity of blood
   c. Congestive heart failure
      1) Tachypnea, dyspnea
      2) Exercise intolerance
      3) Tachycardia (above 160 BPM)
      4) Diaphoresis
      5) Hepatomegaly and edema (late signs)
5. Increased risk of bacterial endocarditis

C. Diagnosis

1. Cardiac catheterization
2. Echocardiography

D. Comparison of Acyanotic and Cyanotic Defects
(see tables IV-3. & IV-4.)

E. NURSING INTERVENTIONS

1. Correct knowledge deficit related to:
   a. Cardiac catheterization
      1) Consider developmental level of child when planning teaching strategies
      2) Explain to parents that procedure is done under conscious sedation
      3) Be alert to postprocedural concerns (same as adult)
   b. Anticoagulant therapy
      1) Explain why this is necessary for children who have prosthetic valves or increased blood viscosity
      2) Instruct parents to be alert for signs of increased bleeding: excessive bruising, epistaxis, hematuria, bloody stools
      3) Explain need for bleeding precautions
   c. Preoperative preparation
      1) Promote parental involvement to decrease anxiety
      2) Include description of what child will feel during procedure, surgery (based on developmental level)
2. Altered cardiac output related to failure of the myocardium to meet the demands of the body

TABLE IV-3.
REVIEW OF ACYANOTIC CONGENITAL HEART ANOMALIES

ANOMALY	HEMODYNAMICS	CLINICAL MANIFESTATIONS	TREATMENT
Patent Ductus Arteriosus (PDA): A vascular channel between the L main pulmonary artery and the descending aorta, as a result of failure of the fetal ductus arteriosus to close	- Shunt of oxygenated blood from the aorta into the pulmonary artery - Increased left ventricular output and work load	- Usually asymptomatic, but frequent impairment of growth or CHF - "Machinery murmur" - Wide pulse pressure	- Medical: administration of indomethacin (*Indocin*) (prostaglandin inhibitor) is effective in some newborns and premature infants - Surgical: ligation of patent ductus (in infancy)
Ventricular Septal Defect (VSD): Defect is in membranous muscular portion of the ventricular septum; may vary from small to large defect	- Shunt of oxygenated blood from L to R ventricle - Leads to R ventricular hypertrophy - Needs surgical repair - Bi-directional shunting may occur with very large defect (Eisenmenger Syndrome)	- May be asymptomatic - Heart murmur is heard in 1st week of life (systolic) - Growth failure, feeding problems during 1st year of life; FTT; frequent respiratory infections - CHF is common	- Some small defects may close spontaneously - Open heart: direct closure suturing with plastic prosthesis (usually at preschool age, may be done earlier in infancy for large defects)
Atrial Septal Defect (ASD): Malfunctioning foremen ovale; or abnormal opening between the atria	- Shunting of oxygenated blood from L to R atrium - Increased R ventricular output and work load - May develop pulmonary hypertension (in adulthood, if not surgically treated in childhood)	- Acyanotic; asymptomatic - Soft blowing systolic murmur - Thin and asthenic - Frequent episodes of pulmonary inflammatory diseases - Poor exercise tolerance	Open heart with direct closure or suturing with plastic prosthesis (usually at pre-school age)
Coarctation of Aorta: - Preductal constriction of the aorta between subclavian artery and ductus arteriosus - Postductal constriction of aorta directly beyond the ductus	- Obstruction of the flow of blood through the constricted segments - Increased L ventricular pressure and work load - Extensive collateral circulation bypasses coarctated area to supply lower extremities with blood	- Hypertension in upper extremities with decreased BP in lower extremities - Weak or absent pulsations in lower extremities - CHF - May be asymptomatic; occasionally fatigue, head-aches, leg cramps, epistaxis	- Surgical resection of coarctate area with direct anastomosis or use of a graft - Correction usually done by 2 years of age to prevent permanent hypertension

TABLE IV-4.
REVIEW OF CYANOTIC CONGENITAL HEART ANOMALIES

ANOMALY	HEMODYNAMICS	CLINICAL MANIFESTATIONS	TREATMENT
Tetralogy of Fallot: combination of four defects: 1) Pulmonary stenosis 2) Ventricular septal defect (VSD) 3) Overriding aorta 4) Hypertrophy of R ventricle	- Obstruction to outflow of blood from R ventricle into pulmonary circuit and increased pressure in the R ventricle leads to R to L shunting of unoxygenated blood thru the VSD directly into the aorta - Severity of defect depends on degree of pulmonary stenosis and size of VSD	- Acute cyanosis at birth - Cyanosis developing during early months that increases with physical exertion - Clubbing of fingers and toes - Systolic murmur - Acute episodes of cyanosis and hypoxia called "tet spells" or hypercyanotic episodes occur if oxygen supply cannot meet demand (for example, with crying, exertion, exercise, feeding) - Squatting - Growth retardation	- Surgical: Blalock-Taussig Procedures-provides blood flow to pulmonary arteries from the L or R subclavian artery - Repair: open heart closure of VSD and resection of stenosis Usually performed in first two years of life
Transposition of Great Vessels (TGV): the aorta originates from the R ventricle and the pulmonary artery from the L ventricle	- Two separate circulations without mixture of oxygenated and unoxygenated blood except through shunts - Mixture of blood may occur through one or more septal defects: - Ventricular septal defect (VSD) - Atrial septal defect (ASD) - Patent ductus arteriosus (PDA)	- Usually deep cyanosis shortly after birth or after closing of ductus - Early clubbing of toes and fingers - Poor growth and development, FTT - Rapid respirations; fatigue - Congestive heart failure	- Medical: administration of IV prostaglandin until surgical repair - Repair: arterial switch is treatment of choice; must be done within first few days of life; great vessels reimplanted under complete circulatory arrest - Several other types of repair are all multiple stage approaches

a. Promote reduced energy expenditures by providing adequate rest periods, planning care to reduce interruptions, and recognizing signs of fatigue; infant seat very helpful; avoid temperature extremes

b. Administer and monitor medications that will promote cardiac function

   1) Digitalis (*Digoxin*) (same as adult) except:

     a) Check apical heart rate one full minute prior to administering-hold digitalis (*Digoxin*) if heart rate is below: 100 for infants; 80 for toddlers and preschoolers; 60 for children and adolescents

     b) Administer medication on an empty stomach; do not give with food or juice; do not repeat dose if child vomits

     c) Therapeutic range for children 0.8 – 2.0 m/l

   2) Diuretics: furosemide (*Lasix*), chlorothiazide (*Diuril*), ethacrynic acid (*Edecrin*)

     a) Monitor potassium levels and supplement losses; observe for hypokalemia - increases risk of digitalis (*Digoxin*) toxicity

     b) Include daily weights, intake/output, and respiratory assessment in daily care

3. Altered nutrition: less than body requirements related to congestive heart failure; "Cardiac" infants usually have a weak suck, become cyanotic during feedings, tire easily, and may fall asleep while feeding

    a. Small, frequent feedings using soft nipple with large hole

    b. Administer 24 kcal/oz formula in order to increase caloric intake

    c. Limit oral feedings to 20 minutes; gavage feed the remainder

4. Altered parenting related to chronic aspects of cardiac problems

    a. Discipline is the most difficult area of parenting due to feelings of guilt and powerlessness

    b. Parents need help remembering child should be treated as normally as possible

    c. Counsel family regarding possibility of developmental delays; include infant stimulation in teaching

    d. Assist with potential grieving: loss of "perfect" infant

Neurological Defects

A. Hydrocephalus

1. Characteristics

    a. Definition: imbalance in either absorption or production of cerebrospinal fluid within intracranial cavity

    b. Classification: either congenital or acquired

    c. Usually diagnosed at birth or within two to four months of life

    d. Often associated with other neural tube defect (example: myelomeningocele)

    e. Clinical manifestations (categorized by age)

       1) Infant: increased head circumference, tense bulging anterior fontanel, distended scalp veins, high pitched cry, irritability, feeding problems, discomfort when held

       2) Older child: headache, vomiting (especially in the morning), diplopia, blurred vision, behavioral changes, decreased motor function, decreased level of consciousness, seizures

2. Diagnosis

    a. May be detected on prenatal sonogram

    b. Clinical signs

       1) Increasing intracranial pressure

       2) Increasing head circumference

    c. CT or MRI scan confirms diagnosis; shows excessive fluid in ventricles (brain)

3. Treatment

    a. Pressure relieved by surgical insertion of a shunting device

    b. Components of a shunt include: catheter, reservoir, pumping device with one-way valve, distal tubing with regulator valve

    c. Most common type of shunt is ventriculoperitoneal

    d. Complications include shunt failure and infection

    e. Shunt will require revision (lengthening of tubing) as child grows

    f. Early treatment necessary to prevent progressive mental retardation

 4. **NURSING INTERVENTIONS**

    a. Risk for injury related to increased intracranial pressure

       1) Preoperatively measure head circumference by obtaining occipito-frontal measurement

       2) Postoperatively

          a) Perform frequent neurologic assessment with daily head circumference

          b) Position on non-operative site; check anterior fontanel to determine positioning of the head; do not pump shunt without order

          c) Monitor for signs and symptoms of shunt failure: lethargy, vomiting, and irritability

          d) Institute seizure precautions

    b. Risk for infection

       1) Monitor for signs of shunt infection: elevated vital signs, decreased LOC, vomiting, feeding problems

       2) Assess incision site frequently for manifestations of inflammation or leakage

    c. Additional nursing diagnoses

       1) Alteration in nutrition (less than body requirements): frequent small feedings; planned rest periods after feeding; daily weight

       2) Knowledge deficit: instruct parents regarding manifestations of shunt failure; encourage infant stimulation to help maximize child's potential

B. Myelomeningocele: most common of neural tube defects

1. Definition: type of Spina Bifida, a fissure in spinal column leaving meninges and spinal cord exposed

2. Characteristics

a. Failure of posterior laminae to fuse with herniation of saclike cyst of meninges, CSF, and spinal nerves
b. Usually associated with other neurologic defects (example: hydrocephalus) *~neuro*
c. Unknown etiology *~neuro*
d. May be prevented by folic acid supplementation by women of childbearing age prior to conception and through first trimester

3. Pathology *~ medical research or finding*
   a. Partial to complete paralysis determined by location of defect (usually lumbosacral)
   b. Musculoskeletal problems such as club foot, scoliosis, congenital hip dysplasia
   c. Sensory disturbances parallel motor dysfunction
   d. Bowel and bladder problems including constipation, incontinence, neurogenic bladder

4. Diagnosis
   a. Amniocentesis: 98% accurate; elevated alpha fetoprotein (AFP), confirmed by prenatal sonogram
   b. Apparent at birth: visible sac

5. Treatment
   a. Decision to correct the defect or not is difficult as well as controversial
   b. Early surgical closure is advocated to preserve neural function, reduce risk of infection, control hydrocephalus

 6. **NURSING INTERVENTIONS**
   a. Risk for infection
      1) Preoperatively, the main goal is to prevent rupture of the sac, which would predispose the newborn to infection
         a) Keep infant in prone position
         b) Cover sac with 4 x 4s moistened with sterile saline
         c) Check sac for tears or cracks
         d) Do not cover sac with clothing or diapers (places pressure on the sac)
         e) Perform perineal care to prevent contamination of sac
         f) Monitor for manifestations of meningitis (irritability, anorexia, fever, seizures)
      2) Postoperatively, the main goal is to promote healing and reduce neurological complications
         Lpriority a) Place infant in prone position with head slightly lower than body
         b) Place protective barrier across incision to prevent contamination
         c) Be aware of long-term problems of infection related to urinary retention,

reflux, chronic urinary tract infections
      (1) Teach parents the Credé maneuver
      (2) Encourage independent intermittent self-catheterization (can be performed as early as 5–6 years of age)
      (3) Stress hydration and early recognition of UTIs
      (4) Explain to parents that urinary diversion procedures are often required
   b. Risk for injury related to increased intracranial pressure secondary to hydrocephalus
      1) Perform neurologic checks with daily head circumference
      2) Monitor for manifestations of increased intracranial pressure
   c. Ineffective parental coping
      1) Parents will need help dealing with the issue of "chronic sorrow" as well as the long-term aspects of the condition
      2) Remember that every family's method of coping is different: offer options in nonjudgmental manner; provide supportive environment that will help families make the most appropriate choices
   d. Risk for injury related to latex exposure: recognize that children with neural tube defects are at increased risk for latex allergy and that exposure to common medical (or other) products containing latex should be avoided (for example: vinyl gloves, balloons)
   e. Additional nursing problems
      1) Risk for impaired skin integrity: frequent position changes, keep perianal area clean of dribbling urine and stool
      2) Impaired mobility: position changes, range-of-motion activities, physical therapy

C. **Cerebral Palsy**
   1. Characteristics
      a. Early onset, permanent, non-progressive disability
      b. Impaired movement and posture, with abnormal muscle tone and coordination
      c. May be accompanied by language and cognitive deficits
      d. Causes undetermined; may be related to prenatal, perinatal or postnatal factors
      e. Increased risk in neonates with an Apgar score of 5 or less
   2. Diagnosis

a. Classified by nature and distribution of neuro-muscular dysfunction
b. May not be diagnosed until child is several months old
c. Confirmed by physical evaluation, or supplemental tests (for example: EEG, tomography, or metabolic screening)
d. Early clinical signs
   1) Persistent primitive reflexes
   2) Hyper or hypotonicity (stiff or floppy arms and legs)
   3) Poor hand control, body control
   4) Feeding difficulties
   5) Irritability
   6) Delayed attainment of developmental milestones
3. Treatment (based on degree of disability)
   a. Physical therapy (active and passive)
   b. Anticonvulsants: phenobarbital or phenytoin (*Dilantin*)
   c. Modified toys or equipment to enhance development
   d. Surgery (to correct contractures or spastic deformities)

 4. **NURSING INTERVENTIONS**
   a. Risk for injury related to neuromuscular and perceptual impairment
      1) Teach family and child safe use of adaptive devices
      2) Modify environment to enhance safety
      3) Institute seizure precautions if appropriate
      4) Encourage physical safety techniques (examples: aspiration precautions, adequate rest)
   b. Self-care deficit related to impaired physical capabilities
      1) Encourage self-care activities to foster independence and confidence
      2) Modify environment, devices to enhance development and increase functional abilities
   c. Risk for communication deficit related to physical or perceptual impairment
      1) Refer to OT and speech therapy for evaluation and development of verbal and non-verbal communication skills
      2) Teach caregivers alternative communication methods to facilitate positive adjustments of child and family

Musculoskeletal Defects

A. Congenital Dysplasia of the Hip (CDH)
1. Characteristics
   a. Refers to imperfect development of the hip of varying degrees
   b. Etiology unknown; familial tendency; females are 8 times more likely to develop
   c. Manifestations: shortening of affected leg, asymmetrical gluteal folds, limited abduction, Ortolani's sign (audible "click" as examiner slips femoral head forward)
   d. Early detection critical: if untreated will lead to lordosis, scoliosis, "duck waddle"
2. Pathology
   a. The head of the femur must be properly located within the acetabulum for correct development of the hip joint
   b. As ossification proceeds, correcting the hip defect becomes more difficult
   c. Once child begins to walk, prognosis questionable
   d. Most common type is subluxation (incomplete dislocation of hip)
3. Diagnosis
   a. Assessment techniques with newborn (Ortolani's "click")
   b. X-rays difficult to read in early infancy because ossification of femoral head does not occur until 3–6 months of life
4. Treatment
   a. If diagnosed within first 2–3 months of life, the hip joint abduction is maintained via double diapering, Frejka pillow, splint, or Pavlik harness
   b. Once adductor muscles contract, traction and/or casting may be used; usually by 6 months (once the child is standing and walking) both methods are used in conjunction with surgery (Bryant's traction if below 2 years)

 5. **NURSING INTERVENTIONS**
   a. Risk for injury related to impaired neurovascular function
      1) Frequent neurovascular checks: CMS (circulation, motion, sensation)
      2) Casts: routine cast care; if hip spica cast is used, teach parents not to use abductor stabilizer bar as a "handle" when moving child
      3) Bryant's traction: legs are elevated at 90 degree angle to body; child's weight provides countertraction; correct amount of traction is applied if child's buttocks are elevated slightly above bed
   b. Risk for impairment of skin integrity: assess skin for irritation or pressure areas
   c. Impaired physical mobility related to cast or traction: need to consider problems of immobility (for example: pulmonary, renal,

eliminative, musculoskeletal); diet should include increased roughage, fluid, calcium, protein, carbohydrates
    d. Knowledge deficit related to home care: Pavlik harness should be worn 24 hours/day; infant with hip spica cast will require special car seat
    c. Same developmental tasks (reinforce with parents)

B. Congenital Clubfoot (Talipes Equinovarus)
1. Characteristics
    a. Forefoot adducted, heel tilted inward (varus), plantar flexion at ankle
    b. Important to differentiate between positional and true clubfoot (true clubfoot cannot be positioned in normal alignment with ROM)
2. Diagnosis and treatment
    a. Apparent at birth; longer treatment postponed, more soft tissue changes occur and correction more difficult
    b. Serial casting is employed to gradually manipulate the foot into normal position; casts are changed at weekly intervals; as each new cast is applied, the foot is re-manipulated and recasted
    c. Dennis-Brown splint may be used to maintain position once casting is completed

3. **NURSING INTERVENTIONS**
    a. Risk for injury related to neurovascular impairment; teach parents to do CMS checks
    b. Knowledge deficit related to cast care or exercise regimen: compliance is critical if defect is to be corrected; encourage follow-up visits as well as meeting child's developmental needs within imposed limitations; parents must be able to perform neurovascular checks at home on casted limb due to infant's growth-rate

Gastrointestinal Defects

A. Cleft Lip *Hare lip*
1. Characteristics
    a. Definition: failure of the maxillary processes to fuse with the nasal processes (may be unilateral or bilateral)
    b. Etiology: unknown, but strong genetic or environmental factors
    c. More common in males
    d. May or may not be accompanied by cleft palate
2. Pathology
    a. Prone to ear, nose, and throat infection
    b. Long-term problems include speech, hearing, and dentition problems

3. Diagnosis and treatment
    a. Defect apparent at birth
    b. Surgical repair initiated within first three months of life
    c. Staggered z-shaped suture line used to minimize scarring
4. **NURSING INTERVENTIONS**
    a. Alteration in nutrition: less than body requirements
      1) Preoperatively: be aware of feeding difficulties related to sucking problems; infants also swallow a great deal of air during feeding; burp frequently; use adaptive feeding devices
        a) Large soft nipples
        b) Breck feeder (syringe with rubber tubing)
        c) Breast feeding
        d) Habermann feeder (soft squeezable nipple attached via diaphragm to bottle to allow formula to be "squirted" into infant's mouth with each sucking attempt
      2) Postoperatively: sucking places undue pressure on the suture line so feeding may present difficulties; use medicine dropper or Breck feeder; begin this type of feeding preoperatively
    b. Risk for injury related to trauma or pressure on the suture line
      1) Restrain infant to prevent pulling or tugging on the suture line (elbow restraints)
      2) Do not position on abdomen
      3) Do not use pacifier (strongly encourage parents to avoid using pacifier preop)
      4) Apply a topical ointment such as bacitracin (BACI-IM), as ordered, to suture line as needed to prevent infection
      5) Apply Logan bar, as ordered, to reduce tension on the suture line
    c. Ineffective airway clearance: infant is at risk for aspiration so positioning is very important; infant should be repositioned frequently to prevent stasis of secretions; side to side or infant seat only acceptable positions
    d. Ineffective family coping: birth of a child with "physical problems" elicits anger, disbelief, denial; parents will encounter "chronic sorrow"; be supportive and encouraging while helping parents overcome their concern; focus should be on bonding; convey attitude of acceptance; show "before and after" photos of other infants

B. Cleft Palate

1. Characteristics
   a. Failure of palatine processes to fuse
   b. More common among females
   c. Defect may include both hard and soft palate
   d. Major problems are similar to cleft lip: feeding; aspiration; ear, nose, and throat infections
   e. May or may not be associated with cleft lip

2. Diagnosis and treatment
   a. Repair usually completed by 12–18 months of age to prevent speech problems
   b. Surgery may be performed in stages

3. **NURSING INTERVENTIONS**
   a. Alteration in nutrition: less than body requirements
      1) Preoperatively: feeding difficulties related to sucking problems; infants also swallow a great deal of air during feeding (burp frequently); use of adaptive feeding devices (see cleft lip)
      2) Postoperatively: nothing can be placed in the child's mouth; child is fed liquefied diet through a cup; spoon cannot be inserted into mouth as it can damage suture line; soft diet maintained until palate healed
   b. Risk for injury related to trauma or pressure on the suture line
      1) Use elbow restraints to keep the child's hands away from the mouth; remove periodically one at a time for ROM
      2) May position on abdomen
      3) Do not allow child to put objects into mouth: child may not suck (no pacifier); small toys or objects must be kept out of the child's reach; child may drink from a cup or sip from the side of a large spoon; oral hygiene after eating is essential to reduce problems with infection
   c. Ineffective airway clearance: child will be at risk for breathing problems during the first 48 hours; new breathing patterns must be established; croupette may be ordered
   d. Ineffective family coping (see cleft lip)

NURSING CARE OF THE CHILD WITH AN ACUTE ILLNESS

Common Problems Associated with Acute Illness

A. Fever

1. Characteristics
   a. Classified as temperature in excess of 100.4°F (38°C)
   b. Not always related to severity of illness; varies from child to child
   c. Always consider
      1) Age of child: below six months, more serious concern *dehydration / more body water*
      2) If child is immunosuppressed or receiving chemotherapy
   d. Most fevers in children are viral, self limiting; may play a role in recovery from infection

2. Diagnosis
   a. Feeling a child's skin for warmth is not an accurate indicator
   b. Always investigate family epidemiology and take a careful history for exposure to communicative diseases
   c. Remember that diet, activity level and behavioral changes are subtle diagnostic clues
   d. Laboratory tests may include complete blood count (CBC), urinalysis (UA), chest film (CXR) and blood cultures. A "septic work-up" includes all of the above with the addition of a lumbar puncture (LP) and urine culture.

3. Treatment
   a. Fever management is questionable because fever is considered a part of the body's defense mechanism *unwrapped infant*
   b. Antipyretic, such as acetaminophen (*Tylenol*) or ibuprofen (*Motrin*) in weight appropriate dose
   c. Do not give aspirin *< 12 Reyes syndrome*

4. **NURSING INTERVENTIONS**
   a. Febrile seizures
      1) Usually seen in children between six months and three years old; related to sudden rise of temperature (above 102°F); child usually has a respiratory or gastrointestinal infection
      2) Therapeutic treatment includes diazepam (*Valium*), antipyretics
      3) Risk for injury related to febrile seizure
         a) Maintain a patent airway

        b) Protect the child from injury (do not restrain child or put objects in mouth, remove toys and sharp objects from bed, institute seizure precautions if history of seizures)

        c) Observe the seizure

    b. Risk for fluid volume deficit related to dehydration:

Teaspoon. every 20 minutes

      1) Assess the child for manifestations of dehydration (examples: sunken eyes, depressed anterior fontanel, dry mucous membranes, poor tissue turgor); specific gravity will be elevated

      2) Encourage clear fluids if child not vomiting

      3) Check to ensure the child is voiding in adequate amounts

    c. Altered body temperature related to infection

      1) Monitor child's temperature every 3 to 4 hours

      2) Employ environmental measures: remove excessive clothing, encourage clear fluids

    d. Knowledge deficit related to home care

      1) Educate parents regarding seizure precautions, methods to control fever, how to prevent dehydration

      2) Address parental fears about fevers

B. Vomiting

1. Characteristics

    a. Assessment includes: amount, color, consistency, time of day emesis occurs, relationship to eating

    b. Vomiting causes a loss of hydrochloric (HCl) acid, which leads to metabolic alkalosis

2. Diagnosis

    a. Frequently child is dehydrated and looks emaciated (*dead*)

    b. Diagnostic procedures for prolonged or unusual emesis may include: upper GI series (UGI), barium enema, abdominal ultrasound, CT of abdomen, pH probe, esophagoscopy

    c. If metabolic alkalosis, may appear lethargic, poorly perfused, hyperventilating

3. Treatment

    a. It is essential to correct both the fluid and acid-base imbalance

    b. If the vomiting is predictable and of brief duration, antiemetics may be ordered to depress the vomiting center, for example: promethazine HCl (*Phenergan*), chlorpromazine HCl (*Thorazine*), metoclopramide HCl (*Reglan*), trimethobenzamide (*Tigan*)

    c. Gastroesophageal reflux is treated with drugs that promote gastric mobility and emptying, such as metoclopramide (*Reglan*) or omeprazole (*Prilosec*); take gastroesophageal reflux precautions (for example: positioning with HOB elevated, especially after meals or feeding)

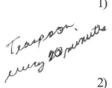 4. **NURSING INTERVENTIONS**

    a. Risk for fluid volume deficit related to loss of fluid and electrolytes secondary to vomiting:

      1) Administer replacement therapy per order; determined by type (for example: isotonic, hypotonic) and degree of dehydration (for example: 5%, 10%)

      2) Monitor potassium (KCl) replacement closely

      3) Measure and record all fluid losses

      4) Assess for signs and symptoms of dehydration

    b. Alteration in nutrition: less than body requirements related to persistent vomiting

      1) Feed infant with a history of vomiting slowly while being held in an upright position; all activities such as bathing or medication administration, should be done prior to feeding

      2) Initiate refeeding following a period of NPO slowly to observe response to PO fluids

    c. Additional nursing problems

      1) Risk for repeated injury related to aspiration: position on abdomen or side-supported; never position supine; may leave infant with gastroesophageal reflux upright in infant seat after feeds

      2) Ineffective parenting: support parents regarding special care and feeding needs

C. Gastroenteritis (Diarrhea)

1. Characteristics

    a. Defined as an increase in fluid, frequency and volume of stool; usually results from increased rate of peristalsis; stools are watery, acidic, green in color, expelled forcefully; Na^+, K^+, and bicarbonate are also lost via the stool

    b. Diarrhea is serious in young children because:

      1) The extracellular space is larger so greater amounts of fluid will be lost

      2) Younger children have a greater body surface area and GI surface areas in relation to body weight

      3) Younger children have a higher basal metabolic rate (BMR) so the fluid and electrolyte balance is unstable

    c. Weight is a critical indicator of fluid loss in young children; 1 gram of weight equals 1 mL of body fluid, a weight loss or gain of 1 kg in a 24-hour period represents a fluid shift of 1,000 mL; the loss of fluid and electrolytes in the diarrhea stool results in dehydration and electrolyte depletion

   d. Causative factors: bacteria (salmonella, shigella), viral (rotavirus), allergies, emotional disturbances, dietary and malabsorption problems

   e. Chronic nonspecific diarrhea (CNSD) or irritable bowel syndrome is the most common form of chronic diarrhea in children:
     1) Diarrhea persists longer than 3 weeks
     2) Normal growth and development
     3) No evidence of enteric pathogens

2. Diagnosis
   a. Serum electrolytes, CBC and blood cultures may be ordered
   b. Antibiotic therapy is a common cause of diarrhea
   c. Obtain a thorough history including dietary habits, family history, recent travel or exposures to contagious illness

3. Treatment
   a. Mild dehydration (2–9%) without hypernatremia; generally treated with oral rehydrating solutions (ORS); critical behaviors that demand immediate attention are persistent diarrhea, weight loss, bloody stools, or physiological changes such as deep breathing, listlessness, reduced urinary output
   b. A secondary lactose intolerance may occur following gastroenteritis; child may be maintained temporarily on a lactose-free diet
   c. Severe dehydration (greater than 10% weight loss) is an acute medical emergency; the child is NPO (12–48 hours), parenteral fluids are administered

4. **NURSING INTERVENTIONS**
   a. Risk for fluid volume deficit related to dehydration
     1) Assess for manifestations of dehydration, weigh daily
     2) Monitor potassium replacement (KCl) closely; administer no more than 4 mEq/Kg/day to correct hypokalemia
     3) Monitor intravenous infusions for correct infusion rate
     4) Monitor laboratory values: BUN/creatinine ratio, serum electrolytes, arterial blood gases; collect urine and stool specimens as needed
   b. Risk for infection related to diarrhea
     1) Isolate client; promote good handwashing
     2) Teach self-care precautions if child is old enough
   c. Alteration in nutrition (less than body requirements):
     1) Initiate refeeding following a period of NPO slowly: offer small amounts of clear fluids every 10 to 20 minutes; initially offer oral rehydration solutions (*Pedialyte*) as tolerated; limit apple juice (causes diarrhea)
     2) Advance diet as tolerated as diarrhea resolves; offer easily digested foods such a breast milk, half-strength soy based formula, applesauce, bananas, rice cereal (ABC diet), dry toast, and saltine crackers; for older children try BRAT diet (bananas, rice cereal, applesauce and toast): after 48 hours, eggs, milk, cheese, and boiled meat; stay away from high-fat food; lactose intolerance may persist for several weeks following diarrhea; use soy-based formulas.
   d. Additional nursing problems
     1) Risk for alteration in skin integrity: change diapers frequently; expose diaper area to air (unless explosive diarrhea) or heat lamp (no closer than 18 inches) for 20 minutes
     2) Knowledge deficit: instruct parents regarding fluid and dietary protocols, infection control

D. Respiratory Infections
1. Acute otitis media (most prevalent childhood disease)
   a. Characteristics
     1) Middle ear infections are common in children under age 5: (breast fed infants have decreased incidence)
       a) Eustachian tube is shorter, wider and straighter,
       b) Organisms from nasopharynx have easier access to middle ear,
       c) Tonsils and adenoids are usually enlarged
       d) Young child has poorly developed immune mechanisms
       e) Infants and toddlers are supine a large portion of the day
     2) Usually follows an upper respiratory infection (URI) during which the swollen mucosa close off the eustachian tube; the growth of the organism along with the fluid retention in the ear combine to cause the infection
     3) Most frequently seen bacterial infection in young children; most serious long-term problem associated with otitis is conductive hearing loss, tinnitus or vertigo
     4) Clinical manifestations: fever; irritability; pulling, tugging or rubbing the affected ear; anorexia; signs of a URI; older children may complain of earache or pain

when chewing or sucking; purulent discharge may be present

b. Diagnosis
  1) Otitis media: otoscopy reveals an intact tympanic membrane that appears inflamed, bulging, and without a light reflex
  2) Chronic otitis media: otoscopy reveals dull, gray membrane with visible fluid behind eardrum

c. Treatment
  1) Oral antibiotics; therapy should last 10–14 days
  2) Oral decongestants such as sympathomimetics (vasoconstriction) or antihistamines (reduce congestion) may be used; analgesics may be ordered to reduce pain, discomfort
  3) Following completion of the antibiotic regimen, treatment effectiveness should be evaluated
  4) Children with recurrent otitis media should be tested for hearing loss
  5) Myringotomy (surgical incision of the ear drum) and insertion of PE (pressure equalizing) tubes may be ordered in cases of recurrent chronic otitis media

d. **NURSING INTERVENTIONS**
  1) Pain
    a) Administer analgesics such as acetaminophen (*Tylenol*) as needed; apply warm compresses to affected ear; avoid foods that require chewing
    b) Assess for nonverbal signs of discomfort; changes in behavior can be an early indicator of pain; humidity, clear PO fluids may also be helpful
  2) Knowledge deficit
    a) Instruct parents regarding the importance of antibiotic compliance; medication should be taken for 10–14 days (even after manifestations have gone away)
    b) Instruct parents in feeding techniques to reduce the incidence of ear infection: upright when feeding; breast feeding offers protection against pathogens
    c) Eliminate tobacco smoke and known or potential allergens from environment
    d) Educate parents following myringotomy and PE (pressure equalizing) tubes insertion, that some drainage from the ears is expected; report obvious bleeding and an abrupt rise in temperature; the ear should be kept dry; avoid activities that require sub-

merging the head in water (use ear plugs for bathing)

2. Epiglottitis
  a. Characteristics
    1) Definition: acute bacterial infection of the supraglottic structures resulting in obstructive airway problems
    2) Seen primarily in children 2–8 years of age; considered a medical emergency, immediate treatment must be initiated
    3) Most common causative organism: H. influenza, type B
    4) Clinical manifestations: abrupt onset with rapid progression to severe respiratory distress, sore throat, stridor, high fever (102°–104°F), drooling, dysphagia, muffled voice; tripod position (sit upright, lean forward with mouth open and tongue protruding)
  b. Diagnosis
    1) Throat is red, inflamed with a cherry-red epiglottis; under no circumstance should an inspection of the throat be initiated unless emergency equipment is available (for example: Trach setup, ET tube); do not take a throat culture
    2) Lateral neck film (for example: soft-tissue x-ray) reveals swollen epiglottis
  c. Treatment
    1) Parenteral therapy with IV antibiotics is begun immediately; PO antibiotics for 10–14 days following IV therapy
    2) Steroid therapy: frequently used for anti-inflammatory effects
    3) Intubation or tracheostomy usually necessary to prevent obstruction; extubation may occur within 3–4 days
    4) Vaccine prevention: H influenza type B conjugate vaccine effective against H influenza epiglottitis (see immunization schedule, table IV-10)
  d. **NURSING INTERVENTIONS**
    1) Ineffective breathing patterns related to airway obstruction and pulmonary changes secondary to infection
      a) Assess respiratory effort every 1–2 hours or prn; be alert for manifestations of increasing respiratory distress (examples: increased retractions, stridor, cyanosis, irritability, nasal flaring, use of accessory neck muscles to breathe)
      b) Have oxygen and suction equipment at bedside
      c) Keep client in mist tent warm and dry; have sides of tent tucked securely

around tent, provide appropriate supportive care (examples: toys, encourage rooming-in)

2) Other nursing problems
   a) Anxiety related to respiratory distress: do not leave child unattended; encourage parents to stay with child as much as possible
   b) Risk for fluid volume deficit: parenteral fluids while NPO; monitor for dehydration

3. Laryngotracheobronchitis (croup)
   a. Characteristics:
      1) Most common form of croup; peak age is below 5 years of age; because of smaller airway diameter, child is more prone to significant airway narrowing
      2) May begin as an upper respiratory infection, proceed to lower respiratory structures
      3) Most common causative organisms: parainfluenza viruses
      4) Clinical manifestations are the result of inflammation and subsequent narrowing of airway: hoarseness, barking or "seal-like" cough, inspiratory stridor, increasing respiratory distress
   b. Diagnosis
      1) Clinical manifestations are diagnostic
      2) Lateral or soft-tissue x-rays of neck may be ordered
   c. Treatment
      1) Humidity with cool mist provides relief by reducing inflamed mucosa
      2) Aerosol epinephrine (*Racepinephrine*) may also be used if client is hospitalized
      3) Corticosteroids may be used for their anti-inflammatory effect
   d. **NURSING INTERVENTIONS**
      1) Ineffective breathing pattern related to inflammation
         a) Educate parents about home care of the child with mild croup: use of cool-mist humidifier; monitor for impending distress; nocturnal and spasmodic coughing episodes may be relieved by taking child into cool night air or humid, warm bathroom (shower running and door closed)
         b) Continuous observation of hospitalized child during periods of respiratory distress; be alert to signs of impending respiratory failure: nasal flaring, retractions, increased stridor; place client in cool-air mist tent,

supplemental oxygen may be used

2) Other nursing problems
   a) Anxiety related to respiratory distress: encourage rooming in
   b) Risk for fluid volume deficit: parenteral fluids if NPO

4. Bronchiolitis
   a. Characteristics
      1) Acute viral infection that primarily affects bronchioles; most commonly seen in infants between 1–18 months of age; occurs in winter and spring months
      2) Respiratory syncytial virus (RSV) is responsible for half of the documented cases of bronchiolitis; mode of transmission is hand to nose, droplet infections; reinfection common in all ages
      3) Bronchiolar obstruction leads to hyperinflation and air trapping
      4) The younger the client, the greater the chance of severe lower respiratory disease requiring hospitalization; infants at high risk for severe RSV infection include: premature infants, infants with underlying cardiac or respiratory conditions, immune deficient infants
      5) Clinical manifestations: initial manifestations of URI that progress to tachypnea; paroxysmal coughing, increased restlessness; nasal flaring, fever, cyanosis intercostal and substernal retractions, wheezing, and decreased breath sounds indicate severe lower respiratory tract disease
   b. Diagnosis
      1) Manifestations are clinically diagnostic
      2) RSV is diagnosed using enzyme linked immunosorbent assay (ELIZA) from nasal secretions
      3) Chest film will reveal areas of consolidation that are difficult to differentiate from bacterial pneumonia; areas of hyperinflation
   c. Treatment
      1) Treated symptomatically; humidity, rest, adequate hydration are main therapeutic interventions; can be successfully treated at home in most cases
      2) Rationale for hospitalization: tachypnea (> 70 breaths/min), severe retractions, change in behavior, hydration problems; at-risk children with chronic or debilitating diseases should be hospitalized
      3) In serious cases, steroids and inhaled bronchodilators will be administered
      4) With severe RSV infection, ribavirin (*Virazole*), an anti-viral aerosol, may be administered via oxygen tent or hood; ter-

atogenic effects have been reported, so pregnant caregivers are at-risk, strict guidelines exist for use

d. **NURSING INTERVENTIONS**
   1) Ineffective airway clearance:
      a) Assess respiratory effort every two hours an as needed (respiratory rate, rhythm and depth, retractions, color, cough, chest auscultation for rales, rhonchi, wheezing)
      b) Administer oxygen therapy via oxyhood or cool air mist tent
      c) Use ABGs and pulse oximetry to determine response to treatment
      d) Elevate head of bed
      e) Keep infant NPO if tachypneic
   2) Risk for fluid volume deficit related to insensible water loss secondary to tachypnea: monitor hydration status by daily weight, strict intake and output, urine specific gravity; parenteral fluids if NPO
   3) Impaired gas exchange: increased secretions in lower airway place infant at risk for hypoxia; be alert for manifestations of increasing distress.
   4) Risk for infection: due to age of infant immune system poorly developed; increased risk for superimposed infection; risk for nosocomial spread is high: respiratory isolation and strict handwashing necessary; if RSV positive, child can only room with another child with RSV.

SECTION V

NURSING CARE OF THE SURGICAL CHILD

A. **Preoperative Preparation** (see also Unit I, Section III)
1. Assess parents' and child's level of understanding
2. Teaching based on developmental level
3. Involve parents and allow discussion
4. Gather baseline data

B. **Common Surgical Problems**
1. Tonsillectomy and adenoidectomy (T&A)
   a. Tonsils help protect body from infections; typically enlarged in children *Lymph tissue*
   b. Rationale for surgery
      1) Chronic tonsillitis (controversial)
      2) Massive hypertrophy that interferes with breathing (obstructive apnea)
   c. Preoperative care
      1) Assess bleeding and coagulation time

2) Confirm client is free from current infection
3) Preparation

d. **NURSING INTERVENTIONS** (postoperative)
   1) Hemorrhage: greatest risk first 48 hours, then 5–7 days later; manifestations: frequent swallowing or clearing of throat, bright red emesis, oozing from capillary bed, shock (late sign, indicates significant blood loss); prevention: avoid coughing, sneezing, sucking on straw
   2) Impaired swallowing related to inflammation and pain: advance diet as tolerated; cool liquid diet first 24 hours; no acidic foods, milk products, or red colored fluids; advance to regular diet when tolerated
   3) Pain: administer analgesics regularly first 24 hours – acetaminophen (*Tylenol*); may require rectal or parenteral route due to throat pain; may return to school in 1–2 weeks

2. Pyloric stenosis
   a. Congenital hypertrophy of pyloric sphincter
   b. Clinical manifestations
      1) Insidious vomiting occurring 2–3 weeks after birth, increasing in intensity until forceful and projectile (no bile) by about 6 weeks of age
      2) Small olive-size mass in right upper quadrant
      3) Weight loss, dehydration
      4) Chronic hunger
   c. Diagnosis
      1) History and physical signs
      2) Upper GI series
      3) Barium swallow under fluoroscopy
   d. Treatment
      1) Correct dehydration, metabolic alkalosis
      2) Pylorus resected

e. **NURSING INTERVENTIONS**
   1) Preoperative: NPO; daily weights; NG tube for gastric decompression; monitor intake, output and specific gravity; monitor emesis
   2) Postoperative: position on right side to prevent aspiration; begin oral feedings 4–6 hours postoperatively after bowel sounds return; maintain in upright position after feeding in infant seat; start with small, frequent feeds of oral rehydration solution (*Pedialyte*); monitor for emesis; advance feeding as tolerated

3. Appendicitis
   a. Inflammation of vermiform appendix
   b. School-age problem
   c. Characteristics

1) Periumbilical pain radiating to right lower quadrant; rebound tenderness
2) Low-grade temperature
3) Nausea and vomiting
4) White blood cell count typically 12,000–15,000 x 10³ NL
5) May perforate and lead to peritonitis; sudden relief of pain followed by increased pain and rigid abdomen; high fever

d. **NURSING INTERVENTIONS**
1) Preoperative
a) Pain: medicate, position for comfort
b) Risk for infection: obtain baseline vitals, monitor WBC, administer antibiotics, observe for peritonitis
c) Fluid volume deficit: NPO with parenteral fluids, monitor hydration; keep NPO until bowel sounds return postoperatively
2) Postoperative
a) Impaired skin integrity: if perforated, wound left to heal by secondary intention; dressing changes; administer antibiotics
b) Pain, risk for infection, fluid volume deficit: as preoperative
c) Knowledge deficit: educate parents in dressing changes, if applicable

4. Intussusception
a. Telescoping of the bowel
b. Characterized by
1) Colicky pain with knees drawn up
2) Currant jelly stools
c. Treatment
1) Barium enema: diagnostic; may reduce intussusception by hydrostatic pressure
2) Bowel resection if barium enema does not reduce
d. **NURSING INTERVENTIONS**
1) Prepare for procedure
2) Routine postoperative abdominal surgery care

5. Hirschsprung's disease (megacolon)
a. Congenital absence of parasympathetic ganglion in distal colon
b. Bowel proximal to a ganglionic section becomes enlarged
c. Characterized by
1) In newborn: failure to pass meconium within 24 hours after birth
2) In older child: recurrent abdominal distension; chronic constipation with ribbon-like stools; diarrhea; bile-stained emesis

d. Treatment
1) Cleansing enemas with antibiotics preoperatively
2) Temporary colostomy
3) Bowel resection to remove aganglionic portion
e. **NURSING INTERVENTIONS**
1) Colostomy care: same as adult client
a) Check stoma for color
b) Change dressings frequently (abdominal, perineal)
c) Monitor accurate intake and output
d) Avoid incision irritation (keep diapers low)
2) Parent and child instruction
a) Encourage independence of based on age of child
b) Discuss diet and hydration

6. Hernias
a. Most common: inguinal and umbilical
b. Always consider developmental level (example: mutilation fears) when preparing child
c. Usually repaired in ambulatory surgery setting
d. **NURSING INTERVENTIONS:** instruct parents:
1) Surgical site care
2) Manifestations of infection

SECTION VI

NURSING CARE FOR PEDIATRIC ACCIDENTS

A. **Ingestions**
1. General information
a. Emergency care: ABCs
b. Identify substance, save evidence of poison
c. Call poison control center for treatment advice
d. Removal of substance
1) Syrup of ipecac
(a) Emetic
(b) 15 mL with 200–300 mL of water
(c) Save emesis
(d) Contraindications
(1) Unconscious
(2) Convulsing
(3) Ingested hydrocarbon, lye, strychnine
2) Activated charcoal
3) Gastric lavage
4) Administer specific antidote
e. Provide supportive therapy
f. Educate parents about childproof environment
g. Provide anticipatory guidance

1) Infants and toddlers: at risk because everything goes into the mouth
2) Adolescents: at risk for intentional ingestion
2. Types of ingestions (see table IV-5.)

B. Pediatric Medication Administration

1. General information
   a. Consider age and developmental level of child
   b. Identify any contraindications to oral route (for example: poor swallow, no gag reflex, oral surgery)
   c. Evaluate child's ability to cooperate and understand
2. Preparation
   a. Caution with calculation and administration; especially IV meds
   b. Nearly all medications are administered to pediatric clients by calculating the desired amount of medication according to the child's weight (for example: mg per kg)
   c. Use vastus lateralis for IM injections
   d. Place med in, or on nipple and allow infants to suck
   e. If administering via oral syringe, never squirt directly into back of throat

C. Burns (see also Unit I, Section XIII)

1. Characteristics of burns in children
   a. Due to the difference in proportions of head, trunk and limbs, burn percentages are rated differently for children
   b. Due to the high percentage of extracellular fluids in the child, fluid loss can quickly lead to hypovolemic shock
2. Treatment
   a. Similar to adult
   b. Children are likely to resist eating enough calories to sustain healing and growth needs. Parenteral or enteral feedings are usually necessary
3. Rehabilitation
   a. Incorporate play into the PT and OT regimens for improved success
   b. Consider psychosocial needs of the child
   c. Adjustment and transition back to school may be very difficult for the child who has sustained a disfiguring burn

D. Fractures (see also Unit I, Section V)

1. Characteristics of fractures in children
   a. Due to immaturity of bones and incomplete ossification, greenstick (incomplete) fractures are commonly seen

TABLE IV-5.
OVERVIEW OF COMMON ACCIDENTAL INGESTION

INGESTION	CLINICAL MANIFESTATIONS	NURSING TREATMENT	INTERVENTIONS
Salicylate (Aspirin)	- Tinnitus - Hyperpyrexia ↑ temp - Seizures - Bleeding - Hyperventilation	- Emesis - Hydration - Vitamin K - Activated charcoal	- Anticipatory guidance - Bleeding precautions - Counseling if suicide attempt
Acetaminophen (Tylenol)	Liver necrosis in 2–5 days; nausea; vomiting; pain in R upper quadrant; jaundice; coagulation abnormalities, hepatotoxic	- Emesis Mucomyst (antidote) ↓ oral dose precaution	- Counseling if suicide attempt Liver assessment ↓ binding to the food
Lead (paint, also in soil near heavily trafficked roadways, households dust)	- Developmental regression - Impaired growth (encephalopathy) - Irritability - Increased clumsiness	- Chelation therapy: - EDTA - BAL - Child must be well hydrated	- Neuro assessment - Diet high in calcium, iron - Educate parents to wash child's hands, toys, frequently to remove lead dust - Lead abatement
Hydrocarbons (kerosene, turpentine, gasoline)	- Burning in mouth - Choking and gagging - CNS depression	- DO NOT INDUCE EMESIS! - Activated charcoal - Gastric lavage	If vomiting, reduce aspiration
Corrosives (drain or oven cleaner, chlorine bleach, battery acid)	- Burning in mouth - White swollen mucous membranes - Violent vomiting	- DO NOT INDUCE EMESIS! - Dilute toxin with water - Activated charcoal	Keep warm and inactive

b. Fractures to the epiphysis (growth plate) are of greater concern as growth in limb can be stunted depending on the amount of injury

2. Treatment
    a. Similar to adult, although pediatric fractures often have shorter healing times
    b. May use cast (plaster or more commonly, fiberglass) soft splint, traction, or bracing

E. Child Abuse (see also Unit II, Section X)

1. Types
    a. Physical neglect: failure to provide necessities of life
    b. Physical abuse: deliberate infliction of injury
    c. Emotional neglect: failure to provide emotional nurturing
    d. Emotional abuse: deliberate assault on child's self-esteem
    e. Sexual abuse: use of child to meet adult's sexual needs
    f. Munchausen syndrome: fabrication of illness in child by parent (usually mother) to obtain medical treatment and focus attention on parent ← *Dysorderly gain*

2. Risk factors
    a. Parental
        1) Poor self-esteem
        2) Abused as a child
        3) Lack of knowledge
        4) Lack of support system, poor coping skills
    b. Child
        1) Unwanted pregnancy or sex
        2) Difficult temperament, hyperactive
    c. Environment
        1) Chronic stress
        2) Socioeconomic factors

3. Recognition of abuse and neglect
    a. Physical neglect
        1) Failure to thrive: disruption in maternal-infant bonding; poor feeding behaviors; mother does not respond to infant's cues; weight less than 5th percentile; developmental delay
        2) Poor health care, lack of immunizations
        3) Failure to meet basic needs: malnutrition, poor hygiene
    b. Physical abuse
        1) Bruises: not on bony prominences, in varying degrees of healing; with patterns
        2) Burns: with immersion lines, in patterns
        3) Fractures: spiral, twisting
        4) Shaken baby: unconscious infant with retinal hemorrhage and no external signs of trauma
        5) Conflicting stories given by parents, child or others

6) History incompatible with physical findings or developmentally improbable
7) Delay in seeking medical attention

c. Emotional neglect and abuse
    1) Extremes of behavior
    2) Poor self-esteem
d. Sexual abuse
    1) Bruising of the genitalia
    2) STD
    3) Sudden change in behavior, regressive behavior
e. Munchausen syndrome
    1) Abusive parent has medical knowledge
    2) Illness only occurs in parent's presence
    3) Parent "enjoys" hospital environment

4. **NURSING INTERVENTIONS**
    a. Risk for injury: prevent further abuse; report suspicions to child protective authorities: refer family to supportive services
    b. Anxiety: consistent caregiver; do not interrogate child; allow child to grieve loss of parents
    c. Altered parenting: role model parenting behaviors; teach appropriate discipline methods, normal growth and development

SECTION VII

NURSING CARE OF THE CHILD WITH CHRONIC OR LONG-TERM PROBLEMS

A. Immune Disorders

1. Eczema
    a. Known as atopic dermatitis
    b. May be associated with bronchial asthma; often family history of asthma or atopy
    c. Due to hypersensitivity to:
        1) Food (examples: milk, egg white)
        2) Pollen
        3) Environmental
        4) Psychological (element of anxiety)
    d. Characteristics
        1) Papules are red and oozing; predominantly on face and extensor surfaces in infants, flexural areas in children (for example: knees, wrists, antecubital fossa)
        2) Lesions eventually become scaly
        3) Pruritus may lead to secondary infection
    e. Treatment
        1) Topical steroids: triamcinolone (*Kenalog*); avoid chronic use
        2) Diphenhydramine HCl (*Benadryl*) or hydroxyzine HCl (*Atarax*): reduces itching
        3) Elimination diet (for example: milk, eggs, chocolate, wheat)

4) Antibiotics if secondary infection occurs
f. **NURSING INTERVENTIONS**
   1) Impaired skin integrity:
      a) Educate parents in methods to control dry skin to minimize itching
         (1) Use non-soap cleanser
         (2) Apply lubricating creams
      b) Advise that the child may be more comfortable in cotton, long-sleeve clothing
      c) Instruct parents to launder with a non-soap or hypoallergenic cleanser
      d) Fingernails and toe nails should be kept short to prevent scratching
   2) Assess developmental needs; hypoallergenic diet
   3) Provide parental support and education
2. Bronchial asthma (see also Unit I, Section II)
   a. Also known as reactive airway disease (RAD)
   b. Usually begins before 5 years of age
   c. Pathology and etiology
      1) Chronic condition with acute exacerbations
      2) In response to allergen or trigger, acute hyperactive changes occur in reactive (lower) airways
         a) Spasm of smooth muscle
         b) Edema of mucous membranes
         c) Thick, tenacious mucous
         d) Severe sudden dyspnea
      3) Potential triggers
         a) Foods
         b) Inhalants (for example: secondhand smoke)
         c) Infection
         d) Vigorous activity
         e) Stress, anxiety
         f) Allergens (examples: pet dander, dust)
         g) Cold air
   d. Characterized by
      1) Paroxysmal, hacking nonproductive cough
      2) Prolonged expiratory phase with expiratory wheeze
      3) Respiratory distress, anxiety
   e. Complications
      1) Pneumonia
      2) Atelectasis
   f. Treatment
      1) Chronic (home) management of child
         a) Medications via nebulizer or metered dose inhaler
            (1) Bronchodilators: albuterol (*Proventil*) useful for acute attack; salmeterol (*Serevent*) for chronic daily use, not for acute

attack
            (2) Inhaled corticosteroids: effective in reducing airway hyperreactivity; for chronic daily use, not acute attack; avoid chronic oral steroids since they can stunt growth
            (3) Cromolyn sodium (*Intal*): mast cell inhibitor; reduces allergic response; for chronic daily use, not acute attack
      b) **NURSING INTERVENTIONS**
         (1) Avoid allergens and triggers
         (2) Correct use of meter dose inhaler (with spacer device)
         (3) Activities requiring stop and start energy better tolerated
         (4) Use of a peak flow meter to monitor airway compliance
   2) Status asthmaticus: severe respiratory distress requiring hospitalization
      a) Bronchodilators
         (1) Epinephrine (*Adrenalin*): subcutaneous
         (2) Aminophylline (*Phyllocontin*): IV drip
      b) Steroids: IV
      c) Inhalants: bronchodilators - albuterol (*Proventil*), metaproterenol (*Alupent*)
      d) Antibiotics: prophylactic
      e) Hydration
      f) Oxygen therapy
3. Rheumatic Fever: inflammatory disease affecting heart, joints, and central nervous system
   a. Characteristics
      1) Usually occurs 2-6 weeks after an upper respiratory infection with group A beta hemolytic strep
      2) Sequelae includes scarring and damage to mitral valve
   b. Diagnosis
      1) Elevated or rising Antistreptolysin O (ASO) titer with elevated erythrocyte sedimentation rate (ESR)
      2) Jones Criteria (presence of 2 major, or one major and 2 minor manifestations
      3) Signs and symptoms include: arthralgia; fever; hot, red, swollen joints (polyarthritis); tachycardia with precordial friction rub; subcutaneous nodules; truncal rash (erythema marginatum).
   c. Treatment
      1) Drug therapy (penicillin, salicylates)
      2) Bed rest in the acute phase for cardiac rest
      3) Prophylactic antibiotics with all dental work

4. Monitor for development of chorea
   a. Sudden, involuntary movements with involuntary facial grimaces
   b. Muscle weakness and speech disturbances
   c. Is transitory; reassure parents that chorea will self resolve

B. Musculoskeletal Disorders
1. Scoliosis
   a. Lateral curvature of the spine
   b. Most common form is idiopathic seen (predominately) in adolescent females; unknown etiology
   c. Acquired scoliosis; associated with deformity resulting from other neuromuscular disorders
   d. Diagnosis
      1) Classic signs: truncal asymmetry; especially noted in hips and shoulders, posture
      2) Screening exam in school: child flexes at waist; one scapula more prominent
      3) Spinal x-ray
   e. Treatment
      1) Mild scoliosis (< 20° curvature): observation, encourage physical exercise
      2) Moderate scoliosis (20°–40° curvature): Milwaukee brace (pelvis to neck), Boston brace (body jacket/TLSO brace)
         a) Goal is to prevent worsening of curve; not a cure
         b) **NURSING INTERVENTIONS**
            (1) Risk for noncompliance: difficult for adolescent due to body image concerns; must wear 23 hours a day (one hour off for hygiene care); wears T-shirt under brace
            (2) Body image disturbance: Boston brace better accepted (can be completely hidden under clothing)
      3) Severe scoliosis (> 40° curvature): surgery
         a) Spinal fusion with instrumentation
         b) Requires prolonged immobilization in cast, brace or body jacket
         c) **NURSING INTERVENTIONS**
            (1) High risk for injury related to spinal manipulation: log roll first 24 hours; neurovascular checks; advance activity as ordered; observe for paralytic ileus
            (2) Pain: adolescent good candidate for PCA pump
2. Juvenile rheumatoid arthritis (JRA)
   a. Autoimmune, inflammatory disease of the joints

   b. Toddler and school-age child more commonly affected
   c. Etiology unknown
   d. Early diagnosis essential due to long-term complications (blindness, contracture); early onset often associated with spontaneous permanent remission
   e. Classification
      1) Systemic (fever, rash, and organomegaly in addition to joint involvement)
      2) Polyarticular (many joints)
      3) Pauciarticular (few joints)
   f. Characterized by:
      1) Swelling, thickening of joint
      2) Pain, stiffness, impaired range of motion
      3) Lethargy, weight loss
   g. Treatment
      1) Medications
         a) Salicylates
         b) NSAID: tolmetin sodium (*Tolectin*)
         c) Gold compounds
         d) Immunosuppressants and steroids: used in severe cases which do not respond to other medications
      2) Supportive treatment to maintain joint mobility
   h. **NURSING INTERVENTIONS**
      1) Impaired physical mobility related to inflamed joints
         a) Rest inflamed joints
         b) Assist with ADLs
         c) Provide heat, splints, passive range of motion
         d) Provide physical therapy
      2) Pain
         a) Administer medication
         b) Observe for side effects
      3) Risk for altered nutrition: less than body requirements
         a) Provide well-balanced diet
         b) Provide anticipatory guidance and parental support

C. Endocrine Disorders
1. Type 1 diabetes mellitus
   (see also Unit I, Section VI)
   a. Etiology
      1) May be autoimmune response to environmental factors
      2) Genetic component: inherit tendency, not disease
      3) School-age child (5–7 years or at puberty)
   b. Characteristics
      1) Onset: rapid with progression to abrupt ketoacidosis
      2) Hypertrophy and hyperplasia of islet cells

occur early

3) Remission (honeymoon) phase
4) Insulin replacement (cannot use oral hypoglycemics)
5) Exercise lowers blood sugar
6) Management difficult due to
   a) Immaturity of child
   b) Lack of insight

c. Developmental needs
   1) Preschool: biggest issues are the fear of injections and poor appetites of preschoolers (difficult to maintain diet); "free diet"
   2) School age: How will they maintain their regular activities (for example: birthday parties, pizza after the soccer game)
   3) Adolescent: Compliance is the problem. They are truly not interested in long-term effects; they want to be like their peers.

D. Hematological Disorders

1. Hemophilia
   a. Characteristics
      1) Impaired coagulation: deficiency of clotting factors
      2) Sex-linked recessive trait more common in males
      3) Factor VIII and IX are most common deficiencies
      4) Hemarthrosis (bleeding into joint cavities), bruises easily
   b. Treatment
      1) Cryoprecipitate (transfusion that replaces missing clotting factor)
      2) Supportive therapy
   c. **NURSING INTERVENTIONS**
      1) Control bleeding
         a) Immobilize joint
         b) Provide ice packs
         c) Administer cryoprecipitate
            (1) Prophylactic cryoprecipitate for invasive procedures
            (2) Risk for AIDS, hepatitis is decreased because of screening, but does still exist
      2) Safety directed toward developmental level to prevent injury, bleeding
         a) Avoid contact sports (difficult with children)
         b) Childproof environment
         c) Avoid aspirin
      3) Provide parental support

TABLE IV-6.
COMPARISON OF INSULIN SHOCK AND DIABETIC COMA GUIDE

	INSULIN SHOCK (HYPOGLYCEMIA)	DIABETIC COMA (HYPERGLYCEMIA)
Causes:	- Too much insulin - Not eating enough food - Taking unusual amounts of exercise - Delayed meals	- Too little insulin - Failure to follow diet - Infection, fever, emotional stress
Clinical Manifestations:	- Onset is abrupt, rapid - Skin is pale, moist - Vertigo (dizzy) - Urine is normal - Tachycardia - Hungry (polyphagia) - Normal urinary output - Normal thirst - Shallow respirations - Breath normal - Level of consciousness: inappropriate behavior, confused	- Onset is slow, insidious - Skin is hot, dry - No vertigo - Urine is positive for sugar and acetone - Normal pulse - Anorexia - Polyuria - Polydipsia - Deep, labored respirations - Acetone breath - Level of consciousness: lethargic, drowsy
What to do:	- Give fast-acting sugar (e.g., candy, orange juice) - Call physician - Do not give insulin - Glucagon if unconscious	- Call physician - Encourage fluids without sugar - Continue to check urine - Give insulin as usual

2. Sickle cell anemia (see also Unit I, Section VII)
   a. Characteristics
      1) Presence of hemoglobin S, which accounts for elongated shape of red blood cells (RBC)
      2) Sickling occurs in response to
         a) Infection, stress
         b) Dehydration
         c) Decreased oxygen
         d) High altitude
      3) Sickling increases blood viscosity, which causes further sickling and RBC destruction
      4) Manifestations
         a) Severe pain
         b) Swelling
         c) Jaundice
      5) Types of crisis
         a) Vaso-occlusive: "hand-foot syndrome" caused by stasis of blood in capillaries; schema and infarction
         b) Sequestration: pooling of large amounts of blood in liver, spleen; hypovolemia and shock
   b. Treatment
      1) Eliminate cause of crisis
      2) Analgesics
      3) Blood transfusions
      4) Monitor complications
         a) Anemia
         b) Splenic sequestration
         c) Cerebrovascular accidents
   c. **NURSING INTERVENTIONS**
      1) Early recognition of crisis
         a) Increasing irritability
         b) Frequent infections
         c) Pallor
         d) Failure to thrive
      2) Provide hydration
      3) Administer analgesics, antibiotics as ordered
      4) Oxygenation
      5) Reduce stress of hospitalization
      6) Provide parental support

E. **Renal Disorders** (see also Unit I, Section IX)
   1. Glomerulonephritis (see table IV-7.)
   2. Nephrotic syndrome (see table IV-7.)

F. **Metabolic Disorders**
   1. Cystic fibrosis (see table IV-8.)
   2. Celiac disease (see table IV-8.)

SECTION VIII

NURSING CARE OF THE CHILD WITH AN ONCOLOGY DISORDER

A. Leukemia
   1. Characteristics
      a. Most common childhood cancer
      b. Peak incidence: 3–5 years of age
      c. Etiology: unknown, may be related to environmental exposures (example: radiation)
      d. Characterized by proliferation of abnormal white blood cells
   2. Pathology
      a. Bone marrow failure secondary to invasion of cancer cells
         1) Temperature and infection from decreased (normal) WBCs
         2) Anemia, pallor and fatigue from decreased RBCs
         3) Petechiae and epistaxis from decreased platelets
      b. Leukemic infiltrate
         1) Limb and joint pain
         2) Lymphadenopathy
         3) Central nervous system (CNS) involvement
         4) Hepatosplenomegaly/bleeding tendencies
   3. Classification
      a. Acute lymphocytic (ALL)
      b. Acute nonlymphoid (ANLL)
   4. Complications (secondary to bone marrow depression)
      a. Infection
      b. Intracranial hemorrhage
      c. Secondary cancer or relapse
   5. Diagnosis: bone marrow aspiration reveals hypercellular marrow, abnormal cells
   6. Treatments
      a. Terminology
         1) Induction, remission
         2) CNS prophylaxis, consolidation
         3) Maintenance
      b. Chemotherapy
         1) Purine antagonists: 6-mercaptopurine (*Purinethol*) (may affect kidneys)
         2) Alkylating agents: cyclophosphamide (*Cytoxan*) (causes chemical cystitis)
         3) Folic acid antagonists: methotrexate (*Folex*)
         4) Plant alkaloid: vincristine sulfate (*Oncovin*) (neuro toxic)
         5) Steroids: prednisone (*Prelone*)
         6) Enzymes: L-asparaginase (*Elspar*)

TABLE IV-7.
RENAL DISORDERS

	NEPHROTIC SYNDROME	ACUTE GLOMERULONEPHRITIS
Other names	Childhood nephrosis	Post-streptococcal glomerulonephritis
Etiology	Cause unknown; may follow the toxic effects of mercury or Tridione exposure or bee sting	Antigen - antibody reaction secondary to infection elsewhere in the body; usually a Group A beta hemolytic streptococcal infection of the upper respiratory tract
Incidence	Average age of onset about 2-1/2 years; more common in boys	2/3 of cases in children under 4–7 years; more common in boys
Pathology	Increased permeability of the glomerular membrane to protein	Inflammation of the kidneys; damage to the glomeruli allows excretion of red blood cells
Clinical manifestations	Edema: appears insidiously; usually first noticed about the eyes and can advance to the legs, arms, back, peritoneal cavity and scrotum; massive proteinuria; anorexia; pallor	Periorbital edema: appears insidiously; tea-colored urine from hematuria; hypertension; oliguria
Blood pressure	Usually normal; transient elevation may occur early	Varying degrees of hypertension may be present; when blood pressure is elevated cerebral manifestations may occur as a result of vasospasm; these may include headache, drowsiness, diplopia, vomiting, convulsions
Laboratory findings	Urine shows heavy albuminuria	Urine contains red blood cells; has a high specific gravity
Blood	Involves reduction in protein (mainly albumin); gamma globulin is reduced; during the active stages of the disease, the sedimentation rate is greatly increased	Blood urea nitrogen value is elevated; anemia (reduction in circulating red blood cells, in hemoglobin or both) tends to develop rapidly
Course and prognosis	Characterized by remissions and relapses; with protection against infection and suppression of proteinuria by steroid therapy, most children can eventually expect a favorable outcome	Recovery from acute glomerulonephritis is to be expected in nearly all children; mild illnesses last as little as 2–3 weeks; in exceptional instances, the disease is progressive and takes on the characteristics of chronic nephritis
Treatments	1. Prednisone (Deltasone) 2. Furosemide (Lasix) 3. Salt-poor albumin	1. Antibiotics for strep infection 2. Anti-hypertensives and diuretics 3. Corticosteroids
Nursing interventions	Control edema; provide skin care; prevent infection; monitor nutrition: low sodium, high protein, high potassium; monitor urine for proteinuria; monitor for side effects from steroid therapy	Bed rest if hypertensive; restrict fluids; monitor neuro status; monitor blood pressure; provide low potassium diet, no added salt; prevent infection

TABLE IV-8.
COMPARISON OF CYSTIC FIBROSIS AND CELIAC DISEASE

METABOLIC DISORDER	CYSTIC FIBROSIS	CELIAC DISEASE
Onset	0–6 months	6–18 months
Characteristics	Production of abnormally viscid secretions of: pancreas, respiratory, salivary, and sweat glands	Intestinal malabsorption; malnutrition; fat and gluten intolerance; dietary intolerance: fat, gluten
Etiology	Autosomal recessive: 25% chance	Inborn error of metabolism
Manifestations	Meconium ileus in newborn; large, fatty foul-smelling stools in older child; chronic respiratory disease; digestive problems; sweat abnormalities	Diarrhea: large bulky stools; anemia; retarded growth; frequent infections; malabsorption of vitamin D
Diagnosis	Sweat test; pancreatic enzymes	Bowel biopsy; sweat test; gluten-free diet

Treatment	- Pulmonary: postural drainage, aerosol therapy, antibiotic
	- Nutrition: pancreatic, enzymes with meals, high calorie, Vitamins A, D, E, K (fat soluble) twice normal dose, free use of salt
	- Lung transplantation (experimental)
		- Gluten free diet:
		  - meat, eggs, milk, fruit, vegetables, gluten-free bread, Vitamins A, D, E, K (fat soluble)
		- Avoid:
		  - BROW: barley, rye, oats, wheat

Nursing interventions	- Avoid infection - Respiratory toilet - Frequent small feedings - Pancreatic enzymes - Developmental issues - Anticipatory grieving	- Avoid infection - Instruct how to implement diet - Developmental issues
Prognosis	Short lifespan 20-25 years	Normal lifespan if follows gluten-free diet

c. Radiation therapy for CNS involvement

 7. **NURSING INTERVENTIONS** (see table IV-9.)

B. **Nephroblastoma** (Wilms' Tumor)
1. Characteristics
   a. Most frequent type of renal cancer
   b. Peak age is 3 years
   c. Most common clinical sign: swelling, mass within the abdomen
   d. May also see: anemia, hypertension, hematuria
2. Pathology
   a. Arises from embryonal tissue
   b. Encapsulated (do not biopsy, will "seed" tumor further)
3. Diagnosis
   a. Intravenous pyelogram
   b. Computerized tomography

c. Bone marrow to rule out metastasis
4. Treatment
   a. Nephrectomy and adrenalectomy
   b. Radiation and chemotherapy determined by staging
5. **NURSING INTERVENTIONS**
   a. Preoperative care
      1) Treatment begun quickly; support parents and keep explanations simple
      2) Monitor blood pressure due to excess renin production
      3) Prevent rupture of encapsulated tumor
         a) Post sign on bed: "DO NOT PALPATE ABDOMEN"
         b) Bathe and handle gently
   b. Postoperative care

1) Problems related to radiation, chemotherapy (see table IV-9.)
2) Large surgical incision
   a) Pain management
   b) Gentle handling
   c) Prepare parents
3) Protect remaining kidney
   a) Monitor blood pressure
   b) Dipstick urine for protein or blood

C. **Neuroblastoma**
1. Characteristics
   a. Most frequently seen below 2 years of age
   b. Frequently called "silent" tumor because by
      the time of diagnosis, metastasis has occurred
   c. Clinical signs include: abdominal mass, urinary
      retention and frequency, lymphadenopathy,
      generalized weakness, malaise
   d. Primary site is abdomen, most often in flank
      area
2. Diagnosis
   a. Computerized tomography
   b. Bone marrow to determine metastasis
   c. Excessive catecholamine production
3. Treatment
   a. Surgery to remove as much of the tumor as
      possible, determine staging

b. Chemotherapy and radiation determined by
   staging of tumor
4. **NURSING INTERVENTIONS** (see table IV-9.)

D. **Hodgkin's Lymphoma**
1. Characteristics
   a. Primarily affects adolescents and young adults
   b. Clinical signs include: painless enlargement of
      lymph nodes (cervical most common), metasta-
      sis related manifestations (persistent cough,
      abdominal pain), systemic problems (pruritus,
      night sweats, fever)
2. Pathology
   a. Malignancy originates in lymphoid system
   b. Metastasis may include spleen, liver, bone
      marrow, lungs
3. Diagnosis
   a. Computerized axial tomography
   b. Lymph node biopsy, exploratory laparotomy
      (to stage)
4. Treatment
   a. Radiation and chemotherapy determined by
      clinical staging
   b. Surgical laparotomy
   c. Splenectomy
5. **NURSING INTERVENTIONS**
   a. See table IV-9.

depleting calcium

TABLE IV-9.
NURSING CARE OF THE CHILD WITH CANCER

MANAGE PROBLEMS RELATED TO CHEMOTHERAPY	PREPARE CHILD/FAMILY FOR RADIATION THERAPY	TERMINAL PHASE—PROVIDE COMFORT CARE
- Nausea and vomiting - Administer antiemetic prior to treatment and regularly administer p.r.n. drugs - Teach guided imagery - Anorexia: difficult to handle with with children - Mucosal ulceration - Stomatitis: bland diet, soft tooth brush, oral hygiene - Rectal ulcers: sitz baths, stool softeners, no rectal temperatures deformities - Neuropathy (vincristine related) Note bowel movements - Instruct parents concerning foot-drop, weakness, numbness and jaw pain - Hemorrhagic cystitis (cyclophosphamide related) - 1½ to 2 times normal fluid intake - Frequent voiding - Administer drug early in day to allow for sufficient oral intake	- Meticulous skin care: avoid exposure to sun; limit use of soap and lotions; do not wash off markings - Radiation to chest and abdomen frequently results in nausea & vomiting, weight loss, esophagitis - Malaise is most frequent complaint of adolescents and prevents peer involvement - Discuss effects radiation therapy has on puberty, fractures and spinal - Could cause sterility	- If poor prognosis, assist family in dealing with life threatening illness - Perception of death - Infant and toddler: different way of life (e.g., "Mommy is sleeping"); major fear is separation - Preschooler: reversible, cannot separate life and death - School-age child and preadolescent: similar to preschooler's reaction until 9-10 years, then adult concept of death; magical thinking may still be evident - Adolescent: adult concept-of all age groups, has most difficulty dealing with death

b. Instruct family on long-term care following splenectomy
   1) Increased susceptibility to infection
   2) Prophylactic long-term antibiotic therapy is necessary (compliance issues)

SECTION IX

NURSING CARE OF THE CHILD WITH AN INFECTIOUS DISEASE

A. Prevention
   1. Immunizations
      a. Contraindications
         1) Acute febrile illness (temperature > 101°F)

   2) No live attenuated vaccines in the presence of:
      a) Pregnancy
      b) Malignancies
      c) Immunosuppressive therapy
      d) Immunodeficiency disorders
      e) Sensitivity to eggs, chicken, neomycin (*MMR*)
      f) Recent administration of immune serum globulin, plasma, blood
   b. Schedule (see table IV-10.)
2. Communicability
   a. Most communicable diseases are most contagious prior to the onset of manifestations or rash and in the early prodromal period
   b. Most require respiratory isolation precautions if the child requires hospitalization
   c. Most are preventable through immunization or other measures
3. Common childhood infections (see table IV-11.)

TABLE IV-10.
RECOMMENDED IMMUNIZATION SCHEDULE

- Birth	- Hep B	
- 2 months	- DTaP, IPV, HIB, Hep B, PCV	**KEY:** **HIB:** H. influenza type B **MMR:** measles, mumps, rubella **DTaP:** acellular pertussis **Hep B:** hepatitis B **IPV:** Inactivated polio vaccine **VZV:** varicella zoster vaccine **Td:** tetanus, diphtheria **PCV:** Pneumococcal **Menomune:** Meningococcal meningitis *note: DTaP and HIB can be given in combination injection
- 4 months	- DTaP, IPV, HIB, PCV	
- 6 months	- DTaP, (IPV) optional, HIB, Hep B, PCV	
- 12 months	- VZV (optional)	
- 15 months	- MMR, HIB	
- 18 months	- DTaP, IPV	
- 4-6 years	- DTaP, IPV, MMR	
- 11-12 years	- Catch-up vaccinations as needed	
- 14-16 years	- Td (every 10 years), Catch-up vaccinations as needed	
- 18 years	- Menomune (college-bound freshman)	
	Note: An optional influenza vaccine can be given yearly after 6 months of age.	

Note: This schedule is accurate as of January 2004. The American Academy of Pediatrics reviews and revises the schedule yearly and as indicated.

TABLE IV-11.
COMMUNICABLE DISEASES GUIDE

DISEASE	INFECTIOUS AGENTS	TRANSMISSION	INCUBATION	CLINICAL MANIFESTATIONS	TREATMENT AND NURSING INTERVENTIONS	PREVENTION
Acquired immuno-deficiency syndrome (AIDS)	Human immuno-deficiency virus (HIV)	Blood and body fluids: in children: most common exposure is maternal-fetal; adolescents: at risk through sexual contacts or IV drug use	Months to years; in children average age of diagnosis is 18 months	In children: FTT, chronic Candida, frequent URI, opportunistic infections (e.g., Pneumocystis carinii pneumonia [PCP])	Supportive and symptomatic care; antivirals and antiretrovirals; Bactrim prophylaxis for PCP	AZT (Retrovir) given to HIV positive woman in pregnancy greatly reduces risks of prenatal transmission
Chicken pox	Varicella zoster virus	Direct contact, droplet spread, and contaminated objects or contact with skin lesions	2–3 weeks (usually 10–14 days)	Prodromal stage: slight fever, malaise and anorexia, first 24 hours; pruritic rash; macule to papule to vesicle to pustule; rash occurs in all different stages; lesions crust over and usually heal without scarring; client is communicable	Do not use aspirin; control itching; prevent secondary infection; acyclovir may lessen severity of outbreak and promote faster healing; strict isolation if child hospitalized	Varicella zoster immunoglobin (Zovirax)
Derma-tophytosis (tinea capitis) (ringworm)	Microsporum audouinii	- Person to person - Animal to person	N/A	Scaly circumscribed patches with alopecia; pruritic, fluorescent green under woods light	Griseofulvin (Fulvicin-U/F) orally or topically; wash hair/hat	Caution children about sharing hair items
Enterobiasis (pinworms)	Enterobius vermicularis	Ingested; inhaled; poor hygiene after toilet; reinfect self	Eggs hatch and mature in 2–4 weeks	Intense perianal itching; young child may present with general complaints (sleep problems, enuresis); tape test	Sanitize bedding; tight diapers and pants; family precautions; mebendazole (Vermox) prevent itching	Handwashing (especially after using toilet)
Fifth's disease (erythema infectiosum)	Human parvovirus 19	Respiratory secretions, blood	7–18 days	Red rash on cheeks: gives face a "slapped cheeks" appearance; followed by "lace-like" rash on extremes that may fade and reappear	Symptomatic treatment only; monitor for anemia	None
Impetigo	Group A beta strep or staph aureus	Direct contact with skin lesion or articles soiled with discharge	N/A	History of trauma or minor injury; honey-colored blisters that rupture and become crusted; lymphadenopathy; highly contagious	Soak lesions; topical ointment; communicability; prevent scratching; family precautions	Good hygiene; short fingernails
Lyme disease	Borrelia burgdorferi	Transmitted by bite of deer tick	3 days–1 month	Initially flu-like manifestations; red rash in bullseye pattern at bite site; later, joint pain, neurologic and cardiac involvement; may become chronic	Antibiotics; remove tick as soon as possible; symptomatic; analgesics; antipyretic	Avoid tick infested areas; dress appropriately in woods (tuck socks into jeans, long sleeves)

TABLE IV-11.
COMMUNICABLE DISEASES GUIDE (CONTINUED)

DISEASE	INFECTIOUS AGENTS	TRANSMISSION	INCUBATION	CLINICAL MANIFESTATIONS	TREATMENT AND NURSING INTERVENTIONS	PREVENTION
Meningitis	Viral or bacterial (H. Influenza: 3 months–3 years; meningococcal meningitis)	Direct invasion via otitis media, URI, head injury	2–10 days	Onset abrupt with fever, headache, irritability, altered LOC, nuchal rigidity, increased ICP; must do lumbar puncture to isolate organism	Isolate; reduce environmental stimuli; monitor hydration; seizure precautions; IV antibiotics	(Rifampin): given to contacts of client with meningococcal meningitis as prophylaxis
Mumps	Viral (paramyxovirus)	Saliva, direct contact or droplet	14–21 days	Prodromal stage: headache, malaise, anorexia, followed by earache; parotitis 3 days later with pain/tenderness	Symptomatic and supportive; analgesics; antipyretics; hydration	MMR
Pediculosis capitis (head lice)	Pediculus humanus capitis	Sharing of personal items, (e.g., hair ornaments, caps, hats)	Eggs hatch in 7–10 days	Intense itching; can visually see nits attached to base of hair shafts; differentiate from dandruff	Pediculocide: shampoo immediately (Kwell, Rid); 7–10 days later; remove nits; spray furniture; family precautions	Caution children about sharing hair items
Pertussis (whooping cough)	Bordetella pertussis	Respiratory droplets and direct contact	7–21 days	Initially "cold" manifestations; progresses to spasms of paroxysmal coughing (whooping cough)	Antibiotics; corticosteroids; supportive care; isolation; stay with child during coughing spells	DTaP
Rabies	Viral	Contact with saliva of infected animal	1–3 months or as short as 10 days	Prodromal: malaise, sore throat followed by hypersensitivity, excitation, convulsions, paralysis; high mortality	Irrigate wound; psychologic follow-up	Avoid contact with wild animals; rabies shot (given after exposure)
Reye's syndrome	Viral	Unknown: proceeded by viral infection and associated with use of aspirin	N/A	Prodromal: malaise cough, URI (upper respiratory infection); 1–3 days after: fever, decreased LOC, hepatic and cerebral dysfunction; high mortality	Monitor liver function; peak age 4–11 years; neuro assessments; intracranial pressure monitoring	Avoid use of aspirin in teens and children
Rheumatic fever	Group A beta-hemolytic strep	Nasopharyngeal secretions; direct contact with infected person or droplet spread	1–3 weeks after acute infection, develops inflammatory disease	Carditis, arthritis, chorea (involuntary ataxic movements), subcutaneous nodules, erythema marginatum (rash)	Bed rest in acute phase to decrease cardiac workload; full course of antibiotics (penicillin/erythromycin); high dose aspirin therapy (monitor for toxicity, tinnitus)	Adequate, prompt treatment of strep infection (Must finish entire course of therapy)

TABLE IV-11.
COMMUNICABLE DISEASES GUIDE (CONTINUED)

DISEASE	INFECTIOUS AGENTS	TRANSMISSION	INCUBATION	CLINICAL MANIFESTATIONS	TREATMENT AND NURSING INTERVENTIONS	PREVENTION
Roseola (exanthem subitum)	Viral (human herpes virus type 6)	Unknown (limited to children 6 months–2 years of age)	Unknown	Persistent high fever for 3–4 days; precipitous drop in fever with appearance of rash (rose-pink maculopapule on trunk, then spreading to neck, face and extremities); lasts 1–2 days	Antipyretics to control temperature and prevent febrile seizures; hydrate	None
Rubella (German measles)	Viral (rubella virus)	Nasopharyngeal secretions: direct contact, indirect via freshly contaminated nasopharyngeal secretions or urine	14–21 days	Prodromal phase; absent in children, present in adults; rash; first face and rapidly spreads downward to neck, arms, trunk, and legs; teratogenic to fetus	No treatment necessary; isolate child from pregnant women; women of childbearing years should have rubella titer drawn	MMR
Rubeola (measles)	Viral	Respiratory-droplets	10–21 days	Prodromal stage: fever and malaise, coryza, conjunctivitis, Koplik spots (spots with blue/white center on buccal mucosa opposite molars); rash: starts on face, spreads downwards, may desquamate (peel)	Antipyretics to control temperature and prevent seizures; dim lights if photophobia; respiratory precautions	MMR
Scarlet fever	Group A Beta hemolytic strep	Nasopharyngeal secretions, direct contact with infected person or droplet spread	2–4 days	Prodromal stage: abrupt high fever, pulse increased, vomiting, chills, malaise, abdominal pain; enanthema: tonsils enlarged, edematous reddened, covered with patches of exudate; strawberry tongue; exanthema: rash appears 12 hours after prodromal signs	Full course of antibiotics (penicillin/ erythromycin); isolate; monitor for rheumatic fever, glomerulonephritis; hydrate	Adequate, prompt treatment of strep infection (Must finish entire course of therapy)
Tetanus	Clostridium tetany	Deep puncture, not contagious, "anaerobic"	7–14 days	Gradual stiffening of voluntary muscles until rigid (i.e., lockjaw, rigid abdomen); sensitive to stimuli; clear sensorium	Eliminate stimuli; monitor respirations, blood gases; muscle relaxants; monitor hydration	DTaP, Td

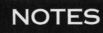

COORDINATED CARE

UNIT CONTENT

SECTION I.   Management 177
SECTION II.   Delegation 179
SECTION III.   Ethical Issues 179
SECTION IV.   Legal Issues 180

SYMBOLS

Key Points

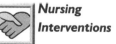
Nursing Interventions

Points to Remember

SECTION I

MANAGEMENT

A. Concepts of Management

1. Leadership
   a. Definition: A way of behaving that influences others to respond, not because they have to, but because they want to. Leaders help others to identify and focus on goals and the achievement of them. Think of leadership as a personal interaction that focuses on the personal development of the members of the group.
   b. Essential components of leadership
      1) Knowledge
      2) Self-awareness
      3) Communication
      4) Energy
      5) Goals
      6) Action
    c. **NURSING INTERVENTIONS:** All nurses need leadership skills to manage other nurses, unlicensed personnel, and their clients. It is essential to the nursing role to identify and implement effective leadership practices.

2. Management
   a. Definition: A problem-oriented process with a focus on the activities needed to achieve a goal. Management involves personal interaction, but the focus is on the group's process. The most effective managers are also effective leaders.
   b. Essential components of management
      1) Planning/organization
      2) Direction
      3) Monitoring
      4) Recognition and reward
   c. Management styles *one person dictates everything*
      1) Autocratic *one thing & other thing*
      2) Laissez-faire
      3) Democratic *everybody works & everybody*
   d. **NURSING INTERVENTIONS:** All nurses need to learn management skills and identify their own personal leadership style. Additionally, the nurse needs to know the differences between being an autocratic and democratic leader. The most effective management style in a health care environment is the democratic leader who uses an interdisciplinary approach that encourages open communication, collaboration and promotes individual autonomy and accountability.

3. Power
   a. Definition: Power is the ability to take action, and having the strength to accomplish goals.

Power can be both inherent and acquired. Everyone has power in different ways and to different degrees.
   b. Types of power
      1) Legitimate
      2) Referent
      3) Reward
      4) Expert
      5) Information
      6) Coercive
      7) Informal
   c. **NURSING INTERVENTIONS:** It is important for the nurse to understand that the power to influence others can originate from a variety of sources. As a practical nurse, the power to influence is aimed at accomplishing goals (for example: use of appropriate delegation to provide quality client care).

4. Teamwork
   a. Definition: A team is a group of individuals working together toward a common goal. Members of the team engage in varying roles supporting achievement of these goals. Each team member's contribution is valued and important to the success of the team as a whole; think collaboration, coordination and communication. Group dynamics are the underlying process that the group engages in during their work as a team. Some of these facilitate and some hinder the progress of the group.
   b. Team roles
      1) Task roles
         a) Initiating
         b) Seeking information
         c) Giving information
         d) Clarifying
         e) Coordinating
         f) Summarizing
      2) Group maintenance roles
         a) Supporting
         b) Mediating
         c) Gate keeping
         d) Following
         e) Tension reducing
         f) Standard setting
      3) **NURSING INTERVENTIONS:** The astute nurse understands the importance of group dynamics and teamwork in the health care environment. The strongest bond in nursing is a shared common purpose or goal (for example: providing client care). In addition, the nurse encourages positive group dynamics that assists in effective clinical decision making and in addressing conflict within groups.

smart, good character

5. Communication
   a. Definition: communication involves sending, receiving, and interpreting both verbal and non-verbal information between at least two people
   b. Components of communication
   c. Basic elements of effective communication
   d. Assertive communication

   e. **NURSING INTERVENTIONS:** Effective communication requires commitment, effort, focus, and cooperation, especially when dealing with complex clinical issues and people with diverse backgrounds and perspectives. It is essential to understand and use effective communication skills to successfully coordinate care.
6. Conflict
   a. Definition: Conflict arises when there are two opposing views, feelings, expectations, and many other issues. It can occur within the individual, between individuals, or between groups and organizations. Conflict can be managed.
   b. Sources of conflict
   c. Conflict resolution
      1) Avoidance
      2) Accommodation
      3) Compromise
      4) Competition
      5) Collaboration
   d. Process of negotiation
   e. Sexual harassment
   f. **NURSING INTERVENTIONS:** The practical nurse's role is to identify the source of conflict, understand the issues that have developed, and work toward conflict-resolution with the other individual. It is essential to address the person with whom you have conflict first before going to his or her superiors (use the chain of command). Remember, the most important conflict strategy involves collaboration that results in a win-win solution for everyone.

B. Continuity of Care
1. Definition: Continuity of care focuses on the experience of the client as the client moves through the health care system. Moving the client through this experience requires coordination, integration, and facilitation of all the events along the continuum.
2. Nursing's role
3. Factors impacting the continuum of care

C. Quality Improvement
1. Definition: a planned process to evaluate the delivery of care and to develop ways to address any problems or difficulties

2. Continuous versus Total Quality Improvement
3. Types of quality indicators
   a. Structure
   b. Process
   c. Outcome
4. Data collection

D. Variances/Incidence/Occurrence Reports
1. Definition: a variance or incident is an event that occurs outside the usual expected "normal" events or activities of the client's stay, unit functioning, or organizational processes
2. Purpose
3. Documentation standards
4. **NURSING INTERVENTIONS:** Incidence or variance reports are not intended to point blame, just document the facts. The purpose is to identify situations or system issues that contributed to the occurrence and to engage strategies to prevent reoccurrence or to correct the situation.

E. Resource Management
1. Healthcare delivery
   a. Retrospective versus prospective payment
   b. Health maintenance organizations
2. Nurse's role in resource management
3. **NURSING INTERVENTIONS:** The nurse must also be aware of economic issues in healthcare. Remember, the more information available to the nurse, the better the decisions and input into long-range planning for the institution.

F. Consultation and Referral
1. Definitions
   a. Consultation: To ask for help in solving a problem or meeting a need of an individual or group. This help is then applied and monitored by the nurse. Often, it is a request for information from someone with specialized knowledge, including peers.
   b. Referral: A request for assistance from someone with specialized knowledge or skills to help in the management of the client's problems. Most often, it is a request for intervention from another professional who has the needed skills and knowledge. The intervention becomes that specialist's responsibility, but the nurse continues to be responsible for the monitoring of the client's response and progress.
2. Common nursing consultation and referral situations
3. Appropriate use of consultation and referral
4. **NURSING INTERVENTIONS:** The processes of consultation and referral are integral for effective utilization of services along the continuum. The

nurse supports the client and families with appropriate consultation and referral to contacts in the community.

SECTION II

DELEGATION

A. Delegation/Supervision
1. Definitions
   a. Delegation: The act of asking another to do some aspect of care, assignment, or work that needs to be accomplished. Delegation can be horizontal to peers, upwardly vertical to management, or downwardly vertical to subordinate.
   b. Supervision: Monitoring the progress toward completion of delegated tasks. The amount of supervision required depends on the direction of the delegation, the abilities of the person being delegated to, and the location of the ultimate responsibility for outcomes.
2. Accountability
3. Components
   a. Tasks
   b. Person
   c. Communication
   d. Feedback
4. **NURSING INTERVENTIONS:** It is very important for the nurse to understand legal responsibilities when managing and delegating nursing care to a wide variety of health care workers. The nurse must delegate activities thoughtfully, taking into account individual job descriptions, knowledge base, and demonstrated skills.

B. Roles and Responsibilities of Levels of Staff
1. Nursing assistant (NA)
   a. May also be called an unlicensed assistant
   b. Training is often on the job
   c. Nursing assistants may complete a certification program (CNA)
   d. Function under the direction of the licensed practical or registered professional nurse
   e. Skills:
      1) Basic hygiene care and grooming
      2) Communication
      3) Assistance with ADLs such as nutrition, elimination and mobility
      4) Emphasis is on maintaining a safe environment and recognizing situations to report to their immediate superior
2. Licensed practical nurse (LPN)
   a. May also be called a licensed vocational nurse (LVN)
   b. Education is approximately 12-18 months in a formal program
   c. LPNs must complete and pass the NCLEX-PN exam for licensure
   d. Function under direction of the registered professional nurse or primary care provider
   e. Skills (all the same as NA with additional skills of):
      1) Meeting health needs of clients
      2) Caring for clients whose condition is considered to be stable
3. Registered professional nurse (RN)
   a. May be diploma, associate degree, baccalaureate degree (or higher)
   b. Education ranges from 2 to 4 (or more) years
   c. RNs must complete and pass the NCLEX-RN exam for licensure
   d. Function under direction of the primary care provider
   e. Skills: all of the skills of the NA and LPN with additional skills as outlined in the nurse practice act for each state. In general, the RN acts as a client advocate and provides care to the client by use of the nursing process
4. Advance practice nurses
   a. May be non-degree or master's degree (or higher)
   b. Education ranges from 18 months to 4 (or more) years (in addition to basic RN program)
   c. Must complete and pass a certification exam (in addition to the NCLEX-RN exam) applicable to the specialty and practice (for example: adult nurse practitioner, diabetic educator)
   d. Functions vary according to the state practice act which may be either autonomously or under the direct or indirect supervision of a physician
   e. Skills: Vary according to the state practice act, may include ability to prescribe, diagnose and treat
5. Primary care provider
   a. May be a physician, physician's assistant, or nurse practitioner
   b. In general, only an attending physician has admitting privileges to an institution, although another care provider in the practice may direct the care given to the client.

SECTION III

ETHICAL ISSUES

A. Ethical Practice
1. Basic ethical principles
   a. Nonmaleficence: the obligation not to harm other people (for example: Hippocrates statement, "First do no harm.")

b.   Beneficence: the obligation to do good for other people

c.   Autonomy/self-determination: the right to make one's own decisions

d.   Fidelity: the obligation to be faithful to the agreements and responsibilities one has undertaken

e.   Justice: obligation to be fair to all people (for example: when allocating limited resources)

f.   Confidentiality: the right to privacy with respect to one's personal life

2.   ANA Code for Nurses: guidelines to use when giving client care which outline the nurse's responsibility to the client, the profession of nursing, and assist the nurse in ethical decision making

3.   Ethical dilemmas: an ethical issue for which two opposing viewpoints can each be supported by sound ethical principle

4.   Ethical decision making: a process in which the nurse, the client, the client's family, and the health care team make decisions taking into consideration personal and philosophical viewpoints, the ANA Code for nurses, and ethical principles

B.   Advanced Directives

1.   Definition: a document in which a competent person is able to express his or her wishes regarding future acceptable health care (including the desire for extraordinary lifesaving measures including resuscitation, intubation, and artificial hydration and nutrition) and/or designate another person to make decisions for the client if the client is physically or mentally unable

2.   Legislative action

3.   Living will

a.   Definition: declaration of what the person finds acceptable or would refuse under identified situations that may occur in the future

b.   Legal standing

c.   Content

4.   Durable power of attorney

a.   Definition: designation of another person to make decisions (often financial) for the client when the client becomes unable to make decisions independently

b.   Legal issues

c.   Purpose

 5.   **NURSING INTERVENTIONS:** it is important for the nurse to identify clients who do not have advanced directives, to inform them of their rights, and to ensure that client with advance directives have copies are placed in their charts

A.   Informed Consent

1.   Definition: consent given by the client that is based on adequate information to consider the risks and benefits of the offered service

2.   Elements of informed consent

3.   Nursing roles and responsibilities

B.   Client Rights

1.   Client Bill of Rights

2.   Americans with Disabilities Act

3.   Nursing role, responsibilities

4.   Legal implications

5.   Confidentiality

C.   Legal Responsibilities

1.   Types of law

2.   Nurse Practice Act

3.   Good Samaritan Law

4.   Mandatory Reporter of Abuse

5.   Malpractice

6.   Negligence

7.   Torts

8.   Breach of duty

9.   Standard of professional practice

D.   Advocacy

1.   Definition: a process by which the nurse assists the client to grow and develop toward self-actualization

2.   Nursing role as advocate

E.   NURSING INTERVENTIONS: The astute practical nurse who recognizes rights and responsibilities in legal matters is better able to protect him/herself against liability or loss of licensure.

POINTS TO REMEMBER:

Remember, the nurse has a duty to intervene when the safety or well being of the client or another person is obviously at risk.

NOTES

NOTES

ALTERNATE
TEST ITEM FORMATS

UNIT CONTENT

SECTION I.   Overview 185
SECTION II.   Fill-in-the-Blank 185
SECTION III. Multiple Response 186
SECTION IV.   Hot Spot 186
SECTION V.   Charts, Tables, & Graphic Images 187

SYMBOLS

Key
Points

Nursing
Interventions

Points to
Remember

SECTION I

OVERVIEW

A. NCLEX Item Types

1. Standard Multiple Choice Question
   (also see Introduction p.5-7)
   a. Traditionally, the format of NCLEX questions
   b. Still the most commonly seen type of question on the NCLEX
   c. Has four options, only one of which is correct ("one best option")
   d. Mastering this format is critical to your success on the NCLEX.
   e. The average standard question takes 60 to 70 seconds to answer.
2. As of April 2003, the NCLEX started including items other than standard multiple choice questions. These items are known as Alternate Test Item Formats.
   a. Fill-in-the-Blank
      1) Calculation
      2) Ordered Response
   b. Multiple Response
   c. Hot Spot
   d. Charts, Tables, Graphic Images
3. The average candidate will be administered only one or two of these alternate items.

POINTS TO REMEMBER:

| ! | You should allot a slightly longer time for alternate test items. |

SECTION II

FILL-IN-THE-BLANK

A. Overview

1. Definition: Fill-in-the-blank items are a type of alternate item that will be primarily numerical. This type of question typically involves either solving a math problem or putting a list of options into the correct sequence.
2. Method of Answer: To answer these questions, you will need to type a number into the answer box on the screen.

B. Types

1. Calculation item
   (also see Appendix A p.191-192)
   a. This type of fill-in-the-blank question typically involves solving a math problem.

b. Method of Answer: To answer these questions, you will need to type a number into the answer box on the screen.
c. Read the question carefully. If you see the question is asking for the answer in a specific unit amount, it is not necessary to put units in your answer.

POINTS TO REMEMBER:

!	1. Write equation down on your scrap paper.
	2. Be certain you are solving for the correct unit value!
	3. Show all of your work.
	4. Bring up drop-down calculator.
	5. Double-check your work

GRAPHIC 6-1.
FILL-IN-THE-BLANK CALCULATION ITEM

There are 13 clients being seen in the emergency room and 5 clients in the waiting room. What is the total number of clients?

Type your answer in the box below.

| 18 |

2. Ordered Response item
   a. This type of fill-in-the-blank question requires you to put a list of options into the correct order.
   b. Method of Answer: To answer these questions, you will need to type a series of numbers into the answer box on the screen.
   c. Read the question carefully. Ordered Response items on the NCLEX may require you to put the options in the order that you would perform them or in order of priority.
   d. It is not necessary to separate the numbers in any way, so do not insert spaces, dashes, commas, slashes or any other spacing device between the numbers.

POINTS TO REMEMBER:

| ! | Remember that there is only one correct sequence that preserves the client's safety at all stages during the procedure. |

GRAPHIC 6-2.
FILL-IN-THE-BLANK ORDERED RESPONSE ITEM

Put the following words in alphabetical order.

1. Pizza
2. Apples
3. Onion
4. Bacon
5. Rice

Type your answer in the box below.

24315

SECTION III

MULTIPLE RESPONSE

A. Overview
1. Definition: Multiple response items are a type of alternate item that require you to choose more than one answer from up to six options. Any number of the options may be correct.
2. Method of Answer: To answer these questions, you will need to click on all the answers that apply.
3. On the NCLEX, you will receive credit only for completely correct answers; there is no "partial credit" given for these item types.

POINTS TO REMEMBER:
Consider each response as you would a true-false question; is that statement true about the question or false? Click on all that you determine are true.

GRAPHIC 6-3.
MULTIPLE RESPONSE ITEM

Which of the following are types of vegetables?

Select all that apply.

☑ 1. Broccoli

☑ 2. Cucumber

☐ 3. Peach

☐ 4. Orange

☐ 5. Grape

SECTION IV

HOT SPOT

A. Overview
1. Definition: Hot spot items are a type of alternate item that will be a "point and click" exercise. Hot spot items will usually require you to identify an anatomical location on a figure.
2. Method of Answer: To answer these questions, you will need to point at an area on the screen with your cursor and click on the correct spot. As you move your mouse around the screen, you will see an arrow. Once you select a spot and click, the arrow will change into a circle with an "X" in it.
3. Read the question carefully, then analyze the image.
4. The NCLEX will allow you to reclick as many times as necessary.

POINTS TO REMEMBER:
It is very important to remember that the screen is NOT a mirror image! If you see that the question is asking for an answer on the right or left side of the body, make sure you are clicking on the correct side.

GRAPHIC 6-4.
HOT SPOT ITEM

The nurse is performing a cardiac assessment. Identify where the nurse will place the stethoscope to best auscultate the apical pulse.

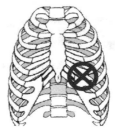

SECTION V

CHARTS, TABLES, & GRAPHIC IMAGES

A. Overview

1. Any of the NCLEX standard multiple choice or alternate items may also include charts, tables or other graphic images that you must analyze and understand in order to correctly answer the question.

2. It is important that you read the question carefully first, then analyze the image.

This graph represents:

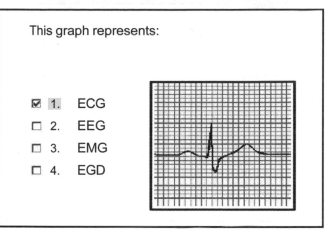

☑ 1. ECG

☐ 2. EEG

☐ 3. EMG

☐ 4. EGD

APPENDICES

UNIT CONTENT

APPENDIX A.   Review of Calculations and Conversions 191
APPENDIX B.   Nutrition 193
APPENDIX C.   Positioning Clients 195
APPENDIX D.   Psychiatric Terms 196
APPENDIX E.   Pharmacology 198

SYMBOLS

 Key Points

 Nursing Interventions

 Points to Remember

APPENDIX A
REVIEW OF CALCULATIONS AND CONVERSIONS

A. Metric System

1 kg = 1,000 gm
1 gm = 1,000 mg
1 mg = 1,000 mcg
1 L = 1,000 mL
1 mL = 1 cc = 1 gm
1 cm = 10 mm

B. Apothecary System - rarely used today

1 dram = 60 grains
1 ounce = 8 drams
1 dram = 60 minims
1 fluid ounce = 8 fluid drams

C. Household System

1 pound = 16 ounces
1 tablespoon = 3 teaspoons
1 ounce = 2 tablespoons
1 cup = 8 ounces
1 pint = 16 ounces
1 quart = 2 pints
1 gallon = 4 quarts

D. Conversions Between Systems

1 grain = 60 mg
1 gm = 15 grains
1 tablespoon = 15–16 mL
2 tablespoons = 1 ounce = 30–32 mL
1 cup = 8 ounces = 240 mL
8 ounces = 240–250 mL
2 cups = 1 pint = 500 mL
1 inch = 2.54 cm
1 kg = 2.2 lbs
1 lb = 454 gms
1 minim = 1 drop
1 mL = 15 minims = 15 drops
60 drops = 1 teaspoon = 1 fluid dram

E. Temperature Conversions

98.6°F = 37.0°C
C = (F - 32) x 5/9
F = (C x 9/5) + 32

F. Calculations for IV Administration

1. # of hours = $\dfrac{\text{mL/hour}}{\text{total volume}}$

2. gtts per min = $\dfrac{\text{total volume x gtts/mL in administration set}}{\text{total number of minutes}}$

G. Calculations for Dosage

$\dfrac{\text{Dosage on hand (H)}}{\text{mL}} = \dfrac{\text{Dosage desired (D)}}{\text{mL}}$

Fill-in-the-Blank question format is a new NCLEX Alternate Test Item Format. Place your answer in the box below the question.

Test Questions

1. A client has the following served for lunch: one cup of tea, one cup of coffee, and 240 mL of milk. The client drinks all of the tea and coffee and half of the milk. The total intake for lunch is:

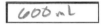

600 mL

2. A client has an order for 0.25 mg of digitalis (Digoxin). You have 0.5 mg tablets of Digoxin. How many tablets should you give the client?

1/2 or 0.5mg tab

3. A client's IV infusion rate is 75 mL per hour. How many hours will a 500 mL bag of IV fluid last?

$$\dfrac{75mL/ht}{500} \qquad \dfrac{500ml}{75ml} \times hu$$

6.6 hrs

4. When the IV rate is 100 mL per hour and the administration set is 15 drops per mL, how many drops per minute should the IV run?

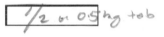

25 gtt/min

$$\dfrac{100mL/ht}{15gtt/m} \qquad \dfrac{1ml\ 15gtts}{100\times 1500}$$

$$\dfrac{100}{60}\times 15=25$$

5. A 4-year-old client is taking 5 mL of ampicillin (*Polycillin Pediatric*) for otitis media every six hours. In preparing for the client's discharge, the nurse should tell the client's mother to give how much ampicillin every six hours at home?

5ml q6hrs

1 teaspoon

6. A client has an order for heparin (Heparin Sodium) 7,000 units IV. The vial contains 10,000 units/mL. How many mL of heparin should be administered?

$\boxed{6.7 \text{ ml}}$

7. The nurse is preparing 300,000 units of procaine penicillin (*Wycillin*). The vial contains 1,500,000 units per 2 mL. How many mL will the nurse administer?

$$\frac{300,000}{1,500,000} \times 2 =$$

$\boxed{0.4 \text{ ml}}$

8. A client weighs 180 pounds and has an order for 0.5 mL of medication per kilogram of body weight. How many mL of medication should he receive?

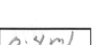

2.2 lbs = 1 kilo   81.82 kg

180 lbs

0.5 ml/kg

$\boxed{4/\text{ml}}$

9. A client is receiving D_5W at 50 mL per hour in one IV and D_5NS 75 mL per hour in another IV. The client also receives IVPB medication every 8 hours prepared in 100 mL of fluid. How much IV fluid will the client receive in 8 hours?

400
600
100

$\boxed{1,100 \text{ ml}}$

10. When the IV administration set delivers 10 drops per mL, the rate of flow in drops per minute for 1,000 mL D_5NS to infuse in 8 hours is:

$$\frac{1,000}{480} \times 10$$

$\boxed{20.83 \text{ gtt/min}}$

11. While measuring a client's output, the nurse has measured 300 mL urine at 8:00 AM, 450 mL liquid stool at 11:30 AM, 225 mL urine at 1:00 PM, and 35 mL emesis at 2:30 PM. What is the client's total output for this shift?

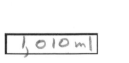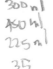

$\boxed{1,010 \text{ ml}}$

300 ml
450 ml
225 ml
35

12. A client receiving an IV infusion has an order for 1,000 mL in 12 hours. Using a micro drip system that delivers 60 micro drops per mL, the nurse should adjust the infusion for how many drops per minute?
   a. 45 drops
   b. 68 drops
   c. 83 drops
   d. 96 drops

$$\frac{1,000}{720} \times 60$$

$\boxed{\text{C. } 83 \text{ gtt}}$

13. A client's temperature is 100°F. What is this temperature in degrees Centigrade?

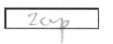

$(F-32) \times \frac{5}{9} = C \quad (68) \times 0.55$

$\boxed{37.4 \text{ °C}} \quad \left(C \times \frac{9}{5}\right) + 32 = F$

14. The nurse has a Tubex marked Demerol 50 mg per mL. To give 35 mg of Demerol, the nurse should give how many mL?

$$\frac{35}{50} \times \text{mls}$$

$\boxed{0.7 \text{ ml}}$

15. A client on fluid restriction may have 800 mL in 8 hours. The IV is running at 50 mL per hour. How much fluid may the client have by mouth?

800 ml in 8 hr

240

$\boxed{2 \text{ cup}}$

Test Answers
1. 600 mL
2. 1/2 tablet
3. 6.6 hours
4. 25 drops
5. 1 teaspoon
6. 0.7 mL
7. 0.4 mL
8. 41 mL
9. 1,100 mL
10. 20 drops per minute
11. 1,010 mL
12. 83 drops
13. 37.7° C
14. 0.7 mL
15. 1 glass and 1 cup

APPENDIX B
NUTRITION

Therapeutic Diets

A. Nutrient Modification

1. Low-protein diet
   a. Indicated for renal impairment, hepatic coma, and advanced cirrhosis
   b. Controls end products of protein metabolism by limiting protein intake
   c. Encourage high-carbohydrate foods
   d. Limit foods high in protein such as eggs, meat, milk, and milk products

2. High-protein diet
   a. Used for tissue building, burns, correction of malabsorption syndromes, mild to moderate liver disease, undernutrition, and pregnancy
   b. Corrects protein loss and/or maintains and re-builds tissues
   c. Encourage high-protein foods such as fish, fowl, organ and meat sources, and dairy products
   d. May include protein supplements

3. Abnormalities in amino acid metabolism
   a. Use for phenylketonuria (PKU), galactosemia, and lactose intolerance
   b. Reduce or eliminate the offending enzyme
   c. Avoid milk and milk products for all three diets
   d. Use substitutes

4. Low-cholesterol diet
   a. Indicated for cardiovascular diseases, diabetes mellitus, high-serum cholesterol levels
   b. Controls cholesterol levels by limiting cholesterol intake
   c. Limit high-cholesterol foods such as egg yolks, shellfish, organ meats, bacon, pork, avocado, olives
   d. Encourage low-cholesterol foods such as vegetable oils, raw or cooked vegetables, fruits, lean meats, and fowl

5. Modified-fat diet
   a. Indicated for malabsorption syndromes, cystic fibrosis, gallbladder disease, obstructive jaundice and liver disease, and obesity
   b. Fat content in the diet is lowered
      1) To stop contractions of the diseased organs
      2) When there is inadequate absorption of fat
      3) To decrease fat storage in the body
   c. To reduce fat intake, avoid gravies, fatty meat and fish, cream, fried foods, rich pastries, whole milk products, cream soups, salad and cooking oils, nuts, and chocolate; allow 2–3 eggs per week, lean meat, butter and margarine
   d. For a fat-free diet, restrict all fatty meats and fat; allow vegetables, fruits, lean meats, fowl, fish, bread, and cereal

6. High-polyunsaturated fat diet
   a. Indicated for cardiovascular diseases
   b. Reduce saturated fats by avoiding foods from animal sources, peanuts, olives, avocados, co-conuts, chocolate, and cashew nuts
   c. Increase polyunsaturated fats by including vegetable sources, margarine, corn/soybean/safflower oil

7. Carbohydrate modification (diabetic diet or ADA diet)
   a. Principles of diabetic diet management
      1) Attain or maintain ideal body weight
      2) Ensure normal growth
      3) Maintain plasma glucose levels as close to normal as possible
      4) Provide 30 calories per kg of ideal body weight
      5) Provide 25% of calories at each meal and 25% for snacks
      6) Provide 20% of calories as protein, 55–60% as carbohydrates, and 20–30% as fats
      7) Include unsaturated fats, high fiber, and complex carbohydrates
   b. Develop meal plans designed for individual needs using exchange lists
      1) Milk exchanges
      2) Vegetable exchanges
      3) Fruit exchanges
      4) Bread exchanges
      5) Fat exchanges

B. Mineral Alterations

1. Potassium-modified diets
   a. Increase potassium intake for diabetic acidosis, thiazide diuretics, 48 hours after burns, vomiting, fevers
   b. Reduce potassium intake for kidney failure
   c. Foods high in potassium include: fruits and fruit juices, (e.g., orange, grapefruit, banana, apple); avocados, prunes, dried apricots; dried beans, soy beans, lima beans, kidney beans, squash, baked potatoes, milk and broiled meats
   d. Foods low in potassium include: breads, cereals, sugar, fats, cranberry and grape juice

2. Sodium-restricted diets
   a. Sodium is restricted in hypertension, congestive heart failure, myocardial infarction, hepatitis, adrenal cortical diseases, kidney disease, lithium carbonate therapy, cystic fibrosis, and conditions such as cirrhosis of the liver and preeclampsia, which cause persistent edema
   b. Mild restriction is 2–3 gm of sodium
   c. Moderate restriction is 1,000 mg of sodium
   d. Strict restriction is 500 mg of sodium

e. Severe restriction is 250 mg of sodium
f. Limit foods high in sodium, such as: potato chips and other salted snack foods, canned soups and vegetables, baked goods that contain baking powder or baking soda, cereals, seafood, beef, processed meats such as bologna, ham, and bacon, dairy products, especially cheese, pickles, olives, and condiments such as soy sauce, steak sauce, Worcestershire sauce, and salad dressings
g. Encourage low-sodium foods such as fresh fruits and vegetables, chicken, salt substitutes, and low-sodium products

3. Iron alterations
a. Increased iron intake is indicated for correction or prevention of iron deficiency anemia, which is most likely to occur in infants, toddlers, adolescents, and pregnant women
b. Food sources high in iron include: fish, meats (particularly organ meats), green leafy vegetables, enriched breads, cereals, and macaroni products, whole grain products, dried fruits, such as raisins and apricots, and egg yolks
c. Vitamin C enhances absorption of iron from the gastrointestinal tract
d. Administration of iron supplements
   1) Oral administration with a straw
   2) Maximum absorption occurs when administered between meals
   3) Fewer GI side effects occur when administered with meals
   4) Injectable iron administered deep IM with Z track

4. Calcium alterations
a. Increased calcium intake is indicated for growing children and adolescents, pregnant and lactating women, and postmenopausal women (prevent osteoporosis)
b. Decreased calcium intake is indicated for kidney stones composed of calcium
c. Food sources high in calcium include: milk and milk products like yogurt and cheese; dark green vegetables, such as collard greens, kale, broccoli; dried beans and peas; and shellfish and canned salmon
d. Some antacids contain calcium
e. Vitamin D enhances absorption of calcium from the gastrointestinal tract

D. **Consistency Modifications**
1. Clear-liquid diet
   a. Indicated for resting the gastrointestinal tract, maintaining fluid balance; immediately postop; for diarrhea, nausea, and vomiting
   b. Includes water, tea, broth, jell-o, apple juice
   c. Not nutritionally adequate
2. Full-liquid diet
   a. When clear liquids are tolerated well, progress to full liquids
   b. Include clear liquids plus milk and milk products, such as custard, pudding, creamed soups, ice cream, sherbet, fruit juices
   c. Can be nutritionally adequate
3. Soft diet
   a. Include full liquids plus pureed vegetables, eggs that are not fried, tender meats, potatoes, cooked fruit
4. Bland diet
   a. Used to promote healing of gastric mucosa by eliminating chemically and mechanically irritating food sources
   b. Indicated for gastric and duodenal ulcers and postoperative stomach surgery
   c. Given in small, frequent feedings to assist in diluting or neutralizing stomach acid; protein foods are good at neutralizing; fat has some ability to inhibit the secretion of acid and delays stomach emptying
   d. Foods usually introduced in stages with gradual addition of foods
   e. Foods allowed include: milk, butter, eggs that are not fried, custard, vanilla ice cream, cottage cheese, cooked refined or strained cereal, enriched white bread, jell-o, homemade creamed, pureed soups, baked or broiled potatoes
5. Low-residue diet
   a. Indicated for ulcerative colitis, postoperative colon and rectal surgery, prep for x-rays and colon surgery, diarrhea, and regional enteritis
   b. Encourage ground meat, fish, skinless broiled chicken, creamed cheeses, warm drinks, refined strained cereals and white bread
   c. Foods high in carbohydrates are usually low in residue
   d. Avoid high-residue foods that have skins and seeds

POSITIONING CLIENTS

TABLE APP-1.

POSITION	DESCRIPTION	INDICATIONS
Semi-Fowler's	Head of bed elevated to 30°	Head injury, postop cranial surgery, respiratory diseases with dyspnea, postop cataract removal, increased intracranial pressure
Fowler's	Head of bed elevated to 45°	Head injury, postop cranial surgery, postop abdominal surgery, respiratory diseases with dyspnea, cardiac problems with dyspnea, bleeding esophageal varices, postop thyroidectomy, postop cataract removal, increased intracranial pressure
High-Fowler's	Head of bed elevated to 90°	Respiratory diseases with dyspnea: emphysema, status asthmaticus, pneumothorax, cardiac problems with dyspnea, feeding, meal times, hiatal hernia, during and after meals
Supine (dorsal recumbent)	Lying on back, head, and shoulders; usually slightly elevated with a small pillow	Spinal cord injury (no pillow), urinary catheterization
Prone	Lying on abdomen, legs extended, and head turned to the side	Immobilized client, amputation of lower extremity, unconscious client, post lumbar puncture 6–12 hours, post myelogram 12–24 hours (oil-based dye), postop T&A
Lateral (side lying)	Lying on side with most of body weight borne by the lateral aspect aspect of the lower ilium	Post abdominal surgery, unconscious client, seizures (head to side), postop T&A, postop pyloric stenosis of lower scapula and the lateral (right side), post-liver biopsy (right side), rectal irrigations
Sims (semi prone)	Lying on side with most of body weight borne by the anterior aspect of the ilium, humerus, and clavicle	Unconscious client, rectal irrigations
Lithotomy	Lying on back with hips and knees flexed at right angles and feet in stirrups	Perineal procedures, rectal procedures, vaginal procedures
Trendelenburg	Head and body are lowered while feet are elevated	Shock
Reverse Trendelenburg	Head elevated while feet are lowered	Cervical traction
Elevate one or more extremities	Elevate legs/feet or arms/hands by adjusting bed or supporting with pillows	Thrombophlebitis, application of cast, edema, postop surgical procedure on extremity

APPENDIX D

PSYCHIATRIC TERMS

TABLE APP-2.

TERMS	DEFINITIONS
ACTING OUT:	The active expression of emotions through actions, not words, that occurs when the client relives the feelings, wishes, or conflicts that are operating unconsciously
AFFECT:	The emotion or mood an individual shows as a response, such as flat affect or inappropriate affect
AMBIVALENCE:	The simultaneous presence of strong, but contradictory or opposite, feelings or ideas about something or someone
ANXIETY:	Fear or apprehension caused by an unknown or unrecognized threat
AUTISM:	A syndrome involving abnormal sensory perception and developmental (usually language and psychosocial) issues
BODY IMAGE:	One's perception of one's body
CATATONIC STATE:	Immobility
COHESIVENESS:	Group togetherness
COMPULSION:	Emotional urge or need to act
CONFABULATION:	A compensatory mechanism for memory loss; filling in the memory gaps with imaginary stories the teller believes to be true
CONFUSION:	Mental bewilderment from disorientation
CRISIS:	A conflict that cannot readily be resolved by using usual coping mechanisms
DEFENSE MECHANISMS:	Mental strategies used to help cope with areas of conflict
DELIRIUM TREMENS:	Alcohol withdrawal syndrome, including restlessness continuing to disorientation, hallucinations, and convulsions
DELUSION:	A fixed false idea
DENIAL:	Unconscious refusal to acknowledge that which is anxiety provoking
DESENSITIZATION:	Gradual systematic exposure of the client to feared situations under controlled conditions
ECHOLALIA:	Repetition by one person of what is said by another
ECHOPRAXIA:	A meaningless imitation of movement
EMPATHY:	Objective and insightful awareness of another's feelings
EXTRAPYRAMIDAL REACTION:	A reversible side effect of some psychotropic drugs characterized by muscle rigidity, drooling, restlessness, shuffling gait, and blurred vision
FAMILY THERAPY:	Treatment that involves the family and explores the relationships among the members
FANTASY:	Daydreams
FLIGHT OF IDEAS:	Rapid shift from an idea to another before the first idea has been concluded
GRIEF:	An emotional response to a recognized loss
GROUP THERAPY:	Application of psychotherapy techniques by a skilled leader to a group of clients
HALLUCINATION:	False sensory perceptions involving any of the senses

TERMS	DEFINITIONS
HOSTILITY:	Feeling similar to anger but of longer duration
IDEAS OF REFERENCE:	Ideas stemming from the incorrect interpretation of incidents as referring directly to self
ILLUSIONS:	Misinterpretation of a real, external sensory experience
INSIGHT:	Self understanding
INTRAPSYCHIC:	Within the mind
LABILE:	Rapidly changing emotions
LIMIT SETTING:	Clear statement of rules with consistent reinforcement
LOOSENESS OF ASSOCIATION:	Ideas appear unrelated or only slightly related
MANIA:	Elated, excited mood state
MANIPULATION:	Control of another's behavior for one's own purposes
MILIEU THERAPY:	Management of the client's environment to promote a positive living experience and facilitate recovery
NEOLOGISM:	Coined word with special meaning to the user
OBSESSION:	Repetitive, uncontrollable thought
PARANOID:	Suspicion, mistrust, without a basis in reality
PHOBIA:	Irrational fear
PREMORBID:	Occurring before development of a disease
PSYCHOSIS:	State in which there is impairment in a person's ability to recognize reality, communicate and relate to others appropriately
RESISTANCE:	Opposition to uncovering unconscious material
ROLE:	Pattern of behavior
SECONDARY GAINS:	Benefits from being ill, such as attention
SELF-ESTEEM:	The degree of feeling worthwhile or valued
SELF-IMAGE:	One's thoughts about one's own self
SOMATIC THERAPY:	Treatment of the emotionally ill by physiological means
STEREOTYPED BEHAVIOR:	Persistent mechanical repetition of speech or motor activity
TRANSFERENCE:	Unconscious phenomenon in which feelings, attitudes, and wishes toward significant others in one's early life are linked to and projected onto others, usually a therapist in one's current life
WAXY FLEXIBILITY:	The extremities remain in a fixed position for a long period of time
WORD SALAD:	Words and phrases having no apparent meaning or logic

APPENDIX E
PHARMACOLOGY
Antimicrobial Agents
PENICILLINS

DRUG: GENERIC/TRADE
- amoxicillin (Polymox)
- ampicillin (D-Amp)
- cloxacillin (Cloxapen)
- dicloxacillin (Dycill)
- nafcillin (Unipen)
- penicillin G (Bicillin L-A)
- penicillin V (Beepen-VK)

ACTION
- Bacteriocidal against microbes by inhibiting cell wall synthesis during cell division

ADVERSE EFFECTS
- Hypersensitivity: rash, urticaria, anaphylaxis

INDICATIONS
- Infections due to gram-positive cocci and some gram-negative cocci

NURSING INTERVENTIONS
- Observe for hypersensitivity
- Teach client to call physician if rash, fever, or chills
- Teach client to take medications as ordered until entire amount taken
- Administer 1–2 hours before meals or 2–3 after meals for best absorption

OTHER INFORMATION
- Resistant strains of bacteria may develop

CEPHALOSPORINS

DRUG: GENERIC/TRADE
- First generation
  - cefazolin sodium (Ancef, Kefzol)
  - cephalexin monohydrate (Keflex)
  - cephalothin sodium (Keflin)
- Second generation
  - cefaclor (Ceclor)
  - cefuroxime (Zinacef)
  - loracarbef (Lorabid)
- Third generation
  - cefixime (Suprax)
  - cefotaxime (Claforan)
  - ceftriaxone (Rocephin)

ACTION
- Bacteriocidal or bacteriostatic
- Inhibits cell wall synthesis

ADVERSE EFFECTS
- Hypersensitivity
- Local irritation at injection site

INDICATIONS
- Infections due to gram-positive cocci and some gram-negative cocci
- Prophylactically before certain operative procedures

NURSING INTERVENTIONS
- Obtain client history
- Change IV sites after 3 days
- Use with caution in clients with renal impairment
- Use with caution on clients with penicillin allergy

OTHER INFORMATION
- Structurally related to penicillin
- May cause false positive urine glucose test
- Excreted unchanged in urine

SULFONAMIDES

DRUG: GENERIC/TRADE
- sulfamethoxazole-trimethoprim (Bactrim, Septra)
- sulfisoxazole (Gantrisin)

ACTION
- Broad spectrum bacteriostatic

ADVERSE EFFECTS
- Hypersensitivity
- Blood dyscrasia-agranulocytosis, aplastic anemia
- Toxic to kidney when output is low
- GI manifestations: nausea, vomiting, diarrhea

INDICATIONS
- Urinary tract infections
- Otitis media
- Sinusitis

NURSING INTERVENTIONS
- Obtain client history
- Monitor CBC routinely
- Teach client to report skin rash, sore throat, fever or mouth sores
- Increase fluid intake to maintain output of 3,000–4,000 mL
- Administer 1 hour before or 2 hours after meals for best absorption

AMINOGLYCOSIDES

DRUG: GENERIC/TRADE
- gentamicin sulfate (Garamycin)
- neomycin sulfate (Mycifradin Sulfate)
- streptomycin sulfate
- tobramycin sulfate (Nebcin)
- vancomycin hydrochloride (Vancocin)

ACTION
- Bacteriostatic or bacteriocidal
- Inhibits protein synthesis

ADVERSE EFFECTS
- Nephrotoxicity
- Ototoxicity (tinnitus, vertigo, hearing loss)

INDICATIONS
- Serious bacterial infections
- Promote bowel sterility prior to GI surgical procedures

NURSING INTERVENTIONS
- Weigh client and obtain baseline renal function studies prior to therapy
- Monitor output for specific gravity, urinalysis, BUN, creatinine, and creatinine clearance
- Monitor peak and trough therapeutic levels for duration of therapy
- Encourage fluids
- Evaluate client's hearing before and during hearing loss therapy

ANTITUBERCULARS

DRUG: GENERIC/TRADE
- ethambutol *(Myambutol)*

ACTION
- Impairs RNA synthesis

ADVERSE EFFECTS
- Vision loss and loss of color discrimination

INDICATIONS
- Pulmonary tuberculosis

NURSING INTERVENTIONS
- Evaluate client's visual acuity and color discrimination before and during therapy

ANTITUBERCULARS

DRUG: GENERIC/TRADE
- rifampin *(Rifadin)*

ACTION
- Impairs RNA synthesis

ADVERSE EFFECTS
- Hepatotoxicity
- Red-orange color to urine and feces
- Drowsiness

INDICATIONS
- Pulmonary tuberculosis

NURSING INTERVENTIONS
- Monitor liver function studies
- Teach client about color changes of body secretions
- Teach client to avoid activities that require alertness

OTHER INFORMATION
- May require increased doses of warfarin, corticosteroids, and oral hypoglycemics

ANTITUBERCULARS

DRUG: GENERIC/TRADE
- isoniazid *(INH)*

ACTION
- Interferes with DNA synthesis

ADVERSE EFFECTS
- Hepatotoxicity
- Peripheral neuropathy

INDICATIONS
- Infection due to tubercle bacilli

NURSING INTERVENTIONS
- Monitor liver function studies
- Teach client to notify physician for loss of appetite, fatigue, malaise, jaundice, and dark urine
- Teach client to avoid alcohol
- Administer pyridoxine *(Vitamin B$_6$) (Beesix)* to prevent peripheral neuropathy

ANTITUBERCULARS

DRUG: GENERIC/TRADE
- para-aminosalicylic acid *(PAS)*

ACTION
- Inhibits folic acid synthesis

ADVERSE EFFECTS
- Hepatotoxicity
- GI symptom: nausea, vomiting

INDICATIONS
- Tuberculosis

NURSING INTERVENTIONS
- Monitor liver function studies
- Teach client to notify physician of loss of appetite fatigue, malaise, jaundice, and dark urine
- Administer with meals or antacid

ANTIFUNGALS

DRUG: GENERIC/TRADE
- amphotericin B *(Fungizone)*
- fluconazole *(Diflucan)*

ACTION
- Alters fungal cell permeability

ADVERSE EFFECTS
- Fever, chills, nausea, vomiting, and headache
- Thrombophlebitis
- Hypokalemia

INDICATIONS
- Systemic fungal infections

NURSING INTERVENTIONS
- Administer acetaminophen *(Tylenol)* and diphenhydramine *(Benadryl)* 1 hour before infusion
- Add hydrocortisone to infusion
- Observe for signs of hypokalemia
- Large doses of potassium may be needed with systemic drugs
- Care with IV administration, can harm tissue

ANTIFUNGALS

DRUG: GENERIC/TRADE
- Nystatin *(Mycostatin)*

ACTION
- Alters fungal cell permeability

ADVERSE EFFECTS
- Rash, urticaria, stinging, burning

INDICATIONS
- Infections due to Candida in the mouth, GI tract, or vagina

NURSING INTERVENTIONS
- Wash hands before and after application

Fluid and Electrolyte Agents
THIAZIDES AND THIAZIDE-LIKE DIURETICS

DRUG: GENERIC/TRADE
- chlorothiazide *(Diuril)*
- hydrochlorothiazide *(Hydro Diuril)*
- chlorthalidone *(Hygroton)*
- quinethazone *(Hydromox)*

ACTION
- Inhibit sodium reabsorption in the kidney
- Increase excretion of sodium and water

ADVERSE EFFECTS
- Hypokalemia
- Altered glucose metabolism

INDICATIONS
- Hypertension
- Edema

NURSING INTERVENTIONS
- Monitor intake and output, weight, and potassium level
- Teach client to increase dietary potassium intake
- Observe for signs of hypokalemia: muscle weakness, cramps, and metabolic alkalosis
- Monitor blood sugar
- Observe for signs of hyperglycemia

OTHER INFORMATION
- Administer in the morning to prevent nocturia
- High risk of digitalis toxicity due to potassium depletion

LOOP DIURETICS

DRUG: GENERIC/TRADE
- furosemide (Lasix)
- ethacrynate sodium (Sodium Edecrin)
- ethacrynic acid (Edecrin)

ACTION
- Inhibit sodium and chloride reabsorption in the kidney
- Increase excretion of sodium and water

ADVERSE EFFECTS
- Fluid and electrolyte imbalances
- Hypocalcemia
- Hypokalemia
- Dehydration
- Hyponatremia
- Orthostatic hypotension
- Hypochloremia

INDICATIONS
- Edema
- Pulmonary edema

NURSING INTERVENTIONS
- Monitor intake and output, weight, and serum electrolytes
- Teach client to increase dietary potassium intake
- Observe for signs of hypokalemia: muscle weakness, cramps, and metabolic alkalosis
- Teach clients to stand up, take the stairs, and move around slowly

OTHER INFORMATION
- Administer in the morning to prevent nocturia
- High risk of digitalis toxicity due to potassium depletion

POTASSIUM SPARING DIURETICS

DRUG: GENERIC/TRADE
- spironolactone (Aldactone)
- triamterene (Dyrenium)

ACTION
- Increased excretion of sodium and water
- Reduces potassium excretion

ADVERSE EFFECTS
- Hyperkalemia

INDICATIONS
- Edema

- Hypertension

NURSING INTERVENTIONS
- Monitor intake and output, weight, and serum electrolytes
- Teach clients to avoid excessive dietary potassium

OTHER INFORMATION
- Used in combination with potassium depleting diuretics

OSMOTIC DIURETICS

DRUG: GENERIC/TRADE
- mannitol (Osmitrol)

ACTION
- Increases osmotic pressure of glomerular filtrate
- Increases excretion of water and electrolytes

ADVERSE EFFECTS
- Fluid and electrolyte imbalances
- Transient plasma volume increase
- Pulmonary edema
- Cellular dehydration

INDICATIONS
- Oliguria
- Edema
- Increased intraocular pressure
- Increased intracranial pressure

NURSING INTERVENTIONS
- Monitor vital signs hourly, including central venous pressure
- Insert Foley, record urine output hourly
- Monitor weight, intake and output, serum sodium and potassium

OTHER INFORMATION
- IV solution may crystallize; dissolve before infusing by warming bottle and shaking

ELECTROLYTE REPLACEMENT DRUGS

DRUG: GENERIC/TRADE
- potassium chloride

ACTION
- Necessary for cardiac contraction, renal function, and transmission of nerve impulses

ADVERSE EFFECTS
- Cardiac arrhythmias, heart block, cardiac arrest
- GI distress

INDICATIONS
- Hypokalemia

NURSING INTERVENTIONS
- Administer IV infusions as dilute solution infuses slowly
- Monitor EKG and serum potassium levels
- Administer oral dose with meals and plenty of fluids
- Monitor for signs of hyperkalemia

Cardiovascular Drugs
CARDIOTONIC GLYCOSIDES

DRUG: GENERIC/TRADE
- digitoxin (Crystodigin)
- digoxin (Lanoxin)
- dobutamine (Dobutrex)

ACTION
- Increases the force of cardiac contraction - positive inotropic
- Decreases heart rate - negative chronotropic

ADVERSE EFFECTS
- Bradycardia, arrhythmias
- Fatigue, muscle weakness, agitation
- Hallucinations
- Signs of toxicity: Anorexia, nausea, yellow-green halos around visual images

INDICATIONS
- Congestive heart failure
- Tachyarrhythmias

NURSING INTERVENTIONS
- Take apical pulse for full minute; record and report significant changes in rate or rhythm. Hold if <60 or >120 in adult client.
- Monitor serum levels of potassium and drug and monitor EKG
- Teach how to take pulse and what signs to report

OTHER INFORMATION
- Narrow range between therapeutic and toxic doses - (0.5-2.0)
- Calcium salts are contraindicated

CORONARY VASODILATORS

DRUG: GENERIC/TRADE
- nitroglycerin (Nitrostat)

ACTION
- Dilate coronary arteries
- Decrease cardiac workload

ADVERSE EFFECTS
- Headache
- Flushing
- Orthostatic hypotension
- Palpitations
- Tachycardia

INDICATIONS
- Angina

NURSING INTERVENTIONS
- Treat headache with acetaminophen (Tylenol)
- Tolerance usually develops
- Monitor vital signs
- Teach to stand up, move slowly
- Teach client to lie down if dizzy

OTHER INFORMATION
- Protect this drug from light, moisture and heat
- Sublingual tablet taken at the first sign of anginal pain
- Client should sit or lie down
- May repeat tablet every five minutes times three if needed
- Call physician if no relief
- Topical drug measured on ruled application paper and applied to non-hairy area

CALCIUM CHANNEL BLOCKERS - ANTI-ANGINAL AND ANTI-HYPERTENSIVE

DRUG: GENERIC/TRADE
- nifedipine (Procardia)
- diltiazem (Cardizem)

ACTION
- Decreases calcium in muscle so dilates coronary arteries and decreases heart rate

ADVERSE EFFECTS
- Bradycardia
- Peripheral swelling
- Coughing
- Hypotension
- GI upsets

INDICATIONS
- Hypertension
- Angina

NURSING INTERVENTIONS
- Assess for bradycardia
- Teach client to be careful when using OTC meds
- Educate client to change positions slowly
- Monitor for swelling

ANTIARRHYTHMICS

DRUG: GENERIC/TRADE
- lidocaine (Xylocaine)
- propranolol hydrochloride (Inderal)
- procainamide hydrochloride (Pronestyl)
- quinidine gluconate (Dura-Tabs)

ACTION
- Decreases cardiac conduction

ADVERSE EFFECTS
- Bradycardia
- Tachycardia - Reflux
- Hypotension

INDICATIONS
- Prevention or treatment of atrial or ventricular arrhythmias including those secondary to MI and digitalis toxicity

NURSING INTERVENTIONS
- Remain with client during infusion, tachycardia
- Monitor EKG, BP, and heart rate and rhythm

OTHER INFORMATION
- Narrow therapeutic index
- Do not confuse lidocaine with epinephrine used for local or topical anesthesia
- IV dose of Inderal much smaller than PO dose

ANTIARRHYTHMICS

DRUG: GENERIC/TRADE
- verapamil (Calan, Isoptin)

ACTION
- Calcium blocker
- Decrease cardiac conduction

ADVERSE EFFECTS
- Headache
- Constipation
- Dizziness
- Heart failure
- Reflux peripheral edema

INDICATIONS
- Atrial arrhythmias

NURSING INTERVENTIONS
- Treat with acetaminophen (Tylenol)

- Increase dietary fiber, fluid intake, and exercise

ANGIOTENSION-CONVERTING ENZYME INHIBITORS (ACE) - ANTIHYPERTENSIVE

DRUG: GENERIC/TRADE
- captopril *(Capoten)*
- enalapril *(Vasotec)*
- benazepril *(Lotensin)*

ACTION
- Prevents production of angiotensin II, causing system vasodilatations

ADVERSE EFFECTS
- Dry cough
- Drop in BP during first 1–3 hours following first dose
- Dizziness, orthostatic hypotension
- No reflux edema

INDICATIONS
- Hypertension
- Management of CHF

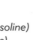 NURSING INTERVENTIONS
- Advise patient to change positions slowly
- Monitor BP, weight, signs to CHF resolution

ANTIHYPERTENSIVES

DRUG: GENERIC/TRADE
- hydralazine hydrochloride *(Apresoline)*
- prazosin hydrochloride *(Minipress)*

ACTION
- Relaxes smooth muscle

ADVERSE EFFECTS
- Tachycardia, palpitation
- Orthostatic hypotension
- Headache, dizziness
- Nausea, vomiting, diarrhea, anorexia
- Weight gain
- Administer diuretic if needed

INDICATIONS
- Hypertension, congestive heart failure

NURSING INTERVENTIONS
- Monitor heart rate and rhythm
- Teach client to stand up and move around slowly
- Treat with acetaminophen (Tylenol); teach client to lie down if dizzy
- Administer with meals
- Weigh daily
- Administer diuretic if needed

OTHER INFORMATION
- Compliance is biggest problem because side effects are worse than the disease - Not used very much today because of this
- Side effects can be minimized by adjusting dose or changing drugs
- Giving drugs daily rather than several times daily may increase compliance

Central Nervous System Drugs
NON-NARCOTIC ANALGESICS

DRUG: GENERIC/TRADE
- aspirin

ACTION
- Analgesic, antipyretic, anti-inflammatory

ADVERSE EFFECTS
- Prolonged bleeding time
- Nausea, vomiting, GI distress

INDICATIONS
- Arthritis
- Mild pain, fever

NURSING INTERVENTIONS
- Teach client who takes large doses for a long time to watch for signs of bleeding
- Administer with meals, milk, or antacids

OTHER INFORMATION
- Contraindicated for children under 18 years old because use has been linked to Reye's syndrome

NON-NARCOTIC ANALGESICS

DRUG: GENERIC/TRADE
- acetaminophen *(Tylenol)*

ACTION
- Analgesic antipyretic

ADVERSE EFFECTS
- Hepatotoxicity only with very large doses

INDICATIONS
- Mild pain, fever

NURSING INTERVENTIONS
- Teach client not to exceed recommended dosage

NON-NARCOTIC ANALGESICS

DRUG: GENERIC/TRADE
- ibuprofen *(Motrin)*
- naproxen *(Naprosyn)*

ACTION
- Anti-inflammatory analgesic

ADVERSE EFFECTS
- GI distress, occult bleeding, allergy

INDICATIONS
- Arthritis, gout
- Pain from inflammation

NURSING INTERVENTIONS
- Administer with meals, milk, or antacids
- Check stool for melena or occult blood
- Treat GI distress

NARCOTIC ANALGESICS

DRUG: GENERIC/TRADE
- codeine sulfate
- meperidine hydrochloride *(Demerol)*
- morphine sulfate

ACTION
- Alter perception of pain

ADVERSE EFFECTS
- Respiratory depression

- Hypotension, bradycardia
- Sedation, clouded sensorium, euphoria
- Nausea, vomiting, constipation

INDICATIONS
- Moderate to severe pain

NURSING INTERVENTIONS
- Monitor respirations before and during treatment
- Monitor BP and pulse
- Teach client to avoid activities that require alertness
- Provide environment that enhances rest

OTHER INFORMATION
- naloxone (Narcan) is used to reverse narcotic-induced respiratory depression

ANTICONVULSANTS

DRUG: GENERIC/TRADE
- phenytoin sodium (Dilantin)

ACTION
- Inhibits spread of seizure activity

ADVERSE EFFECTS
- Ataxia

INDICATIONS
- Tonic/clonic seizure disorder

NURSING INTERVENTIONS
- Determine if ataxia is a manifestation of the disease or a toxic effect of the drug
- Teach client to avoid activities that require alertness
- Use only normal saline solutions for infusion
- Instruct client that good oral hygiene and regular dental care are required
- Monitor therapeutic levels

OTHER INFORMATION
- Do not mix with 5% dextrose because precipitation will occur

Autonomic Nervous System Drugs

CHOLINERGIC BLOCKERS
(Not used as much today because of side effects)

DRUG: GENERIC/TRADE
- benztropine mesylate (Cogentin)
- procyclidine hydrochloride (Kemadrin)
- biperiden hydrochloride (Akineton)
- trihexyphenidyl hydrochloride (Artane)

ACTION
- Parasympatholytic

ADVERSE EFFECTS
- Anticholinergic
- Blurred vision
- Dry mouth
- Constipation
- Urinary retention
- Orthostatic hypotension
- Drowsiness

INDICATIONS
- Parkinson's disease
- Extra-pyramidal manifestations associated with antipsychotics

NURSING INTERVENTIONS
- Provide fluids, hard candy, ice chips
- Increase dietary fiber, fluid intake, and exercise
- Monitor intake and output
- Monitor BP; teach client to stand up slowly
- Teach client to avoid activities that require alertness

OTHER INFORMATION
- Elderly patients particularly sensitive to side effects
- Can produce euphoria and have abuse potential
- Amantadine (Symmetrel) is newer agent for treating Parkinson's disease; not a cholinergic blocker

DOPAMINERGIC THERAPY
(Used more often)

DRUG: GENERIC/TRADE
- levodopa (Sinemet)
- bromocriptine (Parlodel)
- amantadine (Symmetrel)

ACTION
- Increase dopamine

ADVERSE EFFECTS
- Impaired concentration
- Hypotension
- GI upsets

INDICATIONS
- Parkinson's disease

NURSING INTERVENTIONS
- Change positions slowly
- Minimize Vitamin B_6 foods and vitamins (meat, eggs, poultry, sweet potatoes)
- Take with juice, low protein snack

Gastrointestinal Drugs

ANTACIDS

DRUG: GENERIC/TRADE
- aluminum hydroxide (Amphojel)
- aluminum and magnesium hydroxide and simethicone (Mylanta)
- aluminum and magnesium hydroxide (Maalox)
- aluminum magnesium complex (Riopan)
- calcium carbonate (Tums)

ACTION
- Reduce acid in GI tract
- Decrease pepsin activity

ADVERSE EFFECTS
- Constipation
- Hypernatremia
- Hypermagnesemia
- Hypophosphatemia

INDICATIONS
- Peptic ulcers

NURSING INTERVENTIONS
- Record amount and consistency of stools
- Increase dietary fiber, fluid intake, and exercise
- Use laxatives and stool softeners
- Administer Riopan, which has very low sodium content - to client needing salt restriction

- Do not give magnesium containing antacids to clients with renal disease
- When giving aluminum containing antacids, observe for anorexia, malaise, muscle weakness

ANTIEMETICS

DRUG: GENERIC/TRADE
- prochlorperazine maleate *(Compazine)*
- trimethobenzamide hydrochloride *(Tigan)*

ACTION
- Acts centrally by blocking chemoreceptor trigger zone, which acts on vomiting center

ADVERSE EFFECTS
- Drowsiness, dizziness - rare extrapyramidal reaction can occur

INDICATIONS
- Nausea and vomiting

NURSING INTERVENTIONS
- Teach client to avoid activities that require alertness

ANTIEMETICS

DRUG: GENERIC/TRADE
- dimenhydrinate *(Dramamine)*
- scopolamine *(Transderm V)*

ACTION
- Acts centrally by blocking chemoreceptor trigger zone, which acts on vomiting center

ADVERSE EFFECTS
- Drowsiness, dizziness

INDICATIONS
- Prevention of nausea and vomiting associated with motion sickness

NURSING INTERVENTIONS
- Teach client to avoid activities that require alertness

ULCER MEDICATIONS

DRUG: GENERIC/TRADE
- cimetidine *(Tagamet)*
- sucralfate *(Carafate)*
- omeprazole *(Prilosec)*

ACTION
- Tagamet is GI antihistamine; reduces gastric acid secretion
- Carafate coats and protects surface of ulcer
- Omeprazole blocks acid production

ADVERSE EFFECTS
- Abdominal cramps, diarrhea
- Agranulocytosis, increased pro-time

INDICATIONS
- Short-term treatment of duodenal and gastric ulcers, gastroesophageal reflux disease (GERD)

NURSING INTERVENTIONS

- Administer with meals for prolonged drug effect
- Avoid OTC preparations such as aspirin, cough medications
- Report bruising
- Do not crush, chew, or open capsules *(Prilosec)*

OTHER INFORMATION
- Short-term treatment only
- Separate administration of these medications from administration of antacids by one hour

Hormonal Agents

STEROIDS

DRUG: GENERIC/TRADE
- cortisone acetate *(Cortone)*
- dexamethasone *(Decadron)*
- prednisone *(Meticorten)*

ACTION
- Anti-inflammatory

ADVERSE EFFECTS
- Euphoria, insomnia, psychotic behavior
- Hypokalemia
- Hyperglycemia and carbohydrate intolerance
- Peptic ulcer
- Cushingoid symptoms with long-term therapy
- Withdrawal symptoms

INDICATIONS
- Adrenal insufficiency
- Allergic inflammation, edema, immunosuppression

NURSING INTERVENTIONS
- Assess behavior, especially with high doses
- Potassium supplement may be needed
- High-protein diet rich in potassium
- Diabetics may require higher doses of insulin
- Administer with meals
- Teach client manifestations
- Reduce dose gradually, not abruptly

INSULINS

DRUG: GENERIC/TRADE
- Humalog insulin (Ultrarapid acting)
- Semilente regular insulin (Rapid acting)
- Lente NPH (Intermediate acting)
- Ultralente protamine (Long acting)
- Combination Insulin: 70/30 *(70% NPH insulin and 30% regular insulin)*

ACTION
- Facilitates transport of glucose into cells
- Lowers serum glucose level

ADVERSE EFFECTS
- Hypoglycemia
- Hyperglycemia

INDICATIONS
- Insulin dependent diabetes Mellitus

NURSING INTERVENTIONS
- Administer orange juice or candy PO for hypoglycemia
- Administer rapid acting insulin for hyperglycemia
- Monitor capillary blood sugar (CBS) routinely

OTHER INFORMATION
- Refrigeration is recommended for long-term storage
- Do not inject cold insulin

SULFONYLUREAS

DRUG: GENERIC/TRADE
- tolbutamide (Orinase)
- chlorpropamide (Diabinese)
- tolazamide (Tolinase)
- glyburide (Micronase, DiaBeta)

ACTION
- Increases insulin release from the pancreas

ADVERSE EFFECTS
- Hypoglycemia
- Hepatotoxicity

INDICATIONS
- Adult onset, non-insulin dependent
- Diabetes mellitus

NURSING INTERVENTIONS
- Teach client to take in morning to avoid hypoglycemic reaction at night
- Avoid OTC medications and alcohol

Hematologic Agents
HEMATONICS

DRUG: GENERIC/TRADE
- ferrous sulfate (Slow-Fe)

ACTION
- Source of iron replacement

ADVERSE EFFECTS
- Nausea, constipation, black stool

INDICATIONS
- Iron deficiency anemia

NURSING INTERVENTIONS
- Absorption best if given between meals
- For GI upset, give with meals or orange juice
- Teach client to increase dietary fiber, fluid intake, and exercise

OTHER INFORMATION
- Vitamin C may increase absorption

ANTICOAGULANTS

DRUG: GENERIC/TRADE
- heparin sodium (Hep-Lock, Hepalean)
- enoxaparin (Lovenox); low molecular weight heparin

ACTION
- Prevents conversion of fibrinogen to fibrin and prothrombin to thrombin

ADVERSE EFFECTS
- Hemorrhage

INDICATIONS
- Thrombosis
- Pulmonary embolism
- Myocardial infarction (MI)

NURSING INTERVENTIONS
- Monitor platelet count
- Monitor partial thromboplastin time (PTT)
- Avoid salicylates
- Observe for bleeding gums, bruises, nosebleeds, and petechiae

OTHER INFORMATION
- IV absorption is more regular than subcutaneous injection
- PTT should be 1.5–2 times control value
- Antagonist is protamine sulfate

ANTICOAGULANTS

DRUG: GENERIC/TRADE
- warfarin sodium (Coumadin)

ACTION
- Prevents prothrombin formations

ADVERSE EFFECTS
- Hemorrhage

INDICATIONS
- Pulmonary embolism
- Thrombosis, MI, heart valve damage

NURSING INTERVENTIONS
- Monitor PT
- Avoid salicylates
- Observe for bleeding gums, bruises, nosebleeds, and petechiae
- Teach client to use soft toothbrush and electric razor

OTHER INFORMATION
- Oral administration PT should be 1.5–2 times control value
- Antagonist is Vitamin K

ANTINEOPLASTICS

DRUG: GENERIC/TRADE
- methotrexate (Folex, Rheumatrex)
- cisplatin (Platinol)
- bleomycin (Blenoxane)

ACTION
- Act by many different mechanisms, most affect DNA synthesis or function

ADVERSE EFFECTS
- Many cause bone marrow depression, thrombocytopenia, nausea, vomiting, mouth ulcers

INDICATIONS
- Cancer
- Chemotherapy

NURSING INTERVENTIONS
- Assess for signs of infection
- Monitor platelet count
- Monitor IV site carefully, ensure patency; follow protocols for infiltration to prevent tissue ulceration/necrosis
- Wear gloves, masks, gowns while handling or preparing medication; discard equipment in designated containers

Eye Agents
MIOTICS

DRUG: GENERIC/TRADE
- pilocarpine hydrochloride (Carpine)

ACTION
- Pupillary constriction

ADVERSE EFFECTS
- Myopia

- Blurred vision

INDICATIONS
- Glaucoma
- Surgical procedures on the eye

NURSING INTERVENTIONS
- Usually disappears after 10–14 days of treatment

OTHER INFORMATION
- Press inner canthus for a minute or two to decrease systemic absorption

MYDRIATICS

DRUG: GENERIC/TRADE
- atropine sulfate (Atropisol)

ACTION
- Pupillary dilatation, cycloplegia

ADVERSE EFFECTS
- Blurred vision
- Photophobia

INDICATIONS
- Acute inflammation of the eye
- Diagnostic procedure

NURSING INTERVENTIONS
- Warn client about temporary blurring of vision
- Dark glasses
- Teach client not to drive until vision is clear

MYDRIATICS

DRUG: GENERIC/TRADE
- phenylephrine hydrochloride (Neo-Synephrine)

ACTION
- Pupillary dilatation

ADVERSE EFFECTS
- Hypertension
- Blurred vision

INDICATIONS
- Diagnostic procedure

NURSING INTERVENTIONS
- Monitor BP
- Avoid use in clients with hypertension
- Teach client not to drive until vision is clear

ANTILIPIDEMIC AGENTS

DRUG: GENERIC/TRADE
- Bile acid sequestrants: cholestyramine (Questran) lowers LDL and serum cholesterol HMG-COA - lovastatin (Mevacor)

ACTION
- Decreases level of cholesterol in the bloodstream

ADVERSE EFFECTS
- HMG-COA: GI distress
- CNS: headaches, insomnia, fatigue, skin rashes
- Bile sequestrants: constipation, bloating, headache, tinnitus, orange color to urine

INDICATIONS
- Hypercholesterolemia

NURSING INTERVENTIONS
- Fiber supplements, high-fiber diet
- HMG COA - take with meals. Change diet to include low fat and cholesterol.

Antianxiety Agents (Minor Tranquilizers)
BENZODIAZEPINE COMPOUNDS

DRUG: GENERIC/TRADE
- chlordiazepoxide (Librium)
- diazepam (Valium)
- oxazepam (Serax)
- clonazepam (Clonopin)
- clorazepate (Tranxene)
- lorazepam (Ativan)
- alprazolam (Xanax)

ACTION
- CNS depression
- Muscle relaxation
- Anticonvulsant

ADVERSE EFFECTS
- Drowsiness, sedation

LONG-TERM ADVERSE EFFECTS
- Tolerance
- Dependency
- Rebound insomnia/anxiety

INDICATIONS
- Anxiety disorder
- Detoxification alcohol dependence disorder
- Skeletal muscle relaxation
- Premedication operative procedures
- Seizures

NURSING INTERVENTIONS
- Teach client to avoid activities that require alertness, such as driving
- Caution to avoid falls
- Discourage social isolation
- Observe carefully, offer support
- Short-term use only
- Avoid alcohol or other CNS depressant
- Discontinue by slowly tapering off

OTHER INFORMATION
- Avoid during pregnancy and lactation
- Elderly more vulnerable to side effects

SEDATING ANTIHISTAMINES

DRUG: GENERIC/TRADE
- hydroxyzine (Vistaril, Atarax)

ACTION
- CNS depressant (subcortical levels)

ADVERSE EFFECTS
- Convulsions
- Tremors, fatigue
- Dizziness, confusion, depression
- Headache
- Dry mouth

INDICATIONS

- Preoperative medication
- Anxiety disorders

NURSING INTERVENTIONS
- Observe closely, may lower seizure threshold
- Teach client to avoid activities that require alertness

ANXIOLYTICS

DRUG: GENERIC/TRADE
- buspirone *(BuSpar)*

ACTION
- Unknown

ADVERSE EFFECTS
- Depression, stimulation, insomnia
- Tremors
- Hypotension
- Tachycardia, palpitations

INDICATIONS
- Relief of short-term anxiety

NURSING INTERVENTIONS
- Teach 2–3 week lag time before therapeutic effect achieved
- Monitor BP, pulse

OTHER INFORMATION
- No sedative/hypnotic properties or muscle relaxation properties
- Do not use with MAOIs

BETA-BLOCKERS

DRUG: GENERIC/TRADE
- propranolol *(Inderal)*
- clonidine *(Catapres)*

ACTION
- Non-selective B blocker

ADVERSE EFFECTS
- Dizziness, confusion
- Hypotension, bradycardia
- Dry mouth
- Drowsiness, sedation

INDICATIONS
- Anxiety disorders
- Narcotic withdrawal
- Convulsions

NURSING INTERVENTIONS
- Observe carefully
- Monitor when out of bed
- Monitor BP, pulse
- Increase fluids

SEDATIVE-HYPNOTICS

DRUG: GENERIC/TRADE
- flurazepam *(Dalmane)*
- temazepam *(Restoril)*
- triazolam *(Halcion)*

ACTION
- Produces CNS depression and sedation

ADVERSE EFFECTS
- Drowsiness

- Dizziness, lightheadedness

OVERDOSE
- Somnolence
- Confusion
- Impaired coordination
- Coma

INDICATIONS
- Sleep disturbance of anxiety
- Short-term use only

NURSING INTERVENTIONS
- Observe carefully
- Advise caution when out of bed
- Suicide assessment
- Obtain emergency medical treatment

Antipsychotic Agents
ANTIPSYCHOTICS

DRUG: GENERIC/TRADE
- chlorpromazine *(Thorazine)*
- mesoridazine *(Serentil)*
- perphenazine *(Trilafon)*
- chlorprothixene *(Taractan)*
- haloperidol *(Haldol)*
- loxapine *(Loxitane)*
- risperidone *(Risperdal)*
- thioridazine *(Mellaril)*
- fluphenazine *(Prolixin)*
- trifluoperazine *(Stelazine)*
- thiothixene *(Navane)*
- molindone *(Moban)*
- clozapine *(Clozaril)*

ACTION
- Depresses cerebral cortex, which controls activity aggression

ADVERSE EFFECTS
- Sedation
- Extrapyramidal effects
  - Dystonia
  - Akathisia
  - Tardive dyskinesia
- Anticholinergic symptoms
  - Dry mouth
  - Constipation
  - Urinary retention
  - Blurred vision
  - Nasal congestion
  - Hypotension
- Photosensitivity
- Agranulocytosis (esp. *Clozaril*)
- Neuroleptic malignant syndrome
- Weight gain

INDICATIONS
- Schizophrenic disorders
- Bipolar disorder, manic phase
- Agitated organic disorders

NURSING INTERVENTIONS
- Ask physician if entire dose can be given at bedtime
- Report parkinsonian symptoms, dystonia to physician
  - Medication may be changed

- Antiparkinsonian medication may be given
- Discontinue at first sign
- Provide laxatives or diet changes if constipation is a problem
- Provide fluids, sugarless candies, and gum for dry mouth
- Monitor intake, output
- Monitor BP, sitting and standing
- Caution to stand up slowly
- Caution client to use sunscreen, protective clothing for sun sensitivity
- Observe and report signs of infection, discontinue
- Observe and report signs: altered consciousness, unstable blood pressure and pulse, muscle rigidity, diaphoresis, tremors; discontinue medication of present
- Monitor diet, increase physical exercise

OTHER INFORMATION

- Drug Interactions: CNS depressants have additive effects; antacids inhibit absorption
- Lowers seizure threshold
- Clozapine (Clozaril) requires weekly WBC
- Use low doses only for elderly
- Avoid thioridazine (Mellaril) in sexually active males
- Risperidone (Risperdal) also effective on negative manifestations

Antidepressant Agents
TRICYCLIC ANTIDEPRESSANTS

DRUG: GENERIC/TRADE
- imipramine (Tofranil)
- desipramine (Norpramin)
- amitriptyline (Elavil)
- nortriptyline (Aventyl, Pamelor)
- clomipramine (Anafranil)
- doxepin (Sinequan)
- protriptyline (Vivactil)
- trimipramine (Surmontil)

ACTION
- Blocks re-uptake of norepinephrine and serotonin into nerve endings

ADVERSE EFFECTS
- Agranulocytosis
- Hypotension
- Paralytic ileus
- Cardiovascular

INDICATIONS
- Major depressive disorders
- Agoraphobia
- Panic disorders
- Obsessive-compulsive disorder
- Psychogenic pain disorder

NURSING INTERVENTIONS
- Monitor CBC
- Caution to stand up slowly
- Observe for nausea and vomiting
- Use cautiously in clients with known heart disease

TETRACYCLIC ANTIDEPRESSANTS

DRUG: GENERIC/TRADE
- amoxapine (Asendin)
- maprotiline (Ludiomil)

ACTION

- Blocks re-uptake of norepinephrine and serotonin into nerve endings

ADVERSE EFFECTS
- Agranulocytosis
- Hypotension
- Paralytic ileus

INDICATIONS
- Depression

NURSING INTERVENTIONS
- Monitor CBC
- Caution to stand up slowly
- Observe for nausea and vomiting

SELECTIVE SEROTONIN REUPTAKE INHIBITORS (SSRI)

DRUG: GENERIC/TRADE
- trazodone (Desyrel)
- sertraline (Zoloft)
- fluoxetine (Prozac)
- paroxetine (Paxil)
- bupropion (Wellbutrin)
- Venlafaxine hydrochloride (Effexor)

ACTION
- Inhibits serotonin and potentiates behavioral changes

ADVERSE EFFECTS
- Anticholinergic effects
- Dry mouth
  - Constipation
  - Urinary retention
  - Blurred vision
  - Aggravates glaucoma
- Cardiovascular effects
  - Postural hypotension
  - Tachycardia, arrhythmias
- Allergic reactions
  - Rashes
  - Photosensitivity
  - Tremors
- CNS
  - Insomnia
  - Stimulation
  - Sedation
  - Delirium
  - Myoclonic twitches
  - Seizures (especially high doses)
  - Sexual side effects such as impaired libido

INDICATIONS
- Depression
- Anxiety disorders

NURSING INTERVENTIONS
- Increase fluids
- Good oral hygiene
- Bulk diet, exercise, stool softeners
- Monitor intake and outflow, lower dose
- Corrective lenses, large print, change to another anti-depressant
- Ophthalmic consult
- Take BP regularly, sitting and standing
- Use smaller divided doses in conduction defects clients with known heart disease
- Avoid in clients with conduction defects or recent MI
- Do pretreatment EKG

- Sunscreen, protective clothing
- Observe carefully
- Advise to avoid caffeine
- Observe and report; may have to discontinue
- Start at low dose and gradually increase (maprotiline and bupropion) to monitor weight gain

OTHER INFORMATION

- Response rate varies but often takes 3-4 weeks for therapeutic effect
- Allow 14 day waiting period before changing from antidepressant to MAOI and vice versa
- Tricyclics can be fatal with overdose; do suicide assessment
- Drug Interactions:
  - Antihypertensives (unable to control BP)
  - Antacids inhibit absorption
  - Antipsychotics
  - Antiarrhythmics

MAO INHIBITORS (MAOI)

DRUG: GENERIC/TRADE

- isocarboxazid (Marplan)
- phenelzine (Nardil)
- tranylcypromine (Parnate)

ACTION

- Acts on CNS by increasing concentration of epinephrine, serotonin, and dopamine, thereby reducing depression effective

ADVERSE EFFECTS

- Excessive perspiration
- Erection/orgasm difficulty preparation
- Anxiety, restlessness
- Hypertensive crisis
- Anticholinergic manifestations
- CNS effects: drowsiness, fatigue, headache, restlessness, insomnia, constipation
- Orthostatic hypotension
- Insomnia (Parnate)
- Weight gain

INDICATIONS

- Because of dietary restrictions, use as second line antidepressant if other antidepressants not effective

NURSING INTERVENTIONS

- Observe, report, provide comfort measures
- Lower dose or switch to a less anticholinergic preparation
- Teach clients to avoid foods with high tyramine content such as aged cheese, fava or Italian green beans, fermented foods, liver, yeast extracts, bologna, beer, Chianti and red wines; limit sour cream, yogurt
- Teach clients to avoid OTC cold preparations
- See antipsychotic medications
- Some side effects can be expected for a short period
- Treat symptoms medically if not severe
- Monitor BP, sitting and standing
- Single AM dose

OTHER INFORMATION

- Drug Interactions:
  - Tricyclic antidepressants cause hypertensive crisis
  - Cocaine and amphetamines potentiate the action
  - Asthma inhalants
  - Narcotics, especially meperidine
  - Local anesthetics with epinephrine
  - Sinus and nasal decongestants

Mood Stabilizing Agents
MOOD STABILIZERS

DRUG: GENERIC/TRADE

- lithium carbonate (Eskalith, Lithonate, Lithotabs, Lithobid)

ACTION

- Alters Na, K, and ion transport in nerve; interferes with balance of epinephrine and serotonin in CNS, thereby affecting emotional responses

ADVERSE EFFECTS

- Fine tremor
- Transient nausea
- Drowsiness, lethargy
- Diarrhea, abdominal discomfort
- Polyuria
- Thirst
- Weight gain
- Signs of toxicity:
  - Vomiting
  - Diarrhea
  - Lethargy
  - Muscle twitching
  - Ataxia
  - Slurred speech
  - Coma
  - Seizure
  - Cardiac arrest

INDICATIONS

- Bipolar disorder, manic phase
- Major depression
- Aggressive conduct disorder

NURSING INTERVENTIONS

- Teach client that side effects are short in duration
- Observe carefully for changes in manifestations
- Monitor blood levels
- Advise to avoid caffeine
- Keep side rails up
- Teach client to avoid activities that require alertness
- Administer with meals
- Increase fluid intake
- Restrict calories, increase physical exercise
- Assess for edema
- Careful observation for manifestations and monitoring of blood levels as Na decreases and lithium levels increase
- Hold next dose and report STAT
- Pretreatment medical exam with thyroid and kidney function testing and EKG
- Nonsteroidal anti-inflammatory drugs may lead to lithium toxicity

OTHER INFORMATION

- Narrow therapeutic index
  - 0.5-1.5 meg/liter: therapeutic
  - Above 1.5 meg/liter: toxic
  - 2.0 meg/liter: lethal

DRUG INTERACTIONS

- Diuretics increase the risk of lithium toxicity
- Antipsychotics may cause neurotoxicity, especially in the elderly
- Ingestion of excessive salt increases lithium excretion
- Discontinue prior to elective surgery or ECT
- Do not take if pregnant

MOOD STABILIZERS

DRUG: GENERIC/TRADE
- carbamazepine *(Tegretol)*

ACTION
- Affects mood by inhibiting nerve impulses, by limiting Na exchange

ADVERSE EFFECTS
- Skin rash
- Sore throat, mucosal ulcerations
- Low-grade fever
- Drowsiness, ataxia, vertigo
- Diplopia, blurred vision
- Nausea and vomiting, hepatotoxicity

INDICATIONS
- Acute mania and prevention of manic episodes with lithium ineffective
- Temporal lobe epilepsy

NURSING INTERVENTIONS
- Caution when used with lithium and haloperidol (Haldol)

MOOD STABILIZERS

DRUG: GENERIC/TRADE
- valproic acid *(Depakote)*

ACTION
- Increases levels of GABA in brain

ADVERSE EFFECTS
- GI complaints
- Tremor, sedation, ataxia
- Increased appetite, weight gain
- Pancreatitis
- Severe hepatic dysfunction
- Thrombocytopenia

INDICATIONS
- Manic episodes when lithium ineffective (better tolerated)

NURSING INTERVENTIONS
- Administer with food or milk
- Teach client to avoid activities that require alertness
- Monitor liver function test and hematology levels

Obstetrics Setting Agents
OXYTOCICS

DRUG: GENERIC/TRADE
- oxytocin *(Pitocin)*

ACTION
- Stimulates contractions of the uterus

ADVERSE EFFECTS
- Hypotension
- Fetal bradycardia or tachycardia
- Tachycardia
- Decreased urine output

INDICATIONS
- Induction of labor

NURSING INTERVENTIONS
- Monitor uterine contractions, blood pressure, maternal heart rate, and fetal heart rate
- Monitor intake and output

OTHER INFORMATION
- Use only when pelvis is adequate, vaginal delivery is indicted, fetus is mature, and fetal position is favorable

OXYTOCICS

DRUG: GENERIC/TRADE
- methylergonovine maleate *(Methergine)*

ACTION
- Stimulates motor activity of the uterus

ADVERSE EFFECTS
- Headache
- Chest pain
- Nausea
- Palpitations

INDICATIONS
- Postpartum hemorrhage due to uterine atony

NURSING INTERVENTIONS
- Assess uterine contractions following administration
- Monitor vital signs and vaginal bleeding

OTHER INFORMATION
- Contraindicated prior to the fourth stage of labor

UTERINE RELAXANTS

DRUG: GENERIC/TRADE
- isoxsuprine hydrochloride *(Vasodilan)*

ACTION
- Vasodilator

ADVERSE EFFECTS
- Hypotension
- Tachycardia

INDICATIONS
- Premature labor
- Labor contractions too frequent or uncoordinated

NURSING INTERVENTIONS
- Monitor blood pressure and pulse

OTHER INFORMATION
- Contraindicated in immediate postpartum period

UTERINE RELAXANTS

DRUG: GENERIC/TRADE
- ritodrine hydrochloride *(Yutopar)*

ACTION
- Inhibits contraction of uterine smooth muscle

ADVERSE EFFECTS
- Hypotension
- Hypertension

INDICATIONS
- Premature labor

NURSING INTERVENTIONS
- Monitor blood pressure; maternal heart rate and fetal heart rate

UTERINE RELAXANTS

DRUG: GENERIC/TRADE
- terbutaline sulfate *(Brethine)*

ACTION
- Relaxes uterine smooth muscle

ADVERSE EFFECTS
- Nervousness
- Tremors
- Headache

INDICATIONS
- Premature labor

NURSING INTERVENTIONS
- Monitor blood pressure and pulse
- Monitor maternal heart rate and fetal heart rate

OTHER INFORMATION
- Use cautiously in clients with diabetes, heart disease, and hypertension

ANTICONVULSANTS

DRUG: GENERIC
- magnesium sulfate

ACTION
- Anticonvulsant

ADVERSE EFFECTS
- Respiratory depression
- Heart block
- Circulatory collapse
- Increased magnesium

INDICATIONS
- Primary intracerebral hemorrhage (PIH)

NURSING INTERVENTIONS
- Hold drug if respirations less than 16
- Monitor for arrhythmias
- Monitor intake and output
- Observe for neuromuscular or respiratory depression

OTHER INFORMATION
- Antidote is calcium gluconate

ANTIDOTES

DRUG: GENERIC/TRADE
- calcium gluconate

ACTION
- Needed for nervous musculoskeletal enzyme reactions, cardiac contraction, blood coagulation, and endocrine and exocrine secretions

ADVERSE EFFECTS
- Bradycardia
- Arrhythmias
- Venous irritation

INDICATIONS
- Hypermagnesemia

NURSING INTERVENTIONS
- Monitor pulse
- Monitor for arrhythmias
- Assess IV site

OTHER INFORMATION
- Contraindicated in digitized clients

ESTROGENS

DRUG: GENERIC/TRADE
- estradiol *(Estrace)*

ACTION
- Hormone needed for adequate functioning of female reproductive system; inhibits ovulation
- Promotes calcium use in bone structure

ADVERSE EFFECTS
- Hypoglycemia
- Dizziness, hypotension
- GI: nausea, vomiting
- Appetite increase, weight gain
- Embolism

INDICATIONS
- Prevent postpartum breast engorgement

NURSING INTERVENTIONS
- Observe glucose in diabetics
- Monitor weight
- Report headache, chest pain

NARCOTIC ANTAGONISTS

DRUG: GENERIC/TRADE
- naloxone *(Narcan)*

ACTION
- Interferes with narcotic absorption at narcotic receptor sites

ADVERSE EFFECTS
- Rapid pulse
- Drowsiness, nervousness
- Nausea, vomiting

INDICATIONS
- Treatment of narcotic induced depression of neonate

NURSING INTERVENTION
- Monitor respiratory rate and depth of neonate

ANTI-INFLAMMATORY DRUGS

DRUG: GENERIC TRADE
- betamethasone *(Celestone)*

ACTION
- Corticosteroid

ADVERSE EFFECTS
- GI distress, hemorrhage, pancreatitis
- Poor wound healing
- CNS depression, flushing, sweating
- Thrombocytopenia
- Hypertension, circ. collapse, embolism

INDICATIONS
- Stimulate lung development in Infant

NURSING INTERVENTIONS
- Monitor temperature
- Monitor blood pressure, report chest pain

OTHER INFORMATION
- Do not discontinue abruptly; adrenal crisis can occur

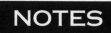

A

abortion, 126
acid-base imbalance, 11
acidosis
    metabolic, 12, 14(t)
    respiratory, 12, 14(t)
acquired immune deficiency syndrome (AIDS), 72
    in children, 171(t)
    in pregnancy, 117
acromegaly, 38
Addison's disease, 39
adenoidectomy, 159
ADHD. *See* attention-deficit and hyperactivity disorder
adolescents
    activity/rest, 144
    developmental stages of, 144
    health maintenance, 145
    language, 144
    motor skills, 144
    nutrition, 144
    physical characteristics, 144
    recreation, 145
adrenal gland, 40(t)
advanced directives, 180
AIDS. *See* acquired immune deficiency syndrome
airflow, factors affecting, 15
alcohol abuse, 100
aldosteronism (Conn's syndrome), 41
alkalosis
    metabolic, 12
    respiratory, 12
alternate test item formats
    fill-in-the-blank item, 185
    multiple response item, 186
    hot spot item, 186
    charts, table, graphic images item, 187
Alzheimer's disease, 104
amniocentesis, 120
amniotic fluid, 113
    emboli, 123
amputation, 36
anemia, 46
    aplastic, 46
    hemolytic, 47
    iron deficiency, 46
        in infants, 136
    pernicious, 47
    sickle cell, 47
        in children, 166

anesthetics, 24
angina, 49
angiography
    cardiac, *See* arteriography
    renal, 57
anorexia, 105, 106(t)
antianxiety agents, 88(t)
antidepressant agents, 96(t), 97(t), 98(t)
antihypertensive agents, 54
antimania agents, 98(t), 99(t)
antipsychotic agents, 92(t), 93(t)
antisocial personality, 100
anxiety
    disorders, 85
    levels of, 86(t)
aortic aneurysm, 53
Apgar score, 128
appendicitis, 159
arterial blood gases, 14
arteriography
    cardiac, 48
    cerebral, 64
arteriosclerosis, 53
arthritis
    rheumatoid, 36(t)
        juvenile, 164
ASD. *See* atrial septal defect
asthma, 16
    in children, 163
atherosclerosis, 53
atrial septal defect (ASD), 148(t)
attention-deficit and hyperactivity disorder (ADHD), 91
autism, 90

B

barium
    enema. *See* lower GI series
    swallow. *See* upper GI series
behaviorist model, 81
benign prostatic hyperplasia (BPH), 61
biopsy
    of kidney, 57
    of liver, 26
bipolar disorder, 94
blood transfusion, 46
    allergic reaction to, 46
    hemolytic reaction to, 46

borderline personality, 100
bowel obstruction, 31
bowel surgery, 31
BPH. *See* benign prostatic hyperplasia
Braxton-Hicks contractions, 114
breast feeding, 124
bronchiolitis, 158
bronchitis, chronic, 16
bronchodilators, 22
bronchoscopy, 15
Buerger's disease, 53
bulimia, 105, 106(t)
burns
    assessment of, 73
    in children, 161
    treatment of, 74

C

CABG. *See* coronary artery bypass graft
CAL. *See* chronic airflow limitation
cancer
    breast, 132
    care of the child with, 169(t)
    cervical, 132
    characteristics of, 70
    chemotherapy, 71, 72(t)
    endometrial, 132
    lungs, 21
    objectives of therapy, 70
    ovarian, 132
    radiation treatment for, 71
    uterine, 132
candidiasis, 131
CAPD. *See* dialysis, continuous ambulatory peritoneal
carbon dioxide narcosis, 17
cardiopulmonary resuscitation (CPR), 56
casts, 35
cataract, 69
catheterization
    bladder, 57
    cardiac, 48
celiac disease, 168(t)
central venous pressure, 48
cerebral palsy, 151
cerebrovascular accident (CVA), 66
Cesarean section, 123
Chadwick's sign, 114
charts, tables, graphic images item, 187
chest physiotherapy (CPT), 21
chest tube, 18
chickenpox, 171(t)

cholangiogram, 26
cholecystectomy, 34
cholecystitis, 33
cholecystogram, 26
cholelithiasis, 33
cholesterol, serum, 48
chorionic villi sampling, 120
chronic airflow limitation (CAL), 16
chronic obstructive pulmonary disease (COPD) *See* chronic
    airflow limitation
cirrhosis, 31
cleft lip, 153
cleft palate, 154
client
    advocacy, 180
    rights, 180
closed chest drainage, 18
clubfoot, congenital, 153
coagulation, tests of, 48
coarctation of the aorta, 148(t)
colic, 138
colonoscopy, *See* sigmoidoscopy
colostomy, 30(t), 31, 32(t)
coma scale. *See* Glascow coma scale
communication
    assertive, 178
    blocks, 85
    therapeutic, 84
computed tomography (CT scan), 63
condyloma, 132
congestive heart failure, 50
Conn's syndrome. *See* aldosteronism
consultation, 178
continuity of care, 178
contraception, 133
contraction stress test, 119
COPD (chronic obstructive pulmonary disease). *See* chronic
airflow limitation
cor pulmonale, 17
coronary artery bypass graft, 50
CPR. *See* cardiopulmonary resuscitation
cretinism, 42
crisis intervention, 82
Crohn's disease, 29(t)
croup. *See* laryngotracheobronchitis
CT scan. *See* computed tomography
Cushing's syndrome, 40
CVA. *See* cerebrovascular accident
cystic fibrosis, 168(t)
cystitis, 58
cystoscopy, 57

D

defense mechanisms, 83

delegation, 179
delirium tremens (DTs), 102
depression, 91 major, 94
dermatophytosis, 171(t)
development
    of the adolescent, 144
    of the infant, 137
    of the preschooler, 141
    of the school-age child, 143
    of the toddler, 140
developmental disabilities, 105
DI. *See* diabetes insipidus
diabetes insipidus, 38
diabetes mellitus, 44
    in children, 164
    in pregnancy, 126
dialysis
    continuous ambulatory peritoneal, 60
    hemodialysis, 60
    peritoneal, 60
diffusion, 11
digitalis (Digoxin) therapy, 51
    in children, 149
dissociative disorders, 89
diverticulitis, 30
diverticulosis, 30
domestic abuse, 107
    in children 162
    signs, 108(t)
DTs. *See* delirium tremens
duodenal ulcer, 28(t)
dwarfism, 38
dysrhythmia
    atrial, 51
    ventricular, 51

E

eating disorders, 105, 106(t)
ECG. *See* electrocardiogram
eclampsia, 127
ECT. *See* electroconvulsive therapy
eczema, 162
EEG. *See* electroencephalogram
EKG. *See* electrocardiogram
electrocardiogram (ECG, EKG), 48
electroconvulsive therapy (ECT), 95
electroencephalogram (EEG), 64
electrolytes, 11; 13(t)
electromyography (EMG), 64
ELISA. *See* enzyme linked immunosorbent assay
EMG. *See* electromyography
emphysema, pumonary,16
empyema, 21
endarterectomy, 66

endometriosis, 132
endoscopy, 26
enterobiasis, 171(t)
enzyme linked immunosorbent assay (ELISA), 73
enzymes, cardiac, 48
epiglottitis, 157
episiotomy, 123
Erikson, psychosocial model, 79, 80(t)
erythema infectiosum. *See* fifth's disease
esophageal varices, 33
esophagogastric duodenoscopy, *See* endoscopy
ethics, 179

F

failure-to thrive syndrome, 162
female reproductive tract, 113
fertilization, 113
fetal
    alcohol syndrome, 131
    assessment, 119
    development, 113, 114
        teratogenic effects on 114
    monitoring, 119
    presentation, 119
fever, in children 154
Fifth's disease, 171(t)
fill-in-the-blank item,
    calculation, 185
    ordered response, 185
flat plate of the abdomen, 26
fluid balance, 11
fluid volume
    deficit, 11
    excess, 11
fractures, 34
    hip, 35
    in children, 161
    pelvis, 36
Freud, psychoanalytical model, 79

G

gallbladder
    disease, 33
    series. *See* cholecystogram
Gardner-Wells traction, 67
gastric
    resection, 30
    secretion analysis, 26
    ulcer, 28(t)
gastroenteritis, 155
gastrointestinal intubation, 27

gastroscopy. *See* endoscopy
German measles. *See* rubella
gestational age
    assessment of, 129
    large for, 130
    small for, 130
gigantism, 38
Glascow coma scale, 63
glaucoma, 69
glomerulonephritis, 58
    in children, 167(t)
Goodell's sign, 114
gout, 37
Graves' disease. *See* hyperthyroidism
gravida, 114
group
    dynamics, 177
    therapy, 82
Guillain-Barré syndrome, 69

H

halo traction, 67
head injury
    basilar skull fracture, 67
    hematoma
        epidural, 67
        subdural, 67
heart block, AV, 52
heart defects, 146
    acyanotic, 148(t)
    cyanotic, 148(t)
Hegar's sign, 114
Heimlich maneuver, 56
hemophilia, 165
hepatitis, 32(t)
hernia, 30
    hiatal, 31
    in children 160
hip dysplasia, congenital, 152
Hirschprung's disease, 160
Hodgkin's lymphoma, 169
hot spot item, 186
hospitalization
    child's reaction to, 145
    family's reaction to, 14
hydatidiform mole, 127
hydrocephalus, 150
hyperbilirubinemia, 131
hyperemesis gravidarum, 126
hyperparathyroidism, 43
hypertension, 54
    pregnancy induced (PIH), 127
hyperthermia, 65
hyperthyroidism (Grave's disease; toxic goiter), 42
hypoparathyroidism, 43

I

ileostomy, 30(t), 31, 32(t)
immunizations, 170(t)
infants
    activity/rest, 138
    developmental stages, 139
    health maintenance, 139
    language development, 139
    motor skills, 138
    nutrition, 137
        guidelines, 138
    physical development, 137
    play, 139
    reflexes, 137
impetigo, 171(t)
incident reports. *See* variance reports
incontinence, 62
infertility, 133
informed consent, 180
insulin
    preparations, 45(t)
    pump, 45
    shock, 165(t)
intermittent positive pressure breathing (IPPB), 22
intracranial pressure, increased, 64
intravenous pyelography (IVP), 57
intussusception, 160
IPPB. *See* intermittent positive pressure breathing
iron preparations, administration of, 47
IVP. *See* intravenous pyelography

K

Kaposi's sarcoma, 73
kidney,
    functions of, 56
    transplantation, 60

L

labor
    analgesia in, 121, 122(t)
    components of, 118
    induction of, 124
    medications used in, 121(t)
    premature, 122
    signs of impending, 120
    stages of, 120- 121(t)

laminectomy, 67
laryngotracheobronchitis, 158
leadership, concepts of, 177
leukemia, 166
lice, head. *See* pediculosis capitis
liver function tests, 27
lipodystrophy, 45
lower GI, 26
LP. *See* lumbar puncture
lumbar puncture (LP), 63
lungs
    cancer of, 21
    function of, 15
    subdivisions of, 15
Lyme disease, 171(t)

M

magnetic resonance imaging (MRI), 64
management
    concepts of, 177
mania, 94
Mantoux test, 15
Maslow, basic needs model, 81, 81(t)
mast cell inhibitors, 22
measles. *See* rubeola
medical-biological theory, 79
Mèniére's disease, 68
meningitis, 172(t)
menopause, 133
mental health continuum, 83
mental retardation, 106
metabolic
    acidosis, 12
    alkalosis, 12
milieu therapy, 82
MRI. *See* magnetic resonance imaging
multiple sclerosis, 67
mumps, 172(t)
Munchausen syndrome, 162
myasthenia gravis, 68
myclogram, 64
myelomeningocele, 150
myocardial infarction, 49
myxedema, 41

N

Nagele's rule, 114
nasogastric suction, 27

nasogastric tube feeding, 27
    NCLEX-PN exam, 3 -7
neonate
    assessment of, 128
    assessment of gestational age, 129
    care of, 130
    initial care of, 128
    large for gestational age, 130
    postmature, 129
    premature, 130
    small for gestational age, 130
nephroblastoma, 168
nephrotic syndrome, 58
    in children, 167(t)
neuroblastoma, 169
neurologic assessment, 63
    "neuro checks", 63
nitroglycerin administration, 49
non-stress test, 119
nurse-client relationship, 84

O

obsessive-compulsive disorders, 87
occurrence reports. *See* variance reports
operative obstetrics
    Cesarean section, 123
    episiotomy, 123
    forceps delivery, 123
    vacuum extraction, 123
organic mental disorders
    delirium, 104
    dementias, 104
osmosis, 11
osteoarthritis, 36(t)
osteoporosis, 35
otitis media, 156
oxygen toxicity, 17

P

pacemaker, 52
pain in children, 146
pancreas, 44(t)
pancreatitis, 34
paracentesis, 26
paraplegia, 67
paranoid personality disorder, 90
parathyroid gland, 43(t)
Parkinson's disease, 68
patent ductus arteriosus (PDA), 148(t)

PDA. *See* patent ductus arteriosus
pediculosis capitis, 172(t)
PEG. *See* percutaneous endoscopic gastrostomy
pelvic inflammatory disease (PID), 132
percutaneous endoscopic gastrostomy (PEG), 27
percutaneous transthoracic cardiac angioplasty (PTCA), 50
pertussis, 172(t)
pH, regulation of body, 12
pheochromocytoma, 41
phobic disorders, 86
PID. *See* pelvic inflammatory disease
PIH. *See* hypertension, pregnancy induced
pinworms. *See* enterobiasis
pituitary gland, 39(t)
placenta
    abruptio, 128
    development, 113
    previa, 128
pleural effusion, 21
pneumonia, 20
pneumothorax, 18
poisoning, 160, 161(t)
polyhydramnios, 126
postoperative care, 24
postoperative complications, 25(t)
postural drainage, 22
power, concepts of, 177
preeclampsia, 127
pregnancy
    ectopic, 127
    emotional adaptations to, 118
    high risk, 125
    induced hypertension (PIH), 127
    molar. *See* hydatidiform mole
    physical adaptations to, 115 - 117(t)
    postpartal adaptations, 124
    postpartum complications
        hemorrhage, 125
        infection, 125
        thromboembolic disease, 125
    signs of
        positive, 114
        presumptive, 114
        probable, 114
prenatal care, 118
preoperative care, 23
    of the child, 159
preschoolers
    activity/rest, 141
    developmental stages, 142
    health maintenance, 142
    language development, 142
    motor skills, 142
    nutrition, 141
    physical development, 141
    play, 142
    sleep disturbances, 141

prostatectomy, 61, 62(t)
prostatitis, 62
psychiatric nursing
    legal aspects of, 109
    overview of, 79
PTCA. *See* percutaneous transthoracic cardiac angioplasty
pulmonary edema, 51
pulmonary toilet, 22
pyloric stenosis, 159

Q

quadriplegia, 66
quality improvement, 178

R

rabies, 172
rape, 108
Raynaud's phenomenon, 53
renal failure
    acute, 59
    chronic, 59
respiratory
acidosis, 12
alkalosis, 12
responsibilities
    of advanced practice nurses, 179
    of licensed practical nurse (LPN), 179
    of primary care provider, 179
    of nursing assistant (NA), 179
    of registered professional nurse (RN), 179
retina, detached, 69
Reye's syndrome, 172(t)
rheumatic fever,163, 170(t)
ringworm. *See* dermatophytosis
roseola, 173(t)
rubella, 173(t)
rubeola, 173(t)

S

scarlet fever, 173(t)
schizophrenia, 89
school age child
    activity/rest, 143
    developmental stages, 143
    health maintenance, 143
    language, 143
    motor skills, 143
    nutrition, 143
    physical development, 143
    play, 143

school phobia, 144
scoliosis, 164
seizure
    disorder, 65
    febrile, 154
Sengstaken-Blakemore tube, 33
shock, 55
SIADH. *See* syndrome of inappropriate secretion of antidiuretic hormone
SIDS. *See* sudden infant death syndrome
sigmoidoscopy, 26
SLE. *See* systemic lupus erythematosus
somatoform disorders, 87
spinal cord injury, 66
sputum examination, 15
steroids, inhaled, 22
stool analysis, 26
substance abuse, 101(t), 102(t), 103
    and the newborn, 131
suctioning, pulmonary, 23
sudden infant death syndrome, 140
suicide, 95
supervision, 179
syndrome of inappropriate secretion of antidiuretic hormone, 38
systemic lupus erythematosus, 37

T

talipes equinovarus. *See* clubfoot, congenital
teratogens, 114
tetanus, 173(t)
tetralogy of Fallot, 149(t)
therapeutic play, 146
thoracentesis, 15
thrombophlebitis, 55
thyroidectomy, 43
thyroid gland, 42(t)
TIA. *See* transient ischemic attacks
tinea capitis. *See* dermatophytosis
toddlers
    activity/rest, 140
    developmental stages, 140
    health maintenance, 140
    language development, 140
    motor skills, 140
    nutrition, 140
    physical development, 140
    play, 140
tonsillectomy, 159
tooth eruption
    permanent, 143(t)
    primary, 137(t)
TORCH syndrome, 117
total parenteral nutrition (TPN), 27

toxic goiter. *See* hyperthyroidism
TPN. *See* total parenteral nutrition
traction, 34
transient ischemic attacks (TIA), 66
transposition of the great vessels, 149(t)
trichomoniasis, 132
tuberculosis, 19
tumors
    classification of, 70
    staging of, 70

U

ulcerative colitis, 29(t)
ulcers, 28(t), 29
ultrasound of the gladder and liver, 26
upper GI, 26
urinalysis, 56
urinary calculi. *See* urolithiasis
urinary diversion, 61
urolithiasis, 58

V

vaginal infections
    candidiasis, 131
    condyloma, 132
    trichomoniasis, 132
valvular disorders, 52
variance reports, 178
varicose veins, 55
ventricular septal defect, 148(t)
vomiting, in children, 155
VSD, *See* ventricular septal defect

W

Wernicke-Korsakoff's syndrome, 104
whooping cough. *See* pertussis
Wilms' tumor (nephroblastoma), 168

X

X-ray
    chest, 15
    KUB, 57